Diagnosis and Treatment of Diabetes and its Complications

Diagnosis and Treatment of Diabetes and its Complications

Editor: Roy Marcus Cohn

AMERICAN
MEDICAL PUBLISHERS
www.americanmedicalpublishers.com

AMERICAN
MEDICAL PUBLISHERS
www.americanmedicalpublishers.com

Cataloging-in-Publication Data

Diagnosis and treatment of diabetes and its complications / edited by Roy Marcus Cohn.
p. cm.
Includes bibliographical references and index.
ISBN 978-1-63927-115-3
1. Diabetes--Diagnosis. 2. Diabetes--Treatment. 3. Diabetes--Complications.
I. Cohn, Roy Marcus.
RC660 .D53 2022
616.462--dc23

American Medical Publishers,
41 Flatbush Avenue,
1st Floor, New York,
NY 11217, USA

ISBN 978-1-63927-115-3 (Hardback)

Contents

Preface

Diabetes is a group of metabolic disorders wherein the blood sugar level is high over a prolonged period of time. Some of its major symptoms are increased thirst, frequent urination and increased appetite. It can cause a large number of complications, if it is not treated in a timely manner. A few of such complications are diabetic ketoacidosis, hyperosmolar hyperglycemic state, stroke, chronic kidney disease, cognitive impairment and damage to the eyes. The diagnosis of diabetes can be conducted by measuring the level of plasma glucose or glycated hemoglobin. The management of diabetes can be done by glucose control and lifestyle changes. This book includes some of the vital pieces of work being conducted across the world, on the diagnosis and treatment of diabetes. It is a valuable compilation of topics, ranging from the basic to the most complex advancements in this field. This book will serve as a reference to a broad spectrum of readers.

After months of intensive research and writing, this book is the end result of all who devoted their time and efforts in the initiation and progress of this book. It will surely be a source of reference in enhancing the required knowledge of the new developments in the area. During the course of developing this book, certain measures such as accuracy, authenticity and research focused analytical studies were given preference in order to produce a comprehensive book in the area of study.

This book would not have been possible without the efforts of the authors and the publisher. I extend my sincere thanks to them. Secondly, I express my gratitude to my family and well-wishers. And most importantly, I thank my students for constantly expressing their willingness and curiosity in enhancing their knowledge in the field, which encourages me to take up further research projects for the advancement of the area.

Editor

1

Principle of Management of Type 2 Diabetes: From Clinical, Public Health and Research Perspectives

Madhur Dev Bhattarai

Abstract

Apart from stopping smoking, controlling hypertension and using statin, losing possible excess bodyweight and regular physical activity and exercise are the cornerstones in diabetes management. There is often need of controlling blood glucose immediately. Approach of '*dynamic dose management of medications likely to cause hypoglycemia*' helps to control high blood glucose immediately as and when required with sulfonylurea or insulin and to taper off their dose later. Anti-hyperglycemic medications which are unlikely to cause hypoglycemia are continued to control hyperglycemia. The diagnosis of gestational diabetes usually made at 24-28 weeks is applicable for clinical management of mother and child and for possible prevention of diabetes later in the mother. From the public health perspectives, however, protection of the susceptible *in utero* population from maternal malnutrition or clinical or subclinical hyperglycemia right from the time of conception itself also needs to be considered to control the diabetes epidemic at the population level. Campaigns and programmes for maintenance of optimal pre-pregnancy body weight as per the recommended body mass index of the respective populations along with regular physical activity and exercise during pregnancy are the essential measures available at hand to prevent the possibility of maternal hyperglycemia right from the early pregnancy.

Keywords: diabetes, CVD, hypertension, high blood pressure, physical activity, exercise, smoking, body mass index, ethnicity, hypoglycemia, acarbose, diabetes epidemiology, diabetes control, maternal health, pre-pregnancy weight

1. Introduction

There are now estimated 415 million adults aged 20–79 with diabetes worldwide and a further 318 million adults are estimated to have impaired glucose tolerance [1]. About half of the

3.7 million deaths due to diabetes and its complications occur before the age of 70 years [2]. Up to 80% of deaths in type 2 diabetes are cardiovascular diseases (CVDs) related. Persons with impaired glucose tolerance are also almost three times more likely to develop coronary heart disease and other major cardiovascular events than people with normal glucose tolerance. In fact, CVDs alone account for nearly 30% of all deaths worldwide and 27% in low-income and middle-income countries [3, 4]. Thus, in one hand, there is a need to prevent and treat diabetes, and on the other hand, considering various possible risk factors, the impaired glucose tolerance itself and CVDs have to be prevented both at individual and population levels.

This chapter will focus on the principles of management of type 2 diabetes at individual and population levels to consider while following the guidelines and managing diabetes and its epidemic. Management is defined as the act or skill of dealing with people or situations in a successful way [5]. The term management in the chapter covers clinical management, research and public health perspectives. Public health is the practice of preventing disease and promoting good health within groups of people, from small communities to entire countries [6]. Primary prevention requires a focus on individuals known to be at risk for disease, i.e. the high-risk strategy with interventions focused on high-risk group, for example on people with glucose intolerance. A large proportion of the reductions in coronary heart disease mortality experienced in many high-income nations since the 1960s have been ascribed to the interventions in people at elevated risk [7]. However, individuals with markedly elevated levels of risk factors are relatively uncommon in the population. The majority of CVD events occur in individuals with average or only mildly adverse levels of risk factors [7, 8]. Therefore, population-wide strategies are also essential. Health promotion and disease prevention strategies must embrace both high-risk and population strategies [7–10].

2. Prevention of CVDs and control of blood pressure (BP)

Seven modifiable well-known risk factors of atherosclerotic CVDs are high BP, glucose intolerance, physical inactivity, tobacco use, dyslipidemia, unhealthy diet and overweight/obesity (**Figure 1**).

2.1. High blood pressure (BP)

Hypertension is the most prevalent risk factor for development of cardiovascular and kidney disease. In 2008, worldwide, approximately 40% of adults aged 25 had been diagnosed with hypertension and its prevalence is predicted to increase by almost 60% in the next 2 decades [11, 12]. Hypertension is responsible for at least 45% of deaths due to heart disease and 51% of deaths due to stroke [11, 12]. High BP is the leading risk factor in the world especially in the non-industrialized countries [13]. In fact there is some increase in cardiovascular risk in patients with BP 120–140/80–90 (i.e. pre-hypertension) than in those with BP less than 120/80 (i.e. normal BP) even in the general population [14]. Untreated BP <120/<80 mmHg (i.e. normal

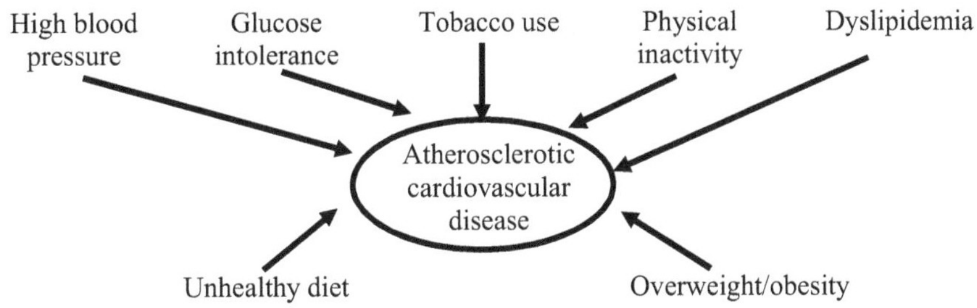

Figure 1. The seven modifiable risk factors of atherosclerotic cardiovascular disease.

BP) is considered as one of the ideal health factors for cardiovascular health [7, 8]. Programmes for controlling high BP in the industrialized countries achieved significant reduction in CVD mortality [7], and tobacco smoking including the second-hand smoke became the leading risk factor [13]. In many non-industrialized countries, such programmes have mostly not been accomplished. As a matter of fact in many such countries due to the inadequate network of the State supported rural and urban health centers/clinics, people often have limited access to blood pressure monitoring and management [15]. It is difficult for the people to regularly visit private clinics or to wait at the long queue in the free medical clinics of public hospitals. In such situations, the patients are more likely to visit hospitals late for crisis management only when the complications (like stroke, coronary heart diseases, kidney failure or pneumonia) develop [15].

2.2. Interaction of high blood pressure and glucose intolerance

Death rate due to CVD, even in the industrialized countries, seems to be on increase again particularly in the relatively younger population [8]. The emerging epidemic of glucose intolerance, another CVD risk factor, seems to be adding up and interplaying with high BP. Among more than 3000 Euro Heart Survey patients with acute and elective coronary heart diseases, only about one-fourth had normal plasma glucose by the WHO criteria [16]. If the American Diabetes Association classification with fasting plasma glucose >5.6 mmol/L (>100 mg/Dl) had also been considered, the proportion of patients with glucose intolerance would perhaps have been more, as reported in another study in patients with acute coronary insufficiency [17]. There are two pertinent points to note in the interaction between high BP and glucose intolerance.

Firstly, hypertension is relatively more common in people with diabetes, about two times more in one study [18], than in those with normal plasma glucose. More than 75% of adults with diabetes have blood pressure (BP) levels ≥130/80 mmHg or are using antihypertensive medication [12]. Secondly, the adverse effects of higher blood pressure are more in people with glucose intolerance than in those with normal blood glucose. Even among people with systolic BP between 120 and 139 mmHg (i.e. at pre-hypertension level), CV mortality rate is about three times more in those with diabetes than in those without diabetes. And the risk is similarly high in different systolic BP ranges from normal to high levels [19]. Mortality is indeed increased 7.2-fold when hypertension is present in patients with diabetes [12]. Lowering 4 mmHg of systolic BP is more effective in reducing cardiovascular events than reducing 1 mmol/L of LDL cholesterol and is about four times more effective than lowering 0.9% of glycated hemoglobin (HbA1c), and thus, in diabetes, BP control is more efficacious and more easy than lowering glucose [20].

Clinical management perspective: The current guidelines recommend to treat hypertension in type 2 diabetes to an systolic BP target of 130–140 mmHg and a diastolic BP target of 80 mmHg and to consider the lower targets if the patients are younger or when additional CV risk factors or microvascular diseases are present [21]. In the studies, the number of antihypertensive drugs required to achieve the systolic blood pressure around 130–140 mmHg are often more than two and even more than three in many patients. Treatment of hypertension in patients with diabetes is lucidly reviewed in the position paper of American Society of Hypertension [12].

Public health perspective: In non-industrialized countries, there is urgent need of establishing the network of the State supported rural and particularly urban health centers/clinics with general practitioners (preferably well trained with residential training in General Practice after medical graduation). It is required (i) for the comprehensive longitudinal health care of the people with diabetes, hypertension, CVD and other conditions, (ii) for supervision of healthcare workers to implement various public health programs including that for hypertension and CVDs and (iii) to provide the State supported diagnostic facilities and antidiabetic, antihypertensive and other CVD drugs and antibiotics (then only it may be possible to restrict the over-the-counter sale of antibiotics and other drugs as the people otherwise would not have any access to such life-saving drugs) [15].

Research perspective: Study of the occurrence of CVD complications in the people with pre-hypertension level of BP and impaired glucose intolerance may indicate the different levels of HbA1c and BP to start antihypertensive treatment. The combined presence of the subclinical or borderline hypertension and glucose intolerance (as 'subclinical or borderline syndrome') may be another CVD risk factor, as a residual risk factor of CVDs, at the population level.

3. Promoting cessation of smoking and tobacco use

The health effects of tobacco use, including on CVD, and various public health measures to control it are well known [2, 10]. Harmful tobacco products also include smokeless tobacco like snuff, gutkha, gul, chimo, mawa, nass, pan masala, tambaku and others [22].

Clinical management perspective: The five A's framework (Ask, Advise, Assess, Assist, Arrange) has been developed to allow physicians to incorporate smoking cessation counseling into busy clinical practices [23]. Others have further added 'Assess again'. There are various pharmacological agents available to help patients quit smoking and tobacco use. However, before such products were available and even now hundreds of thousands of people including health professionals have had stopped tobacco use once they realized the possible complications to them. Physicians' priority, repeated advice and time spent on explaining its importance and its process of quitting play a crucial role for the motivation of the patients to quit tobacco use. Smokers who quit smoking abruptly ('Cold Turkey' method) have been reported to be successful than those who quit gradually [24]. However, the most important well-known point, to emphasize to the patients repeatedly, is that after stopping tobacco use whether abruptly or slowly, it should not be used even once; otherwise the habit is likely to be resumed.

4. Regular physical activity and exercise

Exercise is often classified as aerobic, strength (resistance) and flexibility exercise and each of them has their own utility and limitations. The common recommendation (e.g. 150 minutes or more of moderate-to-vigorous intensity physical activity per week, spread over at least 3 days/week, with no more than 2 consecutive days without activity) is applicable to most adults and help to achieve cardiovascular fitness and other benefits. Brisk walking can be regularly included into the daily life. Two to three sessions/week of resistance exercise on non-consecutive days are also recommended [25]. Increased physical activity is effective in preventing diabetes, and the protective benefit is especially pronounced in persons at the highest risk for the disease [26]. At higher BMI, exercise is protective against diabetes and is dose-dependent. The prevention of diabetes and reduction of hyperglycemia in diabetes occur even without significant weight reduction [27]. American Diabetes Association recommends that prolonged sitting should be interrupted every 30 minutes for blood glucose benefits, particularly in adults with type 2 diabetes [25]. Possible physical activity even while seated (e.g. by leg exercise with or without sit down leg exercise machines) may also help. A more intensive physical activity program including at least 275 minutes per week may be needed to assist weight loss and avoid regain [21]. Higher levels of physical activity before pregnancy or in early pregnancy are associated with a significantly lower risk of developing gestational diabetes mellitus [28]. NICE guideline recommends women with gestational diabetes to take regular exercise (such as walking for 30 minutes after a meal) to improve blood glucose control [29]. **Figure 2** summarizes the potential benefits of regular physical activity and exercise in relation to diabetes.

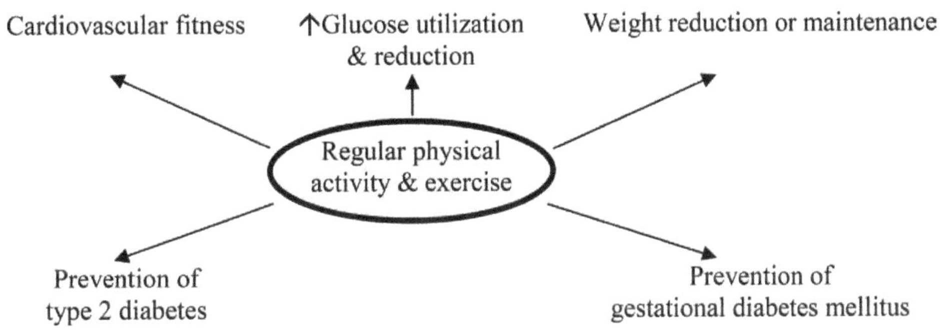

Figure 2. Potential benefits of regular physical activity and exercise in relation to diabetes.

Research perspective: Although type 2 diabetic subjects are insulin resistant, they are not resistant to the stimulatory effects of exercise on glucose utilization [30]. The local cellular and other metabolic adaptations could explain the increase in glucose utilization and improvement in the glucose tolerance in exercise and trained muscles. A major challenge has been to elucidate the molecules or cascade of molecules that act through insulin-independent, exercise-stimulated signaling pathway [30]. If such molecules produced during exercise are secreted in the blood and act like hormones in other tissues, organs, muscles and fat, study of the effect in the resting state by the reuse of serum of blood collected during exercise in the same person may give insight into such actions and the difference in the contents of resting and post-exercise sera may help to elucidate the molecules.

Research perspective: Many overweight older people with diabetes have knee osteoarthritis which may prevent them to walk freely. Exercises to strengthen the quadriceps—for example, quadriceps-setting exercise and straight-leg raises—are effective in reducing pain and improving function in patients with knee osteoarthritis. However, people often may not adhere to the recommended methods of quadriceps strengthening exercises. Regular exercise with a bicycle ergometer in such patients can have beneficial effects not only for knee osteoarthritis but also for diabetes and CVD [31].

5. Use of statin and antiplatelet therapy

The use of statin is the other core element to prevent the premature death and disability in diabetes. The mechanisms of beneficial effects of statins in CVD are not completely understood. Some beneficial effects appear to occur independently of lowering of LDL cholesterol. Thus, most trials of statins and CVD outcomes tested specific doses of statins against placebo or other statins rather than aiming for specific LDL cholesterol goals, suggesting that the initiation and intensification of statin therapy should be based on risk profile [25, 32]. Before starting statin, lipid profile should be required at least once; a fasting sample is not routinely needed [32]. Antiplatelet therapy in diabetes is generally recommended for those with history of CVD and dual antiplatelet therapy is reasonable for up to 1 year after an acute coronary syndrome [25, 32].

Research perspectives: Studies indicate that lower statin doses achieve lipid improvements in Chinese, Japanese and Koreans patients comparable with those observed with higher doses in Caucasians [33]. However as the mechanism of action of statins may not be just related to the lowering of LDL cholesterol, the relation of such observation with cardiovascular events need to be studied.

6. Body weight as per the recommended body mass index (BMI) for the respective populations

The WHO 1998 Consultation on Obesity, based on classifications used in a number of past studies on Europids, indicated BMI of 18.5–24.9 kg/m^2 as normal [34, 35]. A WHO expert consultation on BMI for Asian populations concluded that Asians generally have a higher percentage of body fat than white people of the same age, sex and BMI and that the proportion of Asian people with a high risk of diabetes and CVD is substantial at BMIs lower than the existing WHO 1998 cut-off point for overweight (>24.9 kg/m^2) [36]. The WHO [35], International Diabetes Federation and American Diabetes Association have recommended the upper limit of cut-off point of normal BMI for Asian people as 22.9 kg/m^2 [25, 35, 37]. Similar and variables recommendations for different non-Caucasian populations have been made in various other studies, including those conducted in the Westernized ones.

These recommendations are in agreement with the actual body mass index of the population. The adult mean BMI levels of 20–23 kg/m^2 are found among the general population in Africa and Asia, whereas levels of 25–27 kg/m^2 across North America and Europe in 2002 [10]. The WHO consultation on BMI for Asian populations identified further potential public health action points along the continuum of BMI and indicated that the earlier optimum population range (21–23 kg/m^2) gives some intuitive consistency for policy makers [36]. The risk of insulin resistance and diabetes in adult increases progressively upwards of a BMI of 20–22 kg/m^2 [10]. More than 80% of the people with diabetes live in low- and middle-income countries and nearly two thirds of diabetes globally are attributable to BMI above 21 kg/m^2 [10]. In general, the risk of insulin resistance and glucose intolerance appears to increase once BMI starts rising above the middle of the recommended BMI for the population.

> **Research perspectives:** Compared with the BMI cut point of 30.0 kg/m^2 among Europeans, a similar glucose factor distribution is observed at corresponding BMI cut points of 21.0 kg/m^2 in South Asians, 20.6 kg/m^2 in Chinese and 21.8 kg/m^2 in Aboriginals in Canada [38]. The BMI cut points are, however, higher, for the lipid and blood pressure factors than for the glucose factor in South Asians, Chinese, and Aboriginals in the study [38] pointing out the need to study BMI cut points in different populations similarly considering the glucose, lipid and blood pressure factors separately.

7. Antihyperglycemic medications

Type 2 diabetes is a chronic metabolic condition characterized by insulin resistance and insufficient pancreatic insulin production from beta-cell, resulting in high blood glucose levels [39]. Difficulty in utilizing the available insulin increases the workload of beta-cell. While using antihyperglycemic medications, the issues that need to be considered are shown in **Figure 3**. A few pertinent points are further discussed below.

7.1. Reduction of insulin resistance and beta-cell workload

Beta-cell failure is central to the ultimate development and progression of type 2 diabetes and it antedates and predicts diabetes onset and progression [40]. Subjects with normal glucose tolerance with 2-hour plasma glucose 120–139 mg/dL may have already lost 50% of beta-cell function, whereas subjects with impaired glucose tolerance with 2-hour plasma glucose 180–199 mg/dL have lost up to 80% of beta-cell function. Thus, when the diagnosis of diabetes is made, the patient may have already lost 80% of their beta-cell function [41, 42]. The available clinical studies with appropriate protocols, however, indicate that existing therapy may not reverse or arrest progression of beta-cell dysfunction in type 2 diabetes [40]. Weight loss reduces insulin resistance and beta-cell workload and physical activity increases insulin utilization and also helps to reduce beta-cell workload and bodyweight. Both help to normalize the blood glucose and are also useful for cardiovascular health. Promotion of physical activity and exercise and loss of excess bodyweight for as long as possible are the cornerstones of management in type 2 diabetes. Medications favoring these two aspects are preferred for as long as possible.

7.2. Risk of hypoglycemia

Hypoglycemia can manifest in different ways (**Figure 4**). Insulin is a known cause of hypoglycemia. The risk of hypoglycemia associated with the use of other antihyperglycemic medications is given below [21]:

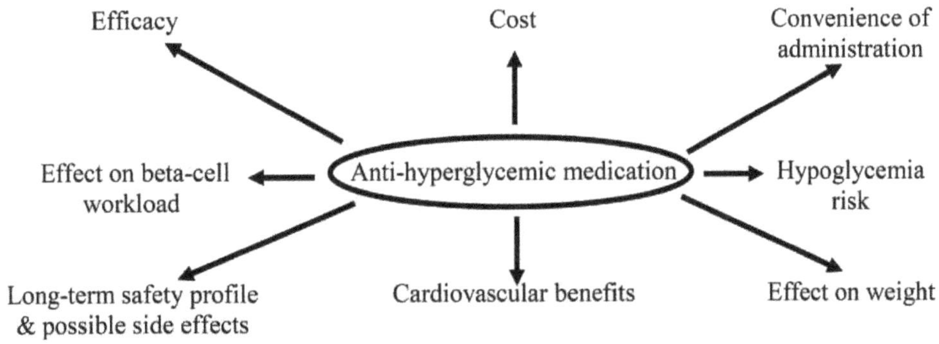

Figure 3. Factors to consider while prescribing antihyperglycemic medications in type 2 diabetes.

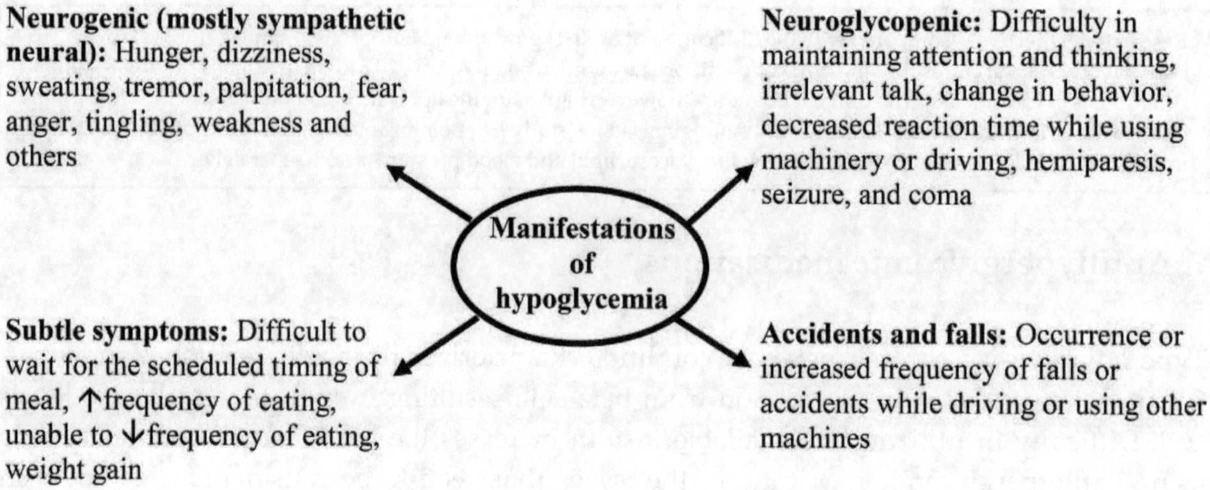

Figure 4. Manifestations of hypoglycemia. *Note:* The patient may not volunteer the information; the healthcare professionals have to ask the leading questions so that the dose of the medications likely to cause hypoglycemia, viz. insulin, sulfonylurea and repaglinides, can be appropriately reduced.

- Metformin, acarbose and other alpha-glucosidase inhibitors, dipeptidyl peptidase-4 inhibitor, glucagon-like peptide-1 receptor agonist and sodium-glucose cotransporter 2 inhibitors are associated with neutral risk of hypoglycemia.

- Sulfonylurea is associated with moderate-to-severe risk and repaglinide moderate risk of hypoglycemia [21].

The patients only on antihyperglycemic treatment unlikely to cause hypoglycemia can check their glycemic control with blood glucose fasting, 2-hour postprandial glucose and HbA1c estimation. If the patients are also on medications, like sulfonylurea, repaglinide and insulin, which can cause hypoglycemia, they need to check their blood glucose also at other time (e.g. before meals and exercise or later in the day or at night) considering the hypoglycemic symptoms and the maximum onset and duration of action of the drugs likely to cause hypoglycemia.

The popular guidelines cover detail aspects of different medications including the monitoring of glucose [21, 25, 39]. As acarbose, an alpha-glucosidase inhibitor, is increasingly used and has relatively longer safety profile, efficacy and other benefits, it can also be considered in the early phase of therapy in glucose intolerance. Four alpha-glucosidase inhibitors currently exist: acarbose, miglitol, voglibose and emiglitate [43]. Acarbose inhibits both alpha-amylase (which breaks down starch to disaccharides) and other alpha-glucosidase (which digests disaccharides), where as voglibose and miglitol inhibit the disaccharide-digesting enzymes well, but have no effect on the starch digesting enzyme alpha-amylase [44]. Acarbose and voglibose are minimally absorbed from the intestine and have very low bioavailability [44] with acarbose having less than 2% systemic availability [45]. Miglitol is almost completely absorbed from the upper part of the intestine [44]. Acarbose was first developed. Among the alpha-glucosidase inhibitors, acarbose is the most prescribed drug and most data and best-outcomes are obtained for it [43].

7.3. Acarbose

Acarbose is an effective drug with relatively long safety profile having various cardiovascular and metabolic beneficial effects, it is not associated with hypoglycemia and it promotes weight loss [43–48]. Different meta-analysis, review articles and more than 350 studies have reported its efficacy (when used alone or in combination with other antihyperglycemic medications, including metformin), safety profile, cardiovascular, weight reduction, metabolic and other benefits [43–48]. Metformin or acarbose is recommended by International Diabetes Federation and American Association of Clinical Endocrinologist when the lifestyle modification strategy is not enough for prevention of type 2 diabetes [21, 49]. Acarbose can also be considered to be used as a first-line antihyperglycemic agent [46, 48].

Gastrointestinal side effects have been an issue with acarbose. The predominant gastrointestinal symptom associated with acarbose is flatulence; however, loose stools and/or abdominal discomfort have also been reported. The side effects occur maximally during the first 2 weeks of therapy and start decreasing. By 12 weeks, 13.7% report flatulence and 2.2% diarrhea, and a 5-year surveillance study of about 2000 patients with diabetes found that gastrointestinal side effects associated with acarbose were reported by only 3.9% of patients [45]. For administration and dose adjustment and for understanding its metabolic benefits, its unique mode of action, not just alpha-glucosidase inhibition, need to be considered.

- The effect of acarbose is to delay the digestion of starch and oligosaccharides in the small intestine so that the release and absorption of glucose takes place over a longer time across the length of the small intestine. In many individuals, alpha-glucosidases are most active in the upper small intestine, and as acarbose treatment continues, there is a compensatory increase in enzyme activity in the lower small intestine and gastrointestinal side effects decrease over time [45].

- Furthermore, exposure of the lower small intestine to undigested carbohydrate leads to an increased quantity and duration of glucagon-like peptide-1 (GLP-1) release [45]. Acarbose also potentiates the reduction of ghrelin [46], thus may help to increase satiety.

- Low glycemic foods are preferred in type 2 diabetes. Low glycemic index foods are created by different processing methods; alpha-glucosidase inhibitors mimic these compounds in that they decrease the glycemic index (as well as the glycemic load) of carbohydrate-rich foods [46].

- Acarbose acts by competitive inhibition of alpha-glucosidase, so it is given at the same time as the ingested carbohydrate [45]. When taken as a tablet, the usual available form, it is less effective than when consumed in powdered form; so it is better to chew the tablet with food than to swallow at the beginning of a meal [47].

- Acarbose blocks and slows the digestion of complex carbohydrate, like starch, and sucrose (table sugar) without affecting the absorption of monosaccharides like glucose and fructose (present in fruits) and disaccharide lactose (present in milk products), which is digested by beta-glucosidase [44–47]. Trials in some countries report a higher incidence of gastrointestinal symptoms when initiating the dose of acarbose [46]. It may be due to the dietary habit of the population using sugar-rich food or soft drinks with or after meals. In any case, while initiating therapy with acarbose, starting with low dose (e.g. 25 mg or in a few cases still lower, once a day after dinner) and with slow stepwise-increasing dose over weeks avoiding the sugar-rich food or soft drinks with or after meals may help the patient to tolerate acarbose. Cochrane review reports that acarbose dosages higher than 50 mg three times daily offer no additional effect on HbA1c but more adverse effects instead. However, the fasting and post-load glucose may benefit from higher dosages [43].

Thus considering the benefits and safety of acarbose, it can be used in the treatment of diabetes next after metformin even if HbA1c is well controlled. With judicious initiation of the drug, most patients may be able to tolerate the drug. As in the case of metformin, those who tolerate the drug will be benefitted.

8. Principles of planning of antihyperglycemic therapy

Apart from various factors (**Figure 3**) to consider while prescribing antihyperglycemic medications, there are other principles to guide planning of antihyperglycemic therapy in type 2 diabetes.

8.1. Possible loss of excess bodyweight for as long as possible and regular physical activity and exercise: The cornerstones of therapy of diabetes

Loss of excess body weight and maintaining regular physical activity and exercise reduce insulin resistance and beta-cell workload and also benefit cardiovascular health and are thus the cornerstones of therapy of diabetes. The medications which support such aspects are preferred.

8.2. Requirement of combination therapy

Combination therapy, even in many newly diagnosed diabetic patients, is often required and it may also allow the use of submaximal doses of each antihyperglycemic medication resulting in fewer side effects [41, 42].

8.3. Need of gradual building up of the doses of metformin and acarbose

The doses of antihyperglycemic medications, particularly of metformin and acarbose having longer history of safety profile and other benefits, have to be built up slowly so that the patients tolerate the drugs; their maximum effect may take some time to be clinically evident.

8.4. 'Dynamic dose management of medications likely to cause hypoglycemia'

There is often need of controlling blood glucose immediately to prevent or treat acute complications [50]. Sulfonylurea and insulin act relatively fast. Insulin remains effective in all situations and it also helps to prevent ketosis. During the infection, other complications or immobility of the patients or the initial stage of diagnosis, rapid control of high blood glucose may thus be required to be done as rescue therapy. However, sulfonylurea, repaglinide and insulin not only cause hypoglycemia but also prevent the patients to lose weight and may even cause weight gain. Normalizing blood glucose is important, but there are other factors to consider as well (**Figure 3**). Moreover, even if sulfonylurea is continued to control the blood glucose, the glucose-lowering effect of sulfonylurea by beta-cell stimulation is not durable and wane over some years [41, 42]. DeFronzo has pointed out that such focus on simply HbA1c reduction with continuous use of sulfonylurea may lead to '*treat to fail*' approach and thus underlying pathophysiology also needs to be considered [41, 42]. The aim in the management of hyperglycemia in type 2 diabetes is to normalize it for as long as possible with the help of antihyperglycemic medications avoiding hypoglycemia and helping the patient to continue regular physical activity and exercise and to reduce excess bodyweight for as long

Phases of therapy	Diet, physical activity and exercise and weight plan	+	Regular use of antihyperglycemic medicines	±	Temporary use of other antihyperglycemic drugs likely to cause hypoglycemia*
1. Initiation of therapy	Recommended diet, reduction of excess body weight and regular physical activity and exercise	+	Gradually building up of metformin dose to the optimum level	±	Short-term temporary use of sulfonylurea or insulin to control hyperglycemia immediately as rescue therapy
2. Once the dose of metformin is optimum & tolerable, next phase of therapy with other 2nd to 4th drugs unlikely to cause hypoglycemia†,‡	Continue above diet, physical activity and exercise and weight plan	+	Addition of acarbose, pioglitazone, dipeptidyl peptidase-4 inhibitor, glucagon-like peptide-1 receptor agonist, sodium–glucose cotransporter 2 inhibitors	±	Short-term temporary use of sulfonylurea or insulin to control hyperglycemia immediately as rescue therapy
3. Regular hypoglycemic therapy	Continue diet and physical activity and exercise plan	+	Repaglinide, sulfonylurea or basal insulin with other drugs	±	Short-term temporary use insulin to control hyperglycemia immediately as rescue therapy
4. Long-term combination insulin therapy phase	Continue diet and physical activity and exercise plan	+	Combination insulin therapy with or without other drugs		

Note: The medications are used if not contraindicated and as per their effectiveness, tolerance by patients and local guidelines.

*'*Dynamic dose adjustment of medications likely to cause hypoglycemia*' aims to taper off the dosage of the drugs like sulfonylurea to continue normalization of HbA1c for long time with diet, regular physical activity and exercise and possible loss of excess bodyweight for as long as possible and with other drugs not likely to cause hypoglycemia.

†Even if HbA1c is well controlled, considering the long-term safety profile, mechanisms of action and negligible systemic absorption, acarbose can be added once the optimum dose of metformin is tolerated. Acarbose is started with low and slow stepwise-increasing dose over weeks or months to the optimum tolerable level. In patients only on antihyperglycemic drugs unlikely to cause hypoglycemia, they may have their major meals two times a day as per their convenience and custom. In such patients, the dose of acarbose can be gradually increased to the optimum tolerable level, e.g. 50–100 mg two times daily with the meals. Whatever the dose the patients tolerate, it is likely to be beneficial considering its unique mode of action and long-term safety profile.

‡Whether to add other new drug even if blood glucose is well controlled and which one to add as 3rd or 4th drug will depend on various factors as discussed in the text and on the guidelines of the local regulatory bodies.

Table 1. A suggested algorithm of antihyperglycemic therapy in type 2 diabetes.

as possible. Physical activity and exercise increases glucose utilization and reduces blood glucose. Thus, there is need of continuous effort to reduce the dose of sulfonylurea, repaglinide and insulin to the lowest possible level as the '*Dynamic dose management of medications likely to cause hypoglycemia*' letting the healthy lifestyle and other non-hypoglycemic antihyperglycemic drugs to maintain the blood glucose [50]. Patient education and guidance from family physicians, diabetes educators and other health care workers will help to achieve such dynamic dose management.

8.5. Long-term safety profile

Geoffrey Rose rightly highlighted 'Safety is paramount with long-term interventions' [9]. There is relatively longer history of safety profile with metformin and acarbose. They are preferred in the prevention and in the early phase of treatment of diabetes so that they can be safely continued for long time.

Based on such principles, a suggested approach of antihyperglycemic therapy is outlined in algorithm in **Table 1**.

Compared to the two agents prescribed separately, combination tablets reduce pill burden and help adherence of patients [49]. However due to the contrasting effect as well as the need of 'dynamic dose adjustment of medications likely to cause hypoglycemia' to the lowest possible dose and of gradual building of the dose of metformin for its continued maintenance at the optimum level, the formulation of fixed dose of combination of such drugs in a single tablet is irrational (**Table 2**) [50]. Availability of such fixed dose combination formulation in the market is likely to lead to the continued usage of sulfonylurea and suboptimal dosage of metformin even right from the time of diabetes diagnosis with all its effects in the patients.

	Metformin	Sulfonylurea or repaglinide
Hypoglycemia risk	Neutral	Moderate to severe
Effect on bodyweight	Slight loss	Gain
Major cardiovascular events	Beneficial	Generally neutral*
Principle of use	To maintain optimum dose	To keep the dose as minimum as possible to minimize hypoglycemia
Administration	Usually after meal	Usually before meal†
Dose adjustment with combination tablet	Difficult and the dose is likely to be suboptimal due to the fear of inducing hypoglycemia	Difficult and likely to cause hypoglycemia if the optimal dose of metformin is targeted or maintained

*Apart from the risk of effect of severe hypoglycemia on heart, it is also advised that use of the sulfonylurea types (glibenclamide, glipizide, glimepiride and others) that bind the sulfonylurea receptor-2 A and B should be avoided in high-risk patients suspected of having significant coronary artery disease [51].

†Sulfonylureas are often advised to be taken at least 15–20 minutes before a meal [51].

Table 2. The contrasting effect and uses of metformin and sulfonylurea and repaglinide making their fixed dose combination formulation irrational.

9. Avoiding unnecessary medicines and products

There is no clear evidence that dietary supplementation with vitamins, minerals, herbs or spices can improve outcomes in people with diabetes who do not have underlying deficiencies, and there may be safety concerns regarding their long-term use [25]. Unnecessary medication or local herbal, traditional or plant products may increase the cost and/or number of tablets to be taken which can affect the adherence to the essential medicines. Any medications or various products are also some form of chemicals and can also cause side effects, affect different organ systems or interact with other medications [52]. It is a famous saying 'Everything under the sun, including the sun, can cause allergy or side-effects'. For example, peripheral edema may occur in up to 16% with pregabalin [53]; however, amlodipine, a useful and essential medicine for hypertension, may instead be inadvertently stopped due to its well-known association with peripheral edema. Symptoms like tingling, numbness or others may need to be investigated. However, if treatment does not change the course of the condition and if symptoms do not affect sleep or daily life of the patients, explanation and reassurance with the required follow-up may be preferred than using unnecessary medications.

Research perspectives: State may develop some support system (e.g. by making available research funds or by involving pharmaceutical companies or other donor agencies) to study the local herbal, traditional or plant products and to identify and isolate the active the pharmacological ingredient of such possible crude products [52].

10. Education to the patient and training of educators

Structured education is an integral part of diabetes care [39]. Lifestyle management is a fundamental aspect of diabetes care and includes diabetes self-management education, diabetes self-management support, nutrition therapy, physical activity, smoking cessation counseling and psychosocial carc [25]. Nurses and other healthcare professionals requires adequate training and certification to work in the health system to fill the gap between medical professionals and patients and thus between the available scientific knowledge and effective application by the patients [50].

Public health perspectives: For the training in the management and education of people with diabetes, the nurses and other healthcare professionals (with minimum of 2 years of professional practice experience) should have at least 1000 hours of practice experience in diabetes self-management education along with various educational activities [54]. In the non-industrialized countries, it may thus entail 1 year of working under the supervision of physicians (as a sort of residential training) in the daily diabetes and other outdoor and indoor services providing care and education to the patients fulfilling the other training requirements (like logbook recordings of case history records, procedure and academic activities, assignments and assessments) [50, 55]. To incorporate such trained personnel in the local health system, the terminology of certification of such training should match with the nomenclatures of other existing healthcare workers and with the various intervention programs being planned and/or implemented [55].

11. Programmes to control diabetes epidemic

There are extensive work done and literature available regarding the diabetes epidemiology, healthy lifestyle, primary prevention of diabetes and effects of gestational diabetes and *in utero* malnutrition and hyperglycemia. Many of them have been cited in the various publications referred in this chapter [1–3, 7, 10, 25, 27, 29, 32, 39, 49, 56, 57, 67, 68]. In this section, the focus is on briefly highlighting the urgent priority public health programmes required to control the diabetes epidemic. The perspectives on controlling the diabetes epidemic in the population as a whole, not just primary prevention of diabetes in individuals, and the implementations of the required programmes are the dire needs today.

11.1. Factors fueling the diabetes epidemic

The epidemic of glucose intolerance in the world is relatively a new phenomenon starting since the latter half of twentieth century and the initial rise in diabetes prevalence has occurred differently in various populations in the world [56, 57]. For example, gradual rise in diabetes prevalence has occurred in Europids in Europe, Canada and the USA since around 1940s with increasing sedentary life, obesity and aging with about a third of their population over 50 years of age. On the top of similar gradual rise, the migrant or urbanized Asian-Indian, Arab, African, Chinese and Hispanic people faced the rapid rise of diabetes prevalence since around 1970s mostly due to the rapid transition in the nutritional status of population leading to dissociation in metabolic states of fetal life (associated with nutritional want) and adult life (with nutritional surfeit) of people. The indigenous people of the USA, Canada, Australia and Pacific region also faced the rapid rise in diabetes prevalence (due to the rapid transition in their nutritional status) since around 1940s and subsequently further faced the accelerated rise mostly due to the addition of the factor of maternal hyperglycemia during pregnancy affecting the *in utero* life of the offspring [56].

Such variations in the rise in diabetes prevalence in different populations can just be ascribed to the effect of ethnic variations leading to a sense of fatalism. The concept of ethnicity does provide self-identification with cultural traditions and social identity and boundaries between groups, but it has dynamic nature [58]. Ethnicity is a sort of surrogate marker for multiple environmental and genetic factors (though genetics playing a relatively small part), in disease causation and for public health policy [56, 59, 60]. In terms of the scientific approach and public health policy, ethnic variations in the prevalence of any disease or condition should lead the humankind to search for such environmental or genetic factors [59]. The different pattern of initial rise in diabetes prevalence in various populations in the world, thus, appears to be related to the various proportions of three groups of risk factors present in different populations. Thus, the three groups of such possible factors to consider are [56]:

- obesity, sedentary life and aging;

- the rapid transition in the nutritional status of population leading to dissociation in metabolic states of fetal life (associated with nutritional want) and adult life (with nutritional surfeit) of people (this factor of *in utero* undernutrition appears to limit the range of normal body mass index in adult life in such population and even in the individual person of any population group) and
- maternal hyperglycemia during pregnancy affecting the *in utero* life of the offspring.

Whatever may be the differences of the initial rise in diabetes prevalence in the world and its pathogenesis, the fact remains that diabetes epidemic is now increasingly affecting the younger and younger population. There is, thus, the need to consider all possible factors to control the epidemic of diabetes in all the populations.

11.2. Healthy diet and weight and regular physical activity and exercise at the population level

Healthy diet with proportionate intake of nutrients, body weight as per the recommended body mass index for the population and regular physical activity and exercise are applicable to general population and people with impaired glucose intolerance, diabetes and CVDs [3, 10, 21, 25, 32, 39, 56].

Public health perspectives: Campaigns and programmes are required to make the people, housewives and children well aware of the recommended bodyweight (as required for the respective population) and the recommendations regarding the daily intake of plain water, fruit, vegetables, salt, sugar, fat (with adequate proportion of mono- and poly-unsaturated and saturated fatty acid) and other nutrient avoiding the trans-fatty acid. Multisectoral population-based approaches, including trade and agricultural policies and the workplace-, school- and other setting-based interventions, for healthy diet and physical activity and exercise need to be considered [2, 3, 10, 56].

Public health perspectives: Pedestrians, cyclists and public transport passengers are the top three hierarchy groups recommended while developing transport and traffic strategies [61]. It is also essential to have campaigns and support system to develop various physical activity and exercise programmes at the community, school and various workplace levels like regular walking, games and sports, marathon running, aerobic dance and others [2, 3, 10, 56].

11.3. Prevention of maternal and childhood malnutrition

Taking a life-course perspective is essential for preventing type 2 diabetes, as it is for many health conditions [2]. Firstborn offspring in the resource poor settings may be at increased risk of glucose intolerance due to the likelihood of possible maternal malnutrition during the first pregnancy as compared to that in later pregnancy [56, 62]. Adequate nutrition and micro- and macronutrient supply before and during pregnancy are the steps to reduce the risk of *in utero* malnutrition and its ill effects [27]. Good nutrition during infancy and childhood and adequate physical activity among children are important for the development of a healthy child and an adult [27].

11.4. Maintenance of optimal pre-pregnancy bodyweight: the key programme required

The diagnosis of gestational diabetes mellitus (GDM) usually made at 24–28 weeks is applicable for the clinical management of the women and their children during and after pregnancy and it may also be useful for the mothers for primary prevention of later development of diabetes. From further public health perspectives to avoid any possible long-term *in utero* effect, prevention of subclinical maternal hyperglycemia right from the time of conception needs to be considered [56]. The sedentary lifestyle, obesity and glucose intolerance affecting relatively younger population are increasing in the community. The risk of maternal hyperglycemia during pregnancy has thus increased (**Figure 5**) [56]. The relative risk of developing overt GDM over the age of 35 years is 2.57 [63]. However, significant increase in the risk of overt GDM is reported even at age >25 years as compared to that in lower age [64].

The exact 'safe' normal level of maternal plasma glucose to prevent relative hyperglycemia *in utero* for fetus appears difficult to define. To find out such level, long period of follow-up is required after birth of offspring with exposure to different levels of maternal plasma glucose correlating with other risk factors [56, 57]. The normal value of neonatal plasma glucose may give some insight. However, the limits of normal plasma glucose defining neonatal hypoglycemia in infants are arbitrary. Neonatal glucose concentrations may decrease after birth, to as low as 30 mg/dL during the first 1–2 hours after birth, and then increase to higher and relatively more stable concentrations, generally above 45 mg/dL by 12 hours after birth [65, 66]. Later, it will gradually rise to adult levels.

Considering the risks of the macrosomia development, the safe normal level of fasting plasma glucose during pregnancy appears to be below 80 mg/dL (4.4 mmol/L), perhaps

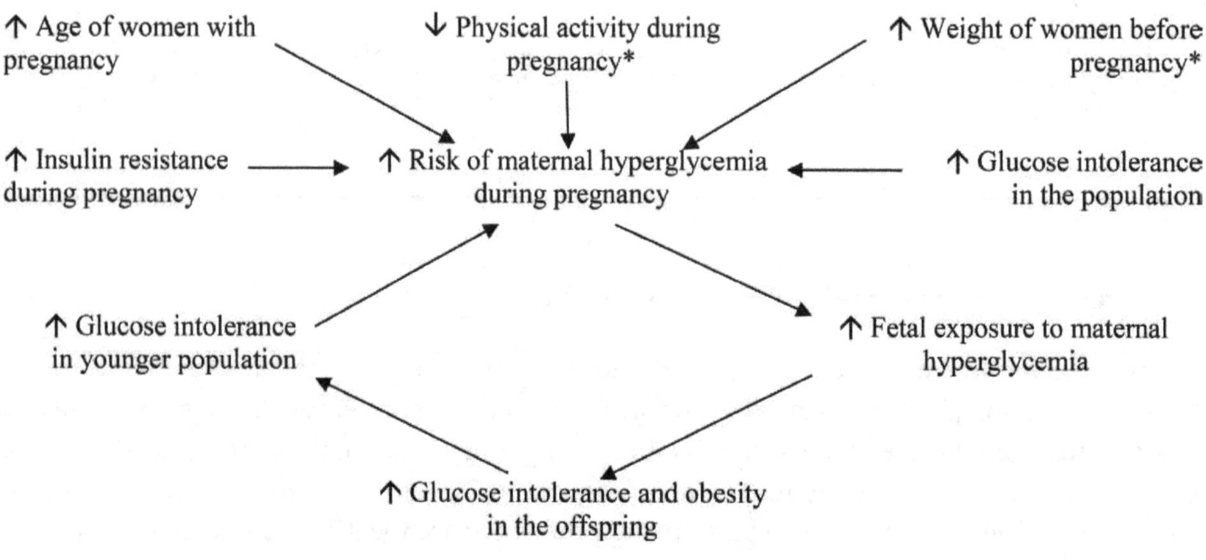

Figure 5. A vicious circle of glucose intolerance in younger population and maternal hyperglycemia during pregnancy. *The two preventable factors from the public health and clinical management perspectives. (Figure published with minor modification with kind permission from *JNMA*2009;48;173 [56]).

even below 75 mg/dL (4.2 mmol/L) [67, 68]. Macrosomia is to a great extent measurable but the fetal programming due to relative maternal hyperglycemia is difficult to assess and is obviously likely to be affected earlier than the overt macrosomia. Weeks 3–8 encompass organogenesis and major malformations in infants of diabetic mother occur during these periods [69]. So to protect the fetus from any possible effect of maternal hyperglycemia, blood glucose during the whole duration, including the early stage, of pregnancy has to be within the safe normal level [56, 57]. As discussed earlier that even in non-pregnant state, the risk of insulin resistance and diabetes in adult increases progressively upwards of a BMI of 20–22 kg/m^2 and more than 80% of the people with diabetes live in low- and middle-income countries and nearly two thirds of diabetes globally are attributable to BMI above 21 kg/m^2 [10]. Considering the inherent insulin resistance during pregnancy and increasing age of mother, the pre-pregnancy bodyweight should preferably around or below the middle of the recommended BMI for the population [56]. In Finland with predominant Europid population, the mean pre-pregnancy BMI of women were 21.9 and 23.7 kg/m^2 in 1960s and 2000, respectively [70]. If it increases to higher level, as in many other populations, the risk of glucose intolerance during pregnancy may also increase. Women who had a child gains extra weight than women who remained nulliparous [71] and the second and subsequent offspring were anticipated about a decade earlier to have increased risk of *in utero* exposure to the maternal clinical or sub-clinical hyperglycemia due to the increased weight of mothers [56]. A recent study indeed reported increased risk of GDM with increasing weight gain from first to second pregnancy [72]. In summary, campaign and programmes for maintenance of optimal pre-pregnancy body weight as per the recommended body mass index of the respective populations along with regular physical activity and exercise during pregnancy are the essential measures available at hand to prevent the possibility of maternal hyperglycemia right from the early pregnancy and are the urgent priority to control diabetes epidemic.

Research perspective: Long-term follow-up study of offspring with exposure to different levels of maternal plasma glucose correlating with other risk factors can be conducted. Possible risk of obesity and early glucose intolerance in both female and male offspring due to the *in utero* hyperglycemia could also be due to the involvement of mitochondrial DNA. Exposure of mitochondrial DNA to reactive oxygen species (ROS) can lead to mitochondrial mutation [73]. Glucose excursions can lead to the formation of ROS, such as superoxide, which leads to oxidative stress in the body [74] and acute hyperglycemia can lead to oxidative stress with increase in the markers of oxidative damage [75–77]. Such oxidative stress due to high glucose level for the fetus during pregnancy can thus be postulated to lead to oxidative damage to fetal mitochondrial DNA and the offspring in this way may later be at increased risk of obesity and glucose intolerance. Superoxide anions, markers of oxidative damage and mediators of subclinical inflammation can be analyzed in the fetal, amniotic and/or maternal samples. If it is such mitochondrial inheritance as postulated, the affected female offspring would transmit the disease to all their children, and affected male offspring, however, would not transmit the disease to their children. The possibility of such pattern can be studied in the populations with high prevalence of type 2 diabetes in young age.

Public health perspectives: Examples of prevention and control programmes in the communicable diseases as a model for similar strategies required at individual and population levels for diabetes epidemic are summarized [78] in **Table 3**. Control programme to protect the other susceptible populations (**Table 3**) is the dire need today to control diabetes epidemic.

	Examples in the communicable disease	Examples in diabetes[†]
Prevention programmes for individuals	• Immunization • Personal protective measures • Chemoprophylaxis	• Population-wide and primary prevention programs with healthy food, physical activity and exercise and weight reduction interventions to prevent impaired glucose tolerance and diabetes • Campaign and programmes to help achieve the body mass index by the people as recommended to the respective populations
Control programmes to protect the other susceptible populations[*]	• Isolation • Quarantine • Vector control (e.g. mosquito control for various diseases, cyclops control for guinea worm, chicken and poultry culling for avian influenza) • Treatment of case (e.g. tuberculosis) and carrier	Campaign and programmes for • Maintenance of optimal pre-pregnancy body weight, as per the recommended body mass index of the respective populations • Nutritional support for the girls and women of childbearing age in rural and poorer sections of the societies

*The vulnerable populations to be protected by the control programme of diabetes include the offspring of malnourished or overweight mothers during their *in utero* life.

†National and international health and diabetes agencies should clearly spell out the control programmes, with appropriate budget allocation, for the control of diabetes epidemic.

Table 3. Examples of prevention and control programmes in the communicable diseases as a model for similar strategies for individuals and susceptible populations in diabetes epidemic (table published with minor modification) [78].

12. Conclusion

Adequate control of blood pressure, use of statin, cessation of tobacco use, regular physical activity and exercise and possible loss of excess bodyweight for as long as possible are the core management aspects in diabetes. Judicious use of antihyperglycemic drugs requires consideration of various factors, especially hypoglycemia and effect on bodyweight and cardiovascular events. The aim should also be to achieve normalization of HbA1c for long time by loss of excess bodyweight for as long as possible, regular physical activity and exercise and using regularly the antihyperglycemic medications not having the risk of hypoglycemia. 'Dynamic dose adjustment of medications likely to cause hypoglycemia' helps to apply such principles by temporary use of sulfonylurea or insulin as rescue therapy. Apart from such clinical management and various research aspects, there are public health approaches to be considered as the top priority for the control of diabetes epidemic in the population. The diagnosis of gestational diabetes usually made at 24–28 weeks is applicable for the clinical management of mother and child and for possible primary prevention of diabetes later in the mother. From the public health perspectives, however, protection of the susceptible *in utero* population from maternal malnutrition or clinical or subclinical hyperglycemia right from the time of conception itself is particularly required to control diabetes epidemic at the population level. There is urgent need of campaigns and programmes for maintenance of optimal pre-pregnancy body weight, as per the recommended body mass index for the respective populations.

Author details

Madhur Dev Bhattarai

Address all correspondence to: mdb@ntc.net.np

Nepal Diabetes Association, Kathmandu, Nepal

References

[1] International Diabetes Federation. Diabetes Atlas. Brussels: IDF; 2015. Available from: https://www.idf.org/e-library/epidemiology-research/diabetes-atlas

[2] WHO. Global Report on Diabetes. Geneva: WHO; 2016. Available from: http://apps.who.int/iris/bitstream/10665/204871/1/9789241565257_eng.pdf

[3] WHO. Preventing Chronic Disease: A Vital Investment. Geneva: WHO; 2005. Available from: http://apps.who.int/iris/bitstream/10665/43314/1/9241563001_eng.pdf

[4] Anderson GF, Chu E. Expanding priorities – confronting chronic disease in countries with low income. New England Journal of Medicine. 2007;**356**(3):209-211. DOI: 10.1056/NEJMp068182

[5] Hornby AS. Oxford Advanced Learner's Dictionary of Current English. Oxford: Oxford University Press; 2010. ISBN 978-0-19-479910-2

[6] American Public Health Association. Fact Sheet: What is Public Health? Washington: APHA, April 23 2015. Available from: https://www.apha.org/~/media/files/pdf/fact-sheets/whatisph.ashx

[7] Lloyd-Jones DM, Hong Y, Labarthe D, et al. American Heart Association special report: Defining and setting national goals of cardiovascular health promotion and disease reduction. Circulation. 2010;**121**:586-613. DOI: 10.1161/CIRCULATIONAHA.109.192703

[8] Greeenland P, Lloyd-Jones D. Time to end the mixed and often incorrect messages about prevention and treatment of atherosclerotic cardiovascular disease. Journal of the American College of Cardiology. 2007;**50**(22):2133-2135. DOI: 10.1016/j.jacc.2007.05.055

[9] Rose G. Strategy of prevention: Lessons from cardiovascular disease. British Medical Journal. 1981;**282**:1847-1851 6786649

[10] WHO. World Health Report 2002: Reducing Risks, Promoting Healthy Life. Geneva: WHO; 2002. Available from: http://www.who.int/whr/2002/en/whr02_en.pdf?ua=1

[11] WHO. A Global Brief on Hypertension: Silent Killer, Global Public Health Crisis. Geneva: WHO; 2013. Available from: http://apps.who.int/iris/bitstream/10665/79059/1/WHO_DCO_WHD_2013.2_eng.pdf?ua=1

[12] Bakris GL, Sowerjs JR. American Society of Hypertension Position Paper: Treatment of hypertension in patients with diabetes – An update. Journal of Clinical Hypertension. 2008;**10**:707-713. DOI: 10.1111/j.1751-7176.2008.00012.x

[13] Lim SS, Vos T, Flaxmon AD, et al. A comparative risk assessment of burden of disease and attributable to 67 risk factors and risk factor clusters in 21 regions, 1990-2010: A systematic analysis for the Global Burden of Disease Study 2010. Lancet, 2012;**380**:2224-2260 DOI: http://dx.doi.org/10.1016/S0140-6736(12)61766-8

[14] Ramchandran SV, Larson MG, Leip EP, et al. Impact of high-normal blood pressure on the risk of cardiovascular disease. New England Journal of Medicine. 2001;**345**:1291-1297. DOI: 10.1056/NEJMoa003417

[15] Bhattarai MD. Facilitation of free residential training inside the country – The fundamental health service responsibility of the Government and its regulatory body. Journal of Nepal Medical Association. 2015;**53**(197):40-69 PMID: 26983048. Available from: http://jnma.com.np/jnma/index.php/jnma/article/view/2704/2239

[16] Bartnik M, Ryden L, Ferrari R, et al. On behalf of the euro heart survey investigators. The prevalence of abnormal glucose regulation in patients with coronary artery disease across Europe: The euro heart survey on diabetes and the heart. European Heart Journal. 2004;**25**:1880-1890. DOI: https://doi.org/10.1016/j.ehj.2004.09.021

[17] Rajbhandari A, Pandeya DR, Bhattarai MD, Malla R. Blood glucose levels in patients with coronary artery disease. Medical Journal of Shree Birendra Hospital. 2012;**11**(1):4-8. Available from: https://www.nepjol.info/index.php/MJSBH/article/viewFile/7758/6339

[18] Shrestha UK, Singh DL, Bhattarai MD. The prevalence of hypertension and diabetes defined by fasting and 2-h plasma glucose criteria in urban Nepal. Diabet Med. 2006;**23**(10):1130-5. DOI: 10.1111/j.1464-5491.2006.01953.x

[19] Stamler J, Vaccaro O, Neaton JD, Wentworth D. The multiple risk factor intervention trial research group. Diabetes, other risk factors and 12-year cardiovascular mortality for men screened in the multiple risk factor intervention trial. Diabetes Care. 1993;**16**:434-444. DOI: https://doi.org/10.2337/diacare.16.2.434

[20] Preiss D, Ray KK. Intensive glucose lowering treatment in type 2 diabetes. British Medical Journal. 2011;**343**:d4243. DOI: https://doi.org/10.1136/bmj.d4243

[21] International Diabetes Federation. Recommendations for managing type 2 diabetes in primary care, 2017. Brussels: International Diabetes Federation. Available from: www.idf.org/managing-type2-diabetes

[22] Piano MR, Benowitz NL, Fitzgerald GA, et al. A policy statement from the American Heart Association - Impact of smokeless tobacco products on cardiovascular disease: Implications for policy, prevention, and treatment. Circulation. 2010;**122**(15):1520-1544. DOI: 10.1161/CIR.0b013e3181f432c3

[23] Lawson PJ, Flocke SA, Casucci B. Development of an instrument to document the 5A's smoking cessation. American Journal of Preventive Medicine. 2009;**37**(3):248-254. DOI: 10.1016/j.amepre.2009.04.027

[24] Lindson-Hawley N, Banting M, West R, Michie S, Shinkins B, Aveyard P. Gradual versus abrupt smoking cessation: A randomized controlled noninferiority trial. Annals of Internal Medicine. 2016;**164**(9):585-592. DOI: 10.7326/M14-2805

[25] American Diabetes Association. Position Statement: Standards of medical Care in Diabetes – 2017. Diabetes Care. 2017;**40**(Suppl 1):S1-S138. DOI: 10.2337/dc17-S001

[26] Helmrich SP, Ragland DR, Leung RW, Paffenbarger RS. Physical activity and reduced occurrences of non-insulin-depended diabetes mellitus. The New England Journal of Medicine. 1991;**325**:147-152. DOI: 10.1056/NEJM199107183250302

[27] Ramachandran A, Chamukuttan S, Shetty S, Nanditha A. Primary prevention of type 2 diabetes in south Asians – Challenges and the way forward. Diabetic Medicine. 2013;**30**: 26-34. DOI: 10.1111/j.1464-5491.2012.03753

[28] Tobias DK, Zhang C, van Dam RM, et al. Physical activity before and during pregnancy and risk of gestational diabetes mellitus: A metanalysis. Diabetes Care. 2011;**34**(1):223-229. DOI: 10.2337/dc10-1368

[29] National Institute for Health and Care Excellence Guideline. Diabetes in pregnancy: management of diabetes and its complications from preconception to the postnatal period. London: NICE, 2015 nice.org.uk/guidance/ng3

[30] Ruderman N, for American Diabetes Association. Handbook of Exercise in Diabetes. New Delhi: Viva Books Private Limited, 2004. ISBN 10: 8176498734 ISBN 13: 9788176498739

[31] Bhattarai MD. Osteoarthritis of the knee. Lancet. 1997;**350**(9087):1328. PMID: 9357435

[32] National Institute for Health and Care Excellence Guideline. Cardiovascular disease: risk assessment and reduction, including lipid modification. London: NICE, 2014 (Updated September 2016). Available from: https://www.nice.org.uk/guidance/cg181

[33] Liao JK. Safety and efficacy of statins in Asians. The American Journal of Cardiology. 2007;**99**(3):410-414. DOI: 10.1016/j.amjcard.2006.08.051

[34] WHO Consultation on Obesity. Obesity: Preventing and Managing the Global Epidemic. Geneva: WHO; 1998. Available from: http://whqlibdoc.who.int/hq/1998/WHO_NUT_NCD_98.1_(p1-158).pdf

[35] World Health Organization, International Association for the Study of Obesity, International Obesity Task Force. The Asia-Pacific Perspective: Redefining Obesity and its Treatment. Sydney: Health Communications; 2000. Available from: http://www.wpro.who.int/nutrition/documents/docs/Redefiningobesity.pdf

[36] WHO Expert Consultation. Appropriate body-mass index for Asian populations and its implications for policy and intervention strategies. Lancet. 2004;**363**:157-163. DOI: 10.1016/S0140-6736(03)15268-3

[37] Alberti G, Zimmet P. The IDF consensus on the prevention of type 2 diabetes. Diabetic Medicine. 2007;**24**(5):451-456. DOI: 10.1111/j.1464-5491.2007.02157.x

[38] Razak F, Anand SS, Shannon H, et al. Defining obesity cut points in a multiethnic population. Circulation. 2007;**115**(16):2111-2118. DOI: 10.1161/CIRCULATIONAHA.106.635011

[39] National Institute for Health and Care Excellence Guideline. Type 2 diabetes in adults: management. London: NICE, 2015 (Updated May 2017). Available from: https://www.nice.org.uk/guidance/ng28

[40] Halban PA, Polonsky KS, Bowden DW, et al. B-cell failure in type 2 diabetes: Postulated mechanisms and prospects for prevention and treatment. Diabetes Care. 2014;**37**(6):1751-1758. DOI: 10.2337/dc14-0396

[41] DeFronzo RA, Eldor R, Abdul-Ghani M. Pathophysiologic approach to therapy in patients with newly diagnose type 2 diabetes. Diabetes Care. 2013;**36**(Suppl 2):S127-S134. DOI: 10.2337/dcS13-2011

[42] DeFronzo RA. From the triumvirate to the ominous octet: A new paradigm for the treatment of type 2 diabetes mellitus. Diabetes. 2009;**58**:773-787. DOI: 10.2337/db09-9028

[43] Van de Laar FA, Lucassen PLBJ, Akkermans RP et al. Alpha-glucosidase inhibitors for type 2 diabetes mellitus. Cochrane Database Syst Rev. 2005;**2**:CD003639. DOI: 10.1002/14651858.CD003639.pub2

[44] Kalra S. Alpha glucosidase inhibitors. The Journal of the Pakistan Medical Association. 2014;**64**(4):4746. PMID: 24864650

[45] Hanefield M. Cardiovascular benefits and safety profile of acarbose therapy in prediabetes and established type 2 diabetes. Cardiovascular Diabetology. 2007;**6**:20. DOI: 10.1186/1475-2840-6-20

[46] DiNicolantonio JJ, Bhutani J, O'Keefe JH. Acarbose: Safe and effective for lowering postprandial hyperglycemia and improving cardiovascular outcomes. Open Heart. 2015;**2**:e000327. DOI: 10.1136/openhrt-2015-000327

[47] Dean W. Anti-aging and life extension medicine. Acarbose: Anti-diabetic, Cardio-protective, Weight loss, and potential Anti-aging agent. Available from: http://warddeanmd.com/acarbose-antidiabetic-cardioprotective-weight-loss-potential-antiaging-agent/ [Accessed: 2017-08-22]

[48] Joshi SR, Ramachandran A, Chadha M, et al. Acarbose plus metformin fixed-dose combination in the management of type 2 diabetes. Expert Opinion on Pharmacotherapy. 2014;**15**(11):1-10. DOI: 10.1517/14656566.2014.932771

[49] Garber AJ, Abrahamson MJ, Barzilay JI, et al. American Association of Clinical Endocrinologists Consensus Statement: AACE' comprehensive diabetes management algorithm 2013 consensus statement. Endocrine Practice. 2013;**19**(Suppl 2):1-35. DOI: 10.4158/EP13176.CSUPPL

[50] Bhattarai MD. Comprehensive diabetes and non-communicable disease educator in the low-resource settings. Journal of the Nepal Medical Association. 2016;**54**(202):94-103. PubMed: 27935933; Available from: http://jnma.com.np/jnma/index.php/jnma/article/view/2828/2548

[51] Bosenberg LH, van Zyl DG. The mechanism of action of oral antidiabetic drugs: A review of recent literature. Journal of Endocrinology, Metabolism and Diabetes of South Africa 2008;**13**(3):80-88. DOI: 10.1080/22201009.2008.10872177

[52] Bhattarai MD. Need of the regulation for profit percentage investment by pharmaceutical companies in new drug discovery research from the various local traditional medicinal and plant systems. Journal of the Nepal Medical Association. 2012;**52**(187):148-150. PMID: 23591178 Available from: http://jnma.com.np/jnma/index.php/jnma/article/view/366/510

[53] Lexicomp®. Pregabalin: Drug information. Waltham: UpToDate, 2017;**19**:3. Accessed on 2017-09-20 from http://cursoenarm.net/UPTODATE/contents/mobipreview.htm?6/4/6223?source=see_link

[54] National Certification Board of Diabetes Educator. Certification Examination for Diabetes Educators. St. Olathe (US): NCBDE; 2015. Available from: https://diabetesed.net/page/_files/NCBDE-Handbook-2015.pdf [Accessed: Aug 22, 2017]

[55] Bhattarai MD. Re: Comprehensive diabetes and non-communicable disease educator in the low-resource settings – As NCD primary care assistant with one year training. Journal of the Nepal Medical Association. 2017;**56**(205):196-197. PubMed: 28598464. Available from: http://jnma.com.np/jnma/index.php/jnma/article/view/2899/2597

[56] Bhattarai MD. Three patterns of rising type 2 diabetes prevalence in the world: Need to widen the concept of prevention in individuals into control in the community. Journal of the Nepal Medical Association. 2009;**48**(174):173-179. PMID: 20387365. Available from: http://jnma.com.np/jnma/index.php/jnma/article/view/240/640

[57] Bhattarai MD. Response to Donovan et al. does exposure to hyperglycaemia in utero increase the risk of obesity and diabetes in the offspring. Diabetic Medicine. 2015. DOI: 10.1111/dme.12980.

[58] Lip GYH, Barnett AH, Bradbury A, et al. Ethnicity and cardiovascular disease prevention in the United Kingdom: A practical approach to management. Journal of Human Hypertension. 2007;**21**:183-211. DOI: 10.1038/sj.jhh.1002126

[59] Pearce N, Foliaki S, Sporle A, Cunningham C. Genetics, race, ethnicity and health. British Medical Journal. 2004;**328**:1070. DOI: 10.1136/bmj.328.7447.1070

[60] Collins FS. What we do and don't know about 'race', 'ethnicity', genetics and health at the dawn of the genome era. Nature Genetics. 2004;**36**(11):S13-S15. DOI: 10.1034/ng1436

[61] UK Parliamentary Business – Select Committee on Environment, Transport and Regional Affairs Eleventh Report. Walking in towns and cities. Available from: URL: http://www.publications.parliament.uk/pa/cm200001/cmselect/cmenvtra/167/16708.htm#n [Accessed: 2017-08-22]

[62] Bajracharya MR, Bhattarai MD, Karki BB, Prajapati S, Karmacharya D, Manandhar S, Rajouria AD. Insulin resistance in firstborn offspring of mother who developed diabetes later in fourth decade: Are both related to possible maternal malnutrition? Journal of Advances in Internal Medicine 2014;**03**(02):56-61. DOI: http://dx.doi.org/10.3126/jaim.v3i2.14065

[63] Wagaarachchi PT, Fernando L, Premachadra P, Fernando DJS. Screening based on risk factors for gestational diabetes in an Asian population. Journal of Obstetrics and Gynaecology. 2001;**21**:32-34. http://dx.doi.org/10.1080/01443610020022087

[64] Thapa P, Shrestha S, Flora MS, Bhattarai MD, et al. Gestational diabetes mellitus – A public health concern in rural communities of Nepal. Journal of Nepal Health Research Council 2015;**13**(31):175-181. ISSN 1999-6217

[65] Adamkin DH, & Committee on Fetus and Newborn, American Academy of Pediatrics. Clinical report – Postnatal glucose homeostasis in late-preterm and term infants. Pediatrics. 2011;**127**(3):575-579. DOI: 10.1542/peds.2010-3851

[66] Canadian Paediatric Society. Checking blood glucose in newborn babies. Paediatrics & Child Health. 2004;**9**(10):731-732. DOI: https://doi.org/10.1093/pch/9.10.731

[67] Metzger BE, Lowe LP, Dyer AR, et al. Hyperglycemia and adverse pregnancy outcomes. The New England Journal of Medicine. 2008;**358**(19):1991-2002. DOI: 10.1056/NEJMoa0707943

[68] International Association of Diabetes and Pregnancy Study Groups Consensus Panel. Recommendations on the diagnosis and classification of hyperglycemia in pregnancy. Diabetes Care. 2010;**33**:676. DOI: 10.2337/dc09-1848

[69] Buchanan TA. Effects of maternal diabetes on intrauterine development. In: LeRoith D, Taylor SI, Olefsky JM, editors. Diabetes Mellitus. Philadelphia: Lippincott-Raven; 1996. p. 684-695

[70] Kinnunen TI, Luoto R, Gissler M, Hemminki E. Pregnancy weight gain from 1960s to 2000 in Finland. International Journal of Obesity and Related Metabolic Disorders. 2003;**27**(12):1572-1577. DOI: 10.1038/sj.ijo.0802471

[71] Bhattarai MD, Singh DL. Excessive weight gain after pregnancy in urban areas: One important area to prevent diabetes. Nepal Medical College Journal. 2005;**7**(2):87-89. PMID: 16519070

[72] Sorbye LM, Skjaerven R, Klungsoyr K, Morket NH. Gestational diabetes mellitus and interpregnancy weight change: A population-based cohort study. PLoS Medicine. 2017;**14**(8):e1002367. DOI: https://doi.org/10.1371/journal.pmed.1002367

[73] Allen JF, de Paula WBM. Mitochondrial genome function and maternal inheritance. Biochemical Society Transactions, 2013;**41**:1298-1304. DOI: 10.1042/BST20130106

[74] Brownlee M. Biochemistry and molecular cell biology of diabetic complications. Nature. 2001;**414**:813-820. DOI: 10.1038/414813a

[75] Marfella R, Quagliaro L, Nappo F, et al. Acute hyperglycemia induces an oxidative stress in healthy subjects. The Journal of Clinical Investigation. 2001;**108**:635-636. DOI: 10.1172/JCI13727

[76] Ceriello A, Bortolotti N, Crescentini A, et al. Antioxidant defences are reduced during the oral glucose tolerance test in normal and non-insulin-dependent diabetic subjects. European Journal of Clinical Investigation. 1998;**28**:329-333. PMID: 9615913

[77] Ceriello A, Quagliaro L, Catone B, et al. Role of hyperglycemia in nitrotyrosine post-prandial generation. Diabetes Care. 2002;**25**:1439-1443. PMID: 12145247

[78] Bhattarai MD. Examining left axis deviation. In:. Interpreting Cardiac Electrograms - From Skin to Endocardium. Michael KA, Ed. Rijeka: Intech, 2017. DOI: 10.5772/intechopen.69435

2

Very Low-Calorie Diets in Type 2 Diabetes Mellitus: Effects on Inflammation, Clinical and Metabolic Parameters

Luis M. Román-Pintos, Geannyne Villegas-Rivera,
Ernesto G. Cardona-Muñoz,
Adolfo D. Rodríguez-Carrizalez, Aldo Moreno-Ulloa,
Nicole Rubin and Alejandra G. Miranda-Díaz

Abstract

Type 2 diabetes mellitus (DM) is a chronic and multifactorial disease strongly linked to a low-grade inflammatory process. Thus far, type 2 DM is generally regarded as an incurable disease by common therapies. However, very low-calorie diet (VLCD) regimens have demonstrated beneficial and rapid effects on glucose metabolism in subjects with type 2 DM. These beneficial effects include improvement of diabetes complications, insulin sensitivity and reduction in glycaemia, glycated hemoglobin (HbA1C), and triglyceride levels. VLCD regimens commonly comprise no more than 800 kcal/day and are therefore associated with rapid weight loss in overweight and obese individuals. This group of diets positively affects local/systemic inflammation and oxidative stress (OS) by modulating inflammatory cytokines, adipokines and endogenous antioxidant levels. The investigation of VLCDs in the field of type 2 DM treatment is progressively augmenting due to the multiple benefits in cardiometabolic health of overweight/obese subjects with type 2 DM. Here, we gather and review the evidence regarding the role of inflammation and OS in individuals with type 2 DM under VLCD regimens.

Keywords: very low-calorie diet, obesity, type 2 diabetes mellitus remission, oxidative stress, adipokines

1. Introduction

Thus far, type 2 diabetes mellitus (DM) is recognized as an incurable metabolic disease by common therapies. Obesity and type 2 DM are intrinsically correlated, and low-grade chronic inflammation at a local and systemic site has been suggested as a key component in the progression toward the disease [1, 2]. In this regard, very low-calorie diet (VLCD) regimens, providing <800 kcal/d, have demonstrated to exert a beneficial and rapid effect on glucose metabolism in individuals with type 2 DM, which are not seen with pharmacological therapies [3]. Since 1970, VLCD has been used to induce rapid weight loss with a favorable safety profile [4]. Benefits of VLCD in T2DM patients with obesity include weight loss, fat mass reduction, reversion of hyperglycemia, elimination of pharmacologic treatment and normalization of both beta cell function and hepatic insulin sensitivity [3, 5]. The main mechanism by which VLCD regimens exert their beneficial effects on metabolism of type 2 DM subjects appears to be their capacity to induce weight loss and modulate inflammation via cytokines and adipokines [6–8]. However, there are considerable limitations of VLCD regimens in certain individuals. The most common issue to resolve in clinical trials evaluating VLCD regimens is noncompliance of patients due to previous dietary patterns, psychological aspects, vitamin deficiency manifestations and renounce to undergo lifestyle changes [9, 10]. In addition, initial weight loss by VLCD treatment is associated with greater weight regain; thus, long-term weight maintenance after VLCD has been an elusive goal when compared to surgical procedures like bariatric surgery [11, 12].

The purpose of the present chapter is to focus on the metabolic and clinical effects of VLCD regimens in type 2 DM subjects as well as on the role of inflammation and oxidative stress (OS).

2. Clinical outcomes with VLCDs in type 2 DM

The most common way to measure effectiveness among different medical treatments is by the assessment of clinical outcomes. A clinical outcome may refer to any measurable variable that is dependent on the assigned treatment [13]. With regard to type 2 DM, the most important and common outcomes evaluated in clinical trials assessing for therapy effectiveness are glycemia, glycated hemoglobin (HbA1C) levels, insulin sensitivity/resistance and elimination of antidiabetic drugs (also known as "diabetes remission"). However, current therapies, other than bariatric surgery, have failed to demonstrate significant effects on the ultimate goal of type 2 DM therapy, disease remission [14, 15]. Hence, this metabolic pathology is commonly referred, thus far, as an incurable and progressive disease.

Obesity is a well-known risk factor for type 2 DM [16]; therefore, several treatment approaches have been implemented to induce weight loss in obese individuals with type 2 DM. It is worth mentioning that since 1970, several studies have documented the capacity of a restricted diet to exert a rapid weight loss in overweight/obese subjects in a positive manner [4]. These types of diets comprise no more than 800 kcal/day and are known as VLCDs. VLCD regimens have been evaluated as diet treatments for type 2 DM based on their capacity to induce rapid weight loss. In 1997, Capstick et al. performed a clinical trial in 14 patients with obesity and type 2 DM aiming to evaluate the effects of a VLCD (425 kcal/day) regimen for 12 weeks on weight and metabolic control. In this clinical trial, body weight (from 108.9 to 94.5 kg), waist circumference (from 116 to 103 cm) and systolic blood pressure (SBP) (−8 mmHg) were reduced. The authors also reported a total reduction in exogenous insulin utilization by 50% in the VLCD cohort individuals who were taking a high dose of insulin per day at baseline, accompanied by a decrease in the number of oral antidiabetic drugs (8–2, median tablets/day). In addition, this regimen was well tolerated with a favorable safety profile [17]. Since then, several studies have implemented a diet treatment for type 2 DM. In 2011, Lim et al. evaluated the clinical effects of a 600 kcal/day VLCD regimen for 8 weeks in 11 middle-aged patients with obesity and type 2 DM. Results showed an average weight loss of 15.3 kg, equivalent to 15% of their initial body weight, with a sustained reduction of 3 kg after a 12-week follow-up [18]. Nevertheless, the majority of these studies have been pursued for <6 months, with limited evidence on their long-term efficacy in the treatment of diabetes.

In regard to the long-term study of VLCD regimens, Paisey et al. compared the clinical effects of a VLCD regimen with an intensive conventional diet plus exercise for 5 years in obese type 2 DM subjects. Fifteen patients in both cohorts finished the program. After 3 years of therapy, subjects in the VLCD regimen lost more body weight (mean ~15 kg weight loss) than their counterparts; however, by 5 years of follow-up, most of the weight was regained. On the other hand, the intensive group had a more sustained and progressive weight loss than the VLCD. The authors demonstrated that VLCD was safe to perform but difficult to follow for more than 6 months and showed a relative low patient compliance rate of ~60% in those individuals [19].

Similarly, Lim et al. showed a persistent beneficial effect on weight control after 6 months of an 8-week VLCD [20]. However, there could be some concerns about the tolerability and safety of VLCD in the long term based on the limited calorie content of these types of diets. Interestingly, Rolland et al. performed a study comparing weight loss and safety in obese subjects of three types of restricted calorie diets: VLCD, low-carbohydrate/high-protein diet and low fat, reduced-energy diet. At 3 months, a greater loss in body weight, total cholesterol, low-density lipoprotein cholesterol (LDL), fasting glucose and diastolic blood pressure in the VLCD cohort was observed. At 9 months, there were no significant differences, with the exception of fasting glucose, among the VLCD (average 550 kcal/day) and low-carbohydrate/high-protein diet (800–1500 kcal/day) regimens. Dropout rates were similar in the VLCD and low-carbohydrate/high-protein diet groups and no adverse effects were reported at 3 and 9 months in both groups [21]. Thus, at least for 9 months, VLCD seems to possess a favorable safety profile compared to less intense restricted calorie diets (>800 kcal/day).

A recent systematic review and meta-analysis compared weight loss following VLCD (<800 kcal/day) and low-energy liquid-formula regimens (>800 kcal/day) in people with and without type 2 DM [5]. The analysis of five studies varying from 4 to 52 weeks in length revealed no significant differences in weight loss among both regimens. Further, data showed that the efficacy on weight loss depended on several factors, including duration of diet and clinical characteristics of the subjects. In addition to effects on body weight, VLCD regimens were associated with a lack of adverse effects.

It is worth mentioning that reduction in body weight by VLCD regimens may trigger beneficial effects on diverse clinical alterations caused by certain pathologies where obesity is linked to their development and/or severity. Indeed, some studies have shown improvements on autonomic nervous system over reactivity (as per changes in heart rate variability) and stage 2 chronic kidney disease (as per changes in glomerular filtration rate) present in obese individuals with type 2 DM by VLCD regimens [22, 23]. Altogether, these studies suggest that weight loss, in the short term, is more rapid and pronounced by VLCD regimens but is also accompanied by more noticeable weight regain in the long term when compared to less restricted calorie diets. However, the long-term effects on body weight by VLCD remain unclear. Weight maintenance and education programs are needed for those individuals willing to follow a VLCD regimen if long-term weight loss is desired.

3. Metabolic parameters with VLCDs

The main goal pursued by pharmacological and nonpharmacological treatments in type 2 DM is to normalize the blood glucose levels. Diabetes remission, defined, as achieving glycemia below the diabetic range in the absence of active pharmacologic or surgical therapy [24] is lamentably rare by common therapies, including exercise, diet and antidiabetic drugs [14]. However, even a small decrease in high blood glucose levels is associated with a significant reduction in microvascular [25] and macrovascular [26] complications in subjects with type 2 DM. Until now, the only therapy that has compelling evidence in inducing long-term (up to 10 years) diabetes remission is bariatric surgery [27]. Interestingly, VLCD regimens have shown metabolic benefits in type 2 DM individuals, in the short term, similar to those observed by bariatric surgery. For instance, in 1979, Savage et al. evidenced a restoration of normal fasting plasma glucose levels by a VLCD regimen (500 kcal/day), for at least 4 weeks, in obese and type 2 DM individuals [28]. Such effects were attributed to the weight loss induced by the diet. Notably, all individuals presented a short duration of diabetes, 2–24 months. In 2004, Jazet et al. performed a clinical trial in 17 obese individuals with type 2 DM, with the purpose to identify the factors that could predict the blood glucose lowering effect induced by a VLCD regimen. After a 30-day treatment with 450 kcal/day, all individuals lost weight, but not all of them (i.e., nonresponders) achieved a reduction in blood glucose levels. But those who did (i.e., responders) had a shorter duration of type 2 DM and preserved the capacity of β-cells to secrete insulin [29]. This evidence provided key information in regard to diabetes remission that was later investigated by other groups. In 2011, the Newcastle Counterpoint study demonstrated reversal in 11 people with type 2 DM (<4 years of diagnosis) using a VLCD consisting of 600–800 kcal/day. A rapid decrease in liver and pancreas fat content derived from weight loss was linked to the glucose-lowering effects elicited by VLCD [18]. Later on, the same group of researchers showed that a higher baseline plasma insulin levels, preserved β-cell function and lower duration of diabetes were linked to diabetes remission following a VLCD regimen (624–700 kcal/day) for at least 6 months [20]. Despite being regarded as progressive and incurable, type 2 DM appears to be reversible by means of VLCD regimens. Nonetheless, long-term diabetes remission remains to be investigated and ongoing clinical trials are in the run [30] to provide more solid and clear evidence, as to if diabetes remission is possible by considerably changing the way people eat, without the necessity of invasive procedures (i.e., bariatric surgery).

4. Cytokines and adipokines in obesity and type 2 DM

Evidence has shown that a prolonged positive energy balance (more calories consumed than those expended) above that required for normal growth and development leads to overweight and obesity [31], which is a well-known risk factor for the development of type 2 DM [16]. Although a high proportion of individuals with type 2 DM are overweight/obese [32], not all of the overweight/obese individuals develop type 2 DM. The anatomical site where the excess calories are preferentially stored as triglycerides plays a pivotal role in the occurrence of metabolic abnormalities [33]. The adipose tissue has been recognized as the main site for lipid accumulation when excess calories are ingested [34]. However, studies have also shown that a positive energy balance over time leads to an increased accumulation of lipids (in the form of triglycerides) in various organs, including the liver, skeletal muscle and pancreas [35]. The abnormal fat accumulation in those organs has been linked to various derangements in the metabolism, including insulin resistance and β-cell failure (core defects of type 2 DM) [3]. Additionally, inflammation is a common feature of both obesity and type 2 DM. Indeed, studies have shown that obese individuals present an increase in adipose tissue macrophages and other immune cell infiltration [1]. These cells are key drivers of inflammation via overproduction of inflammatory cytokines, including interleukin (IL)-1β, tumor necrosis factor-α (TNF-α) and IL-6, which are strongly associated with the progression of the obese phenotype and metabolic traits of type 2 DM [36, 37]. In addition, the abnormal infiltration of immune cells in adipose tissue has deleterious long-term consequences on the biology of this tissue, as adipocytes are major targets of the pro-inflammatory effects of cytokines released by immune cells [38]. It is suggested that adipocytes secrete more than 600 potential hormones and signaling molecules (and the list grows every year), also known as adipokines, some of them are also produced by immune cells [39]. This group of molecules possesses a myriad of effects on diverse tissue/organs, including but not limited to the control of inflammation, fat distribution, insulin sensitivity and secretion, energy balance, appetite and satiety [39–42]. Some of the best studied and relevant adipokines in obesity and type 2 DM are leptin, adiponectin, TNF-α, IL-6, IL-1, resistin, dipeptidyl peptidase IV, apelin, monocyte chemotactic protein-1 (MCP-1), and so on [40, 41]. Interestingly, adipokines can act as either pro-inflammatory or anti-inflammatory signaling molecules. For instance, in lean individuals, adipocytes release anti-inflammatory adipokines (e.g., IL-4, IL-10, IL-13, apelin, etc.), while in obese subjects, pro-inflammatory molecules (e.g., TNF-α, leptin, IL-6, resistin, etc.) are predominantly released. The imbalance of cytokines and adipokines homeostasis in overweight/obese individuals leads to chronic low-grade systemic inflammatory state, a process that is a key driver of insulin resistance and ultimately to the development type 2 DM [2]. Thus, therapeutic strategies targeting cytokine and adipokine levels may favorably influence both obesity and type 2DM.

The most studied adipokines in type 2 DM subjects with VLCD are adiponectin and leptin. Adiponectin is a 244-amino acid hormone synthesized by mature white adipose tissue in subcutaneous, visceral and perivascular adiposity [42]. Adiponectin increases as fat mass decreases, and some of its functions are adipogenesis, adipocyte lipid storage (a "healthy" expansion of adipose tissue) and adipocyte insulin sensitivity via increased GLUT4-mediated glucose uptake [43]. The beneficial metabolic effects of adiponectin are in part related to its capacity to modulate the energy sensor 5′ adenosine monophosphate-activated protein kinase (AMPK) [44]. The regulation of adiponectin is a very complex system; however, low plasma adiponectin levels are associated with overweight, obesity and type 2 DM [43, 45]. The exact mechanisms involved in downregulation of adiponectin are not fully understood. Dietary restriction regimens in all its varieties (e.g., VLCD, calorie restriction, intermittent fasting, etc.) have been documented to exert beneficial metabolic effects in patients with type 2 DM derived from weight loss and concomitant modulation of adipokine levels. VLCD appears to have the most profound and rapid positive effect on weight loss, insulin resistance, β-cell function, inflammation and OS than other calorie-restricted regimens [3, 46–49]. However, the majority of studies performed, thus far, have failed to demonstrate significant changes in adiponectin serum levels after VLCD regimens in obese and type 2 DM individuals, despite improvements on metabolism [6, 8, 50].

Conversely, leptin is a 167-amino acid hormone secreted mainly by white adipose tissue and is positively correlated with body fat content [51]. Leptin regulates energy homeostasis by inhibiting appetite (anorexigenic effects), thereby inducing the weight loss. In obese subjects, circulating levels of leptin are increased [52]. Interestingly, after a three-week regimen with VLCD in obese women, Anderlová et al. demonstrated a significant reduction on leptin serum levels and an increase of soluble leptin receptor levels, with no significant effects on adiponectin [6]. In addition, Lips et al. directly compared the effects between VLCD and bariatric surgery (Roux-en Y gastric bypass) on systemic inflammation markers in obese women. Three months after both interventions such as leptin and adiponectin serum levels were reduced and increased, respectively, by both regimens, although a more favorable inflammatory profile was observed in the VLCD cohort [53]. Noteworthy, VLCD has also been shown to positively affect inflammatory markers in obese type 2 DM subjects. Mraz et al. evidenced that a two-week VLCD regimen (~600 cal/day) decreased body weight and fasting glycemia accompanied by decreased C-reactive protein and IL-6 plasma levels in obese type 2 DM women. Moreover, these subjects experienced a reduction in inflammatory markers at the mRNA level, including chemokine receptors (e.g., CCR-1, CCR-2, CCR-5, IL-6 receptor) in peripheral monocytes and chemokines (CCL-8 and CXCL-10) in subcutaneous adipose tissue [8].

5. VLCD and OS

OS is a condition of imbalance between oxidative species and antioxidant defense [54]. Several lines of evidence suggest a close relationship between inflammation and OS [55–57]. Indeed, various OS markers are up regulated in subjects with type 2 DM [58–60], where a chronic low-grade inflammation state is present. Regimens with calorie-restricted diets have been reported to positively affect OS in obese and type 2 DM individuals via modulation of recognized OS markers. For instance, a study performed with obese individuals (with and without metabolic syndrome diagnosis) evidenced a reduction of oxidized LDL plasma levels after a VLCD for 3 months. In another study, a VLCD regimen for 8 days was associated with improved oxidative status, defined as increase in superoxide dismutase (SOD) and reduction in malondialdehyde (MDA) levels, in obese individuals with and without type 2 DM [61]. Although such effects were only reported in nine patients, surprisingly, a seven-day period was enough to demonstrate significant reductions in those parameters in addition to reductions in fasting plasma glucose, total cholesterol and LDL levels. Likewise, Heilbronn et al. documented reduced DNA damage (a marker of OS) in blood samples from overweight individuals after 6 months of a VLCD regimen compared to individuals who had followed a weight maintenance diet [49]. There exists a link between OS and inflammation in type 2 DM, and in this regard, VLCDs have shown the capacity to attenuate both processes.

6. Future directions and recommendations

There is no doubt about the beneficial metabolic effects linked to VLCD regimens in type 2 DM. Such beneficial effects by VLCD go beyond glycemic and lipid control, since VLCD has shown to reduce OS and inflammation. Perhaps, in addition to its associated safety profile, VLCD regimens are now taking a privileged position in the treatment of type 2 DM, because of their capacity (in part) to exert rapid and substantial weight loss without the common risks associated with bariatric surgery. However, particular points that need to be addressed in VLCD trials are whether these types of diets are viable treatments for long-term diabetes remission and these regimens are applicable in primary care settings. Specifically, there is a need for more evidence related to the VLCD-associated benefits and safety, in longer and larger studies, which fortunately may be available soon because of current ongoing clinical trials evaluating this scenario.

Indeed, the Diabetes Remission Clinical Trial (DiRECT) is an ongoing trial intended to determine whether a weight management program (i.e., consisting in a VLCD regimen, food reintroduction and long-term weigh loss maintenance steps) delivered in a routine primary care setting and is a practical and successful treatment to achieve type 2 DM remission after 2 years [32]. This study started in 2016 and the obtained results are promising.

It has been manifested that individuals under VLCD regimens may suffer from psychological stress (e.g., increase in cortisol levels), which may be associated with weight regain after the discontinuation of VLCD regimens [62]. Interestingly, the Prevention of WEight Regain in diabetes type 2 (POWER) was designed to evaluate the effectiveness of adding a psychological intervention to a VLCD regimen in overweight type 2 DM individuals [63].

Clear recommendations for individuals with type 2 diabetes who would like to improve or reverse their condition by VLCD regimens await further studies. Nevertheless, all individuals with newly diagnosed type 2 DM should be informed about the possibility of reversing their disease by a diet regimen, not commonly offered as a treatment by general practitioners. This will bring hopes and motivation to individuals who are categorized as possessing an incurable disease. It is important to mention that not all individuals are capable to execute a task that comprises a relative drastic change to their lifestyle that has been maintained for years. Hence, structured programs that involve groups of dieticians, nurses, doctors and psychologists are required in order to treat this disease and lead to disease remission. Health Services around the globe will continue to suffer from the cost burden of type 2 DM as its incidence is projected to increase worldwide [64]. Even if a small proportion of type 2 DM individuals reverse their condition, the savings in health programs, particularly in developing countries, will be substantial.

Author details

Luis M. Román-Pintos[1*], Geannyne Villegas-Rivera[1], Ernesto G. Cardona-Muñoz[2], Adolfo D. Rodríguez-Carrizalez[2], Aldo Moreno-Ulloa[3], Nicole Rubin[4] and Alejandra G. Miranda-Díaz[2]

*Address all correspondence to: lmroman@yahoo.com

1 Health & Disease Department, Tonalá University Centre, University of Guadalajara, Guadalajara, Jalisco, México

2 Department of Physiology, Health Sciences, Clinical and Experimental Therapeutics Institute, University Centre, Jalisco, México

3 Biomedical Innovation Department, College Education and Scientific Research Center of Ensenada, Baja California, México

4 Miltenyi Biotec Inc, Auburn, CA, USA

References

[1] Weisberg SP, McCann D, Desai M, Rosenbaum M, Leibel RL, Ferrante AW, Jr. Obesity is associated with macrophage accumulation in adipose tissue. The Journal of Clinical Investigation. 2003 Dec;**112**(12):1796-1808. DOI: 10.1172/JCI200319246

[2] Makki K, Froguel P, Wolowczuk I. Adipose tissue in obesity-related inflammation and insulin resistance: cells, cytokines, and chemokines. ISRN Inflammation. 2013;**2013**(139239):1-12. DOI: 10.1155/2013/139239

[3] Taylor R. Type 2 diabetes: Etiology and reversibility. Diabetes Care. 2013;**36**(4):1047-1055. DOI: 10.2337/dc12-1805

[4] Tsai AG, Wadden TA. The evolution of very-low-calorie diets: An update and meta-analysis. Obesity (Silver Spring). 2006;**14**(8):1283-1293. DOI: 10.1038/oby.2006.146

[5] Leslie WS, Taylor R, Harris L, Lean MEJ. Weight losses with low energy formula diets in obese patients with and without type 2 diabetes: systematic review and metaanalysis. International Journal of Obesity. 2016;**41**(1):96-101. DOI: 10.1038/ijo.2016.175

[6] Anderlová K, Křemen J, Doležalová R, Housová J, Haluzíková D, Kunešová M, Haluzík M. The influence of very-low-calorie diet on serum leptin, soluble leptin receptor, adiponectin and resistin levels in obese women Physiological Research [Clinical Trial] 2006; **55**:277-283

[7] Tumova ESW, Jones PH, Vrablik M, Ballantyne CM, Hoogeveen RC. The impact of rapid weight loss on oxidative stress markers and the expression of the metabolic syndrome in obese individuals. Journal of Obesity. 2013;**2013**(729515):1-10. DOI: 10.1155/2013/729515

[8] Mraz M, Lacinova Z, Drapalova J, Haluzikova D, Horinek A, Matoulek M, Trachta P, Kavalkova P, Svacina S, Haluzik M. The effect of very-low-calorie diet on mrna expression of inflammation-related genes in subcutaneous adipose tissue and peripheral monocytes of obese patients with type 2 diabetes mellitus. The Journal of Clinical Endocrinology and Metabolism. 2011;**96**(4):E606-E613. DOI: 10.1210/jc.2010-1858

[9] Vilchez-López FJ Campos Martín C, Amaya-García MJ, Sánchez-Vera P, Pereira-Cunill JL. Las dietas de muy bajo valor calórico (DMBVC) en el manejo clínico de la obesidad mórbida. Nutrición Hospitalaria. 2013;**28**(2):275-285. DOI: 10.3305/nh.2013.28.2.6285

[10] Group M. Very low calorie diets. Drug & Ther Bull. 2012;**50**(5):54-57

[11] Johansson K, Neovius M, Hemmingsson E. Effects of anti-obesity drugs, diet, and exercise on weight-loss maintenance after a very-low-calorie diet or low-calorie diet: A systematic review and meta-analysis of randomized controlled trials. The American Journal of Clinical Nutrition. 2014;**99**(1):14-23. DOI: 10.3945/ajcn.113.070052

[12] Tsai AG, Wadden TA. The evolution of very-low-calorie diets: An update and meta-analysis. Obesity. 2006;**14**(8):1283-1293. DOI: 10.1038/oby.2006.146

[13] Velentgas P, Dreyer NA, Nourjah P, Smith SR, Torchia MM. Developing A Protocol For Observational Comparative Effectiveness Research: A User's Guide. Rockville (MD); 2013. Available from: https://www.ncbi.nlm.nih.gov/books/NBK126190

[14] Karter AJ, Nundy S, Parker MM, Moffet HH, Huang ES. Incidence of remission in adults with type 2 diabetes: The diabetes & aging study. Diabetes Care. 2014;**37**(12):3188-3195. DOI: 10.2337/dc14-0874

[15] Muller-Stich BP, Senft JD, Warschkow R, Kenngott HG, Billeter AT, Vit G, et al. Surgical versus medical treatment of type 2 diabetes mellitus in nonseverely obese patients: A systematic review and meta-analysis. Annals of Surgery. 2015;**261**(3):421-429. DOI: 10.1097/SLA.0000000000001014

[16] Eckel RH, Kahn SE, Ferrannini E, Goldfine AB, Nathan DM, Schwartz MW, et al. Obesity and type 2 diabetes: What can be unified and what needs to be individualized? The Journal of Clinical Endocrinology and Metabolism. 2011;**96**(6):1654-1663. DOI: 10.1210/jc.2011-0585

[17] Capstick FBB, Burns CM, Zilkens RR, Steinbeck KS, Yue DK. Very low calorie diet (VLCD): A useful alternative in the treatment of the obese NIDDM patient. Diabetes Research and Clinical Practice. 1997;**36**:105-111. DOI: 10.1016/S0168-8227(97)00038-7

[18] Lim EL, Hollingsworth KG, Aribisala BS, Chen MJ, Mathers JC, Taylor R. Reversal of type 2 diabetes: Normalisation of beta cell function in association with decreased pancreas and liver triacylglycerol. Diabetologia. 2011;**54**:2506-2514. DOI: 10.1007/s00125-011-2204-7

[19] Paisey RB, Frost J, Harvey P, Paisey A, Bower L, Paisey RM, al e. Five year results of a prospective very low calorie diet or conventional weight loss programme in type 2 diabetes. Journal of Human Nutrition and Dietetics. 2002;**15**:121-127. DOI: 10.1046/j.1365-277X.2002.00342.x

[20] Steven S, Hollingsworth KG, Al-Mrabeh A, Avery L, Aribisala B, Caslake M, Taylor R. Very low calorie diet and 6 months of weight stability in type 2 diabetes: Pathophysiologic changes in responders and non-responders. Diabetes Care. 2016;**39**(5):808-815. DOI: 10.2337/dc15-1942

[21] Rolland C, Hession M, Murray S, Wise A, Broom I. Randomized clinical trial of standard dietary treatment versus a low-carbohydrate/high-protein diet or the Lighter Life Programme in the management of obesity. Journal of Diabetes. 2009;**1**(3):207-217. DOI: 10.1111/j.1753-0407.2009.00033.x

[22] Lips MA, de Groot GH, De Kam M, Berends FJ, Wiezer R, Van Wagensveld BA, et. al. Autonomic nervous system activity in diabetic and healthy obese female subjects and the effect of distinct weight loss strategies. European Journal of Endocrinology. 2013;**169**:383-390. DOI: 10.1530/EJE-13-0506

[23] Giordani I, Malandrucco I, Donno S, Picconi F, Di Giacinto P, Di Flaviani A, al e. Acute caloric restriction improves glomerular filtration rate in patients with morbid obesity and type 2 diabetes. Diabetes & Metabolism. 2014;**40**(2):158-160. DOI: 10.1016/j.diabet.2013.12.006

[24] Buse JB, Caprio S, Cefalu WT, Ceriello A, Del Prato S, Inzucchi SE, et al. How do we define cure of diabetes? Diabetes Care. 2009;**32**(11):2133-2135. DOI: 10.2337/dc09-9036

[25] Molyneaux LM, Constantino MI, McGill M, Zilkens R, Yue DK. Better glycaemic control and risk reduction of diabetic complications in Type 2 diabetes: Comparison with the DCCT. Diabetes Research and Clinical Practice. 1998;**42**(2):77-83. DOI: 10.1016/S0168-8227(98)00095-3

[26] Mannucci E, Dicembrini I, Lauria A, Pozzilli P. Is glucose control important for prevention of cardiovascular disease in diabetes? Diabetes Care. 2013;**36**(Suppl 2):S259-S263. DOI: 10.2337/dcS13-2018

[27] Sjostrom L, Lindroos AK, Peltonen M, Torgerson J, Bouchard C, Carlsson B, et al. Lifestyle, diabetes, and cardiovascular risk factors 10 years after bariatric surgery. The New England Journal of Medicine. 2004;**351**(26):2683-2693. DOI: 10.1056/NEJMoa035622

[28] Savage PJ, Bennion LJ, Flock EV, Nagulesparan M, Mott D, Roth J, et al. Diet-induced improvement of abnormalities in insulin and glucagon secretion and in insulin receptor binding in diabetes mellitus. The Journal of Clinical Endocrinology and Metabolism. 1979;**48**(6):999-1007. DOI: 10.1210/jcem-48-6-999

[29] Jazet IM, Pijil H, Frölich M, Schoemaker RC, Meinders AE. Factors predicting the blood glucose lowering effect of a 30-day very low calorie diet in obese Type 2 diabetic patients. Diabetic Medicine. 2004;**22**:52-55. DOI: 10.1111/j.1464-5491.2004.01357.x

[30] Leslie WS, Ford I, Sattar N, Hollingsworth KG, Adamson A, Sniehotta FF, et al. The Diabetes Remission Clinical Trial (DiRECT): protocol for a cluster randomised trial. BMC Family Practice. 2016;**17**:20. DOI: 10.1186/s12875-016-0406-2

[31] Hall KD, Heymsfield SB, Kemnitz JW, Klein S, Schoeller DA, Speakman JR. Energy balance and its components: implications for body weight regulation. The American Journal of Clinical Nutrition. 2012;**95**(4):989-994. DOI: 10.3945/ajcn.112.036350

[32] Colosia AD, Palencia R, Khan S. Prevalence of hypertension and obesity in patients with type 2 diabetes mellitus in observational studies: A systematic literature review. Diabetes, Metabolic Syndrome and Obesity. 2013;**6**:327-338. DOI: 10.2147/DMSO.S51325

[33] Sattar N, Gill JM. Type 2 diabetes as a disease of ectopic fat? BMC Medicine. 2014;**12**:123. DOI: 10.1186/s12916-014-0123-4

[34] Choe SS, Huh JY, Hwang IJ, Kim JI, Kim JB. Adipose tissue remodeling: Its role in energy metabolism and metabolic disorders. Front Endocrinol (Lausanne). 2016;**7**:30. DOI: 10.3389/fendo.2016.00030

[35] Szendroedi J, Roden M. Ectopic lipids and organ function. Current Opinion in Lipidology. 2009;**20**(1):50-56. DOI: 10.1097/MOL.0b013e328321b3a8

[36] Xu H, Barnes GT, Yang Q, Tan G, Yang D, Chou CJ, et al. Chronic inflammation in fat plays a crucial role in the development of obesity-related insulin resistance. The Journal of Clinical Investigation. 2003;**112**(12):1821-1830

[37] Coope A, Torsoni AS, Velloso LA. Mechanisms in endocrinology: Metabolic and inflammatory pathways on the pathogenesis of type 2 diabetes. European Journal of Endocrinology. 2016;**174**(5):R175-R187. DOI: 10.1172/JCI19451

[38] Caër C, Christine R, Le Roy T, Poitou C, Aron-Wisnewsky J, Torcivia A, et al. Immune cell-derived cytokines contribute to obesity-related inflammation, fibrogenesis and metabolic deregulation in human adipose tissue. Scientific Reports. 2017;**7**(1):1-11. DOI: 10.1038/s41598-017-02660-w

[39] Lehr S, Hartwig S, Sell H. Adipokines: A treasure trove for the discovery of biomarkers for metabolic disorders. Proteomics Clinical Applications. 2012;**6**(1-2):91-101. DOI: 10.1002/prca.201100052

[40] Freitas Lima LC, Braga VA, do Socorro de Franca Silva M, Cruz JC, Sousa Santos SH, de Oliveira Monteiro MM, et al. Adipokines, diabetes and atherosclerosis: an inflammatory association. Frontiers in Physiology. 2015;**6**:304. DOI: 10.3389/fphys.2015.00304

[41] Dunmore SJ, Brown JE. The role of adipokines in beta-cell failure of type 2 diabetes. The Journal of Endocrinology. 2013;**216**(1):T37-T45. DOI: 10.1530/JOE-12-0278

[42] Bluher M. Clinical relevance of adipokines. Diabetes and Metabolism Journal. 2012;**36**(5): 317-327. DOI: 10.4093/dmj.2012.36.5.317

[43] Balsan GA, Vieira JL, Oliveira AM, Portal VL. Relationship between adiponectin, obesity and insulin resistance. Revista da Associação Médica Brasileira (1992). 2015;**61:**72-80. DOI: 10.1590/1806-9282.61.01.072

[44] Fu Y, Luo N, Klein RL, Garvey WT. Adiponectin promotes adipocyte differentiation, insulin sensitivity, and lipid accumulation. Journal of Lipid Research. 2005;**46**(7):1369-1379. DOI: 10.1194/jlr.M400373-JLR200

[45] Stern JH, Rutkowski JM, Scherer PE. Adiponectin, leptin, and fatty acids in the maintenance of metabolic homeostasis through adipose tissue crosstalk. Cell Metabolism. 2016;**23**:770-784. DOI: 10.1016/j.cmet.2016.04.011

[46] Saltevo J, Laakso M, Jokelainen J, Keinanen-Kiukaanniemi S, Kumpusalo E, Vanhala M. Levels of adiponectin, C-reactive protein and interleukin-1 receptor antagonist are associated with insulin sensitivity: a population-based study. Diabetes/Metabolism Research and Reviews. 2008;**24**(5):378-383. DOI: 10.1002/dmrr.831

[47] Foster-Schubert KE, Alfano CM, Duggan CR, Xiao L, Campbell KL, Kong A, et al. Effect of diet and exercise, alone or combined, on weight and body composition in overweight-to-obese postmenopausal women. Obesity (Silver Spring). 2012;**20**(8):1628-1638. DOI: 10.1038/oby.2011.76

[48] Trepanowski JF, Canale RE, Marshall KE, Kabir MM, Bloomer RJ. Impact of caloric and dietary restriction regimens on markers of health and longevity in humans and animals: A summary of available findings. Nutrition Journal. 2011;**10**:107. DOI: 10.1186/1475-2891-10-107

[49] Heilbronn LK, de Jonge L, Frisard MI, DeLany JP, Larson-Meyer DE, Rood J, et al. Effect of 6-month calorie restriction on biomarkers of longevity, metabolic adaptation, and oxidative stress in overweight individuals: A randomized controlled trial. Journal of the American Medical Association. 2006;**295**(13):1539-1548. DOI: 10.1001/jama.295.13.1539

[50] Garaulet M, Viguerie N, Porubsky S, Klimcakova E, Clement K, Langin D, et al. Adiponectin gene expression and plasma values in obese women during very-low-calorie diet. Relationship with cardiovascular risk factors and insulin resistance. The Journal of Clinical Endocrinology and Metabolism. 2004;**89**(2):756-760. DOI: 10.1210/jc.2003-031495

[51] Kelesidis T KI, Chou S, and Mantzoros CS. Narrative review: The role of leptin in human physiology: Emerging clinical applications. Annals of Internal Medicine. [Review]. 2010; **152**(2):93-100. DOI: 10.7326/0003-4819-152-2-201001190-00008

[52] Klok MD, Jakobsdottir S, Drent ML. The role of leptin and ghrelin in the regulation of food intake and body weight in humans: A review. Obesity Reviews. 2007;**8**(1):21-34. DOI: 10.1111/j.1467-789X.2006.00270.x

[53] Lips MA, van Klinken JB, Pijl H, Janssen I, Willems van Dijk K, et al. Weight loss induced by very low calorie diet is associated with a more beneficial systemic inflammatory profile than by Roux-en-Y gastric bypass. Metabolism. 2016;**65**(11):1614-1620. DOI: 10.1016/j.metabol.2016.07.013

[54] Sies H. Oxidative stress: A concept in redox biology and medicine. Redox Biology. 2015; **4**:180-183. DOI: 10.1016/j.redox.2015.01.002

[55] Salzano S, Checconi P, Hanschmann EM, Lillig CH, Bowler LD, Chan P, et al. Linkage of inflammation and oxidative stress via release of glutathionylated peroxiredoxin-2, which acts as a danger signal. Proceedings of the National Academy of Sciences of the United States of America. 2014;**111**(33):12157-12162. DOI: 10.1073/pnas.1401712111

[56] Holvoet P. Relations between metabolic syndrome, oxidative stress and inflammation and cardiovascular disease. Verhandelingen – Koninklijke Academie voor Geneeskunde van België. 2008;**70**(3):193-219

[57] Cachofeiro V, Goicochea M, de Vinuesa SG, Oubina P, Lahera V, Luno J. Oxidative stress and inflammation, a link between chronic kidney disease and cardiovascular disease. Kidney International Supplement. 2008;**111**:S4-S9. DOI: 10.1038/ki.2008.516

[58] Gradinaru D, Borsa C, Ionescu C, Margina D. Advanced oxidative and glycoxidative protein damage markers in the elderly with type 2 diabetes. Journal of Proteomics. 2013;**92**:313-322. DOI: 10.1016/j.jprot.2013.03.034

[59] Bandeira Sde M, Guedes Gda S, da Fonseca LJ, Pires AS, Gelain DP, Moreira JC, et al. Characterization of blood oxidative stress in type 2 diabetes mellitus patients: Increase in lipid peroxidation and SOD activity. Oxidative Medicine and Cellular Longevity. 2012; **2012**:819310. DOI: 10.1155/2012/819310

[60] Pandey KB, Mishra N, Rizvi SI. Protein oxidation biomarkers in plasma of type 2 diabetic patients. Clinical Biochemistry. 2010;**43**(4-5):508-511. DOI: 10.1016/j.clinbiochem.2009.11.011

[61] Škrha J, Kunešová M, Hilgertová J, Weiserová H, Křížová J, Kotrlíková E. Short-term very low calory diet reduces oxidative stress in obese type 2 diabetic patients. Physiological Research. 2005;**54**(1):33-39

[62] Tomiyama AJ, Mann T, Vinas D, Hunger JM, Dejager J, Taylor SE. Low calorie dieting increases cortisol. Psychosomatic Medicine. 2010;**72**(4):357-364. DOI: 10.1097/PSY.0b013e3181d9523c

[63] Berk KA, Buijks H, Ozcan B, Van't Spijker A, Busschbach JJ, Sijbrands EJ. The prevention of weight regain in diabetes type 2 (POWER) study: The effectiveness of adding a combined psychological intervention to a very low calorie diet, design and pilot data of a randomized controlled trial. BMC Public Health. 2012;**12**:1026. DOI: 10.1186/1471-2458-12-1026

[64] Rowley WR, Bezold C, Arikan Y, Byrne E, Krohe S. Diabetes 2030: Insights from yesterday, today, and future trends. Population Health Management. 2017;**20**(1):6-12. DOI: 10.1089/pop.2015.0181

3

Diabetes and Cancer: Is there a Link?

Andra-Iulia Suceveanu, Adrian-Paul Suceveanu,
Andreea-Daniela Gheorghe and Laura Mazilu

Abstract

Cancer and diabetes are two major health problems worldwide, and incidence is increasing globally for both diseases. Type 2 diabetes is characterized by hyperinsulinemia and insulin resistance and the effect of insulin and insulin growth factor I on cancer development and progression have been demonstrated in animal and human studies. The relationship between diabetes and cancer was reported for more than 60 years. Many epidemiological studies conducted over time suggested the association between diabetes and cancer. Epidemiological studies show an increased risk in type 2 diabetic patients for colon, breast, liver, pancreas, bladder cancers and non-Hodgkin's lymphoma, and a decrease risk for prostate cancer. Lung cancer does not appear to be related to diabetes and for renal cancer data are inconclusive. Diabetes, beside the fact that it is an independent risk factor for different type of cancer, can also have an impact on prognosis of cancer, and studies shown an increased cancer mortality in patients with diabetes.

Keywords: diabetes, cancer, hyperinsulinemia, insulin resistance

1. Introduction

Cancer and diabetes are two major health problems worldwide, and incidence is increasing globally for both diseases. In 2012, 14.1 million new cancer cases and 8.2 million death occurred worldwide, and the number of cases and deaths is expected to grow as populations adopt lifestyle behaviors that increase the cancer risk [1, 2]. Diabetes is also an important health problem associated with severe complications, and its growing worldwide In 2014 was estimated that 422 million adults were living with diabetes, the prevalence of diabetes globally is 8.5% in adult population and caused 1.5 million death in 2012 [3]. Globally, cancer is the 2nd cause of death, and diabetes is 12th cause of death [4]. The economic growth is accompanied by lifestyle westernization, characterized by physical inactivity, high-calorie diet and obesity and may explain this change in incidence and mortality of lifestyle related diseases such as diabetes, cancer and cardiac disease.

The relationship between diabetes and cancer was reported for more than 60 years. Theodore Tuffier, a French surgeon, is probably the first one to hypothesize the existence of a relationship of type 2 diabetes mellitus and cancer risk in the second half of nineteenth century. He observed that patients with type 2 diabetes have a greater risk of certain cancers than those without diabetes and formulated some key questions: could diabetes affect the incidence of cancer? could diabetes influence the natural history of cancer? and could cancer affect the natural history of diabetes? [5].

Many epidemiological studies conducted over time suggested the association between diabetes and cancer. Studies show an increased risk in type 2 diabetic patients for colon, breast, liver, pancreas, bladder cancers and non-Hodgkin's lymphoma [6–12], and a decrease risk for prostate cancer [13]. Lung cancer does not appear to be related to diabetes and for renal cancer data are inconclusive [14].

Diabetes, beside the fact that is an independent risk factor for different type of cancer, can also have an impact on prognosis of cancer, and studies shown an increased cancer mortality in patients with diabetes. A meta-analysis of 23 studies comparing the overall survival in cancer patients with or without diabetes showed that diabetic patient have an increased mortality, HR of 1.41 (95% CI, 1.28 to 1.55) compared to non-diabetic patients in all cancer types [15].

The majority of the studies that explore the relation between diabetes and cancer do not make the difference between type 1 and type 2 diabetes. It is important to make that distinction, because type 1 diabetes is an autoimmune disease and it is caused by destruction of pancreatic β cells with resultant insulin deficiency and hyperglycemia, and on the other hand type 2 diabetes it appears because of peripheral insulin resistance and it is characterized by hyperinsulinemia and β cell hyperplasia. These 2 entities differ also in the age of onset, type 2 diabetes occurs in adults patients, while type 1 diabetes is usually observed in young people. Considering the differences in the physiopathology of these two diseases, it is important to make diagnostic distinction before any conclusion is made about the association of diabetes and cancer. But, the large majority of patients with diabetes have type 2 diabetes and most study have been conducted on patients with diabetes at older age, this can extrapolate that the majority of diabetic patients who develop cancer are patients with type 2 diabetes.

One Swedish study was conducted on patients with type one diabetes, but did not found an increased risk for pancreatic, breast or colorectal cancer in this patients [16, 17].

2. Diabetes and cancer – common risk factors

Diabetes and cancer very often coexist in the same patients; up to 18% of patients with cancer have also diabetes. Risk factors that are common for both diseases, diabetes and cancer are age, obesity and overweight, physical inactivity, smoking [18]. An important problems is whether the association of diabetes with different type of cancer is related to common risk factor for both diseases or diabetes with metabolic modification like insulin resistance and hyperinsulinemia is responsible for the increased risk of cancer. More studies are needed to understand the role of each component of lifestyle independent of other, to understand the relation between diabetes and cancer.

2.1. Age

More than 60% of cancers are diagnosed in patients aged 60 years or more, and the prevalence of diabetes is 17% in this age group; the coexistence of cancer and diabetes is expected to raise as life expectancy increases [19, 20].

2.2. Obesity

Diabetes is known to be related with overweight and obesity, studies shown over the years a strong association between obesity, insulin resistance and type 2 diabetes and early age diagnosis of diabetes is reported to be linked directly to obesity severity [21, 22]. Cancers most frequently associated with obesity and overweight are breast cancer in postmenopausal women, colon, pancreas, endometrium, gallbladder and liver, and may increase mortality in prostate cancer [23, 24].

The association between weight loss and decreased risk of diabetes was strengthened by numerous studies. A randomized, prospective, multicenter Diabetes Prevention Trial, shown that lifestyle intervention and physical activity was associated with 58% reduction in incidence of diabetes in high risk individuals [25].

The relation between weight loss and cancer risk is not that clear, and most data are derived from breast cancer studies, and in this studies association observed was very weak [26]. The Nurses' Health Study shown a statistical significant association between weight loss and decrease incidence of breast cancer, if the weight loss is maintained for more than 4 years [27].

2.3. Physical inactivity

Data from epidemiologic observational studies shown that physical activity is associated with lower risk of colon, breast and endometrial cancers, and may help to prevent lung or prostate cancer, but in this case the link is not yet established [28–31].

A protective role of increased physical activity in diabetes metabolism and outcomes has been demonstrated in studies. Data from observational studies suggest that approximately 30 to 60 minutes of moderate-intensity physical activity, at least 5 days per week reduces substantially, with 25–36%, the risk of developing type 2 diabetes [18, 32].

2.4. Smoking

Smoking is a well-known risk factor for lung cancer incidence and mortality. Other types of cancer that is known to be associated with cigarette smoking are cancer of larynx, upper digestive tract, bladder, pancreas, liver, kidney and uterine cervix. Studies have shown that smoking is an independent risk factor for diabetes, and it is well known to act as an adverse effect on diabetes complications [33, 34].

2.5. Alcohol consumption

Alcohol consumption increases the risk of many type of cancers, oral cavity, pharynx, colon, liver and female breast. For diabetes, increased alcohol consumption is a considered a risk, but moderate consumption was associated with reduced incidence of diabetes in both men and women [35, 36].

3. Mechanisms underlying diabetes and cancer

Carcinogenesis is a very complex process in which normal cells must undergo multiple genetic modification in order to appear malignant phenotype and invasion and metastasis occurs. This process of carcinogenesis is divided in three steps. First step is initiation, this is the irreversible step toward cancer, second step is promotion, the stimulation of growth of initiated cells, and the third step is progression. Any factors that have the capability to affect one of these steps could be associated with cancer incidence and mortality.

Diabetes may have an effect on carcinogenesis process by multiple mechanisms: hyperinsulinemia, either is exogenous due to administration of insulin or endogenous due to insulin resistance, hyperglycemia or chronic inflammation [18].

There are many epidemiologic evidence that support the link between diabetes and cancers. Diabetes and cancer may be related simply because these two diseases share common risk factors such as obesity, diet, physical inactivity, but several biologic mechanism have been described that may strengthen this link between diabetes and cancer.

Information regarding biologic mechanism is from in vivo and in vitro studies, research is ongoing currently to provide more clear understanding of these possible mechanisms, and the information from these studies may be important for prevention of the disease and management of the patient.

3.1. Hyperinsulinemia

Insulin and insulin-like growth factor (IGF) receptors form a complex network of cell surface receptors and majority of cancer cells express these receptors. The A isoform is commonly expressed on cells, and can stimulate insulin-mediated mitogenesis, even in cells that do have a deficiency in IGF-I receptors, and in addition to this function, the insulin receptor is capable to stimulate cell proliferation and to promote metastasis [18, 37, 38]. Interaction of insulin receptors or IGF-I receptors with their ligands activate multiple pathways, that can stimulate proliferation, resistance to apoptotic stimuli, invasion and metastasis. IGF-I have more important anti-apoptotic and mitogenic activities than insulin, and could act as growth factor in pre-neoplastic or cancer cells that express insulin and IGF-I receptors. In cancer cells these receptors are over-expressed and many cancer cell lines have been shown to be very responsive even to the mitogenic effect of normal concentrations of IGF-I [39–41].

High levels of IGF-I have been associated with an increased risk of postmenopausal breast cancer, colon and prostate cancer [18, 42, 43].

It is also possible that hyperinsulinemia may promote carcinogenesis by indirect mechanisms. Insulin reduces the hepatic production of insulin growth factor binding protein (IGFBP) and this will lead to increased levels of circulating free IGF-I.

Hyperinsulinemia have an indirect effect on reduction in hepatic production and blood levels of sex-hormone binding protein, which increase bioavailability of estrogen in both man and women and also increase bioavailability of testosterone in women which is also link to cancer, but not in man [18, 44].

In postmenopausal women, body fat is the primary site of estrogen synthesis, and obesity is related to high levels of serum estrogen this will increase the risk for breast and endometrial cancers in women who do not use hormonal replacement therapy [45].

3.2. Hyperglycemia

The link between effect of hyperglycemia and cancer is still unclear. Hyperglycemia increases production of free radicals which could lead to oxidative damage to DNA and mutation in oncogenes and tumor suppressor genes [18]. Research is still unclear about whether high levels of circulating glucose fuels malignant growth.

The recent interest in Warburg hypothesis emphasize the dependence of many cancers on glycolysis, creating a high requirement for glucose, so called "glucose addiction," because ATP generation glycolysis requires more glucose than oxidative phosphorylation. This is the basis for F-flurodeoxyglucose—positron emission tomography (PET) of cancer, that detects tissues with high glucose uptake [46].

Studies correlating hyperglycemia with cancer do not indicate that the high level of glucose itself mediate this correlation, because chronic hyperglycemia is associated with insulin resistance and often with excess of body fat, and hyperglycemia may act as surogate [18].

3.3. Chronic inflammation

Type 2 diabetes and obesity are characterized by chronic inflammation that increases the production of free radicals. This can disrupt insulin signaling and damage DNA. Adipose tissue is an active endocrine organ and is producing interleukin-6 (IL-6), plasminogen activator inhibitor-1 (PAI-1), adiponectin, leptin and tumor necrosis factor-α (TNF-α). All of these factors may play a role in malignant transformation and cancer progression, and some of these roles are well known [47].

4. Diabetes treatment and cancer

Type 2 diabetes is treated with different types of medications, so it may be a link between these drugs and the risk of cancer. Anti-diabetic medication includes drugs that increase insulin in circulation (insulin and sulfonylureas) and drugs that improve insulin action and decrease insulin levels (metformin, thiazolidinediones). The central goal of diabetes management is glucose control, this minimize morbidity and mortality related to diabetes by reducing diabetes associated complications. When selecting antidiabetic therapies, physician and patients consider several factors, these includes type of diabetes, glucose-lowering potential of the antidiabetic agent, adverse effect of treatment, costs, patient characteristic and comorbidities.

Type 2 diabetes represent the majority of diabetic population and account for 95% of diabetic population and majority of studies were conducted on this patients. It is generally associated with obesity and overweight in almost 80% of cases. In type 2 diabetes insulin resistance and hyperglycemia are progressive [48, 49].

The majority of studies on antidiabetic treatment and cancer risk have limitations, one limitation is that diabetic patients are treated with more than one antidiabetic agent, because of the progressive nature of type 2 diabetes. In this case is very difficult to assess an association between a specific antidiabetic drug and cancer risk [18].

There are 14 diabetes drugs available at this time, and data suggest a higher risk of cancer development with pioglitazone, insulin and insulin secretagogues [50–53]. Metformin have been identified in several studies in the past few years to improve survival in patient diagnosed with cancer and diabetes and to reduced cancer risk [54]. Insulin has been shown in studies to have a direct proliferative effect; for the insulin analogues, further studies are needed to determine the potential role in cancer proliferation.

5. Diabetes and site – specific cancer

5.1. Diabetes and breast cancer

Breast cancer is the leading cause death among females worldwide. An estimated 1.7 million new cases and more than 500,000 deaths occurred in 2012 [2]. Risk factors for breast cancer include age greater than 50 years, family history, genetics, female gender, Caucasian and African American Race, obesity and hormonal factors such as menstrual history, nulliparity and use of hormone replacement therapy [55].

The association of diabetes and breast cancer was studied extensively and appears to be connected via activation of insulin-IGF pathway through hyperinsulinemia and dysregulation of sex hormones [56, 57]. Cell proliferation in both normal human cell and in breast cancer cell has been shown to be influence by insulin. Insulin stimulates cell cycle progression and DNA synthesis of MCF-7 breast cancer cells in vitro [58, 59].

One mode of action of breast cancer gene 1 (BRCA-1) is a tumor suppressor activity which depends on its ability to mimicry a cellular low-energy status, which is also known to block tumor cell anabolism and suppress the malignant phenotype. Studies shown that increased physical activity and normal weight in young women and adolescence have been associated with significantly delayed breast cancer onset for Ashkenazi Jewish women carrying BRCA-1 gene mutations [60].

Similar to animal model, human studies demonstrated a link between hyperinsulinemia and the risk for breast cancer. One study, although was conducted on postmenopausal women without diabetes, the Women's Health Initiative, reported that fasting insulin levels, independent of obesity, were strongly associated with breast cancer risk [61]. Studies conducted on women with diabetes, demonstrated also the association between hyperinsulinemia and risk for breast cancer. The Nurses' Health Study was conducted on women with type 2 diabetes and concluded that women with type 2 diabetes had an elevated incidence of breast cancer, independent of body adiposity and also that the risk was observed on women with estrogen receptor positive breast cancer [62].

Other studies explored the relationship between type 2 diabetes and breast cancer mortality and reported positive association. For example, prospective cohort study conducted by Coughlin et al. [63] showed that diabetic patient had an increased risk of breast cancer mortality in comparison with controls. Several factors may contribute to the increased mortality in diabetic breast cancer patients, these include delayed cancer diagnosis, suboptimal cancer treatments, direct tumor promoting effects of hyperinsulinemia, and adverse effects of diabetes-related comorbidities or certain antidiabetic medications [64].

In conclusion, several studies have demonstrated an increased risk of breast cancer and breast cancer mortality in patients with type 2 diabetes and this may be related to biological effect of diabetic state.

5.2. Diabetes and endometrial cancer

Worldwide in 2012, more than 500,000 women were diagnosed with uterine cancer, and the mortality rate was 1.7 to 2.4 per 100,000 women [65]. In developed countries, uterine cancer is the most common gynecologic neoplasia, counting over 50,000 new cases and over 10,000 deaths from this disease every year [66–68].

An important and well known risk factor for endometrial cancer is obesity. Other risk factors are reproductive factors, hypertension, physical activity, exposure of endometrium to estrogen unopposed by progesterone and diabetes.

In vitro studies have shown that endometrial cancer cells have an increased proliferation by activation of IGF-I, activation of insulin, and through the ovarian steroid hormone signaling pathways, such as estrogen and androgen [68, 69]. Although is not known to exist a direct correlation with insulin or IGF levels in endometrial cancer, additional factors such as ovarian steroid hormones or inflammatory cytokines make difficult to confirm if there is a single effect of insulin or IGF activation through insulin or IGF serum levels. Estrogen can activate IGF-I receptor on endometrial cancer cells, this will increase cellular proliferation through PI3K signaling, a link to IGF-I receptor activation [70]. The androgen receptor (AR) activated by the binding with androgen could also increase the proliferation of endometrial cells by the Notch signaling pathway [66, 71]. Insulin resistance increases C-reactive protein (CRP) levels and was associated with an increased risk of endometrial cancer in postmenopausal women [66, 72]. This show that endometrial cancer could be associated with the chronic inflammation that present in type 2 diabetes.

Obesity is a well-established risk factor form endometrial cancer, and due to close relationship between obesity and type 2 diabetes it is important to distinguish and there a very few studies that examined the effect of diabetes in endometrial cancer by body weight, and the findings in this studies is inconsistent [73]. There are many studies that examine the association between diabetes and the incidence of endometrial cancer, but only three studies adjusted for body mass index (BMI) and one study reported a significant association of endometrial cancer risk and diabetes [74, 75].

Association between diabetes and incidence of endometrial cancer and the potential effect of modification by obesity and physical activity was prospectively examined in the Swedish Mammography Cohort Study. Diabetes was associated with an increased risk for endometrial cancer, and combination of diabetes with obesity and low physical activity was associated with a further increased risk for endometrial cancer [76]. Interventions to reduce body weight and increase physical activity may have important implications in terms of endometrial cancer and future management of diabetic subjects.

5.3. Diabetes and colorectal cancer

In 2012, there were an estimated 1.4 million new colorectal cancer cases and 693,900 deaths. The highest colorectal cancer incidence rates in both males and females are in Japan, followed by Europe, Oceania, and North America. The lowest rates are found in Africa, some Asian countries, and Latin America and the Caribbean [2].

Type 2 diabetes was suggested as a risk factor for colorectal cancer [77]. Mechanisms implicated in this association are a slower bowel transit in patient with diabetes, that lead to increased exposure to toxins, increased production of carcinogenic bile acids and hyperinsulinemia [78].

Hyperinsulinemia has been associated with insulin resistance, increased levels of growth factors, including IGF-1, and alterations in NF-_B and peroxisome proliferator-activated receptor signaling, which may promote colon cancer through their effects on colonocyte kinetics and was explored in most studies.

The Nurses' Health Study shown that patients with type 2 diabetes included in the study had a relative risk for colorectal cancer of 1.43 [79]. Several studies shown an increased risk for colorectal cancer in diabetic patients using insulin therapy [80] and also reported increased mortality in diabetic patients with colorectal cancer aged over 30 [77].

In conclusion, both colorectal cancer risk and mortality appear to be increased in patients with type 2 diabetes and hyperinsulinemia is mediating this association.

5.4. Diabetes and pancreatic cancer

Cancer of the pancreas is one of the deadliest cancer types. Based on the GLOBOCAN 2012 evaluation it is estimated that pancreatic cancer is responsible for more than 330,000 deaths per year, putting pancreatic cancer on the seventh place of leading causes of cancer death in both sexes together. Worldwide, according to data available, more than 330,000 people had pancreatic cancer in 2012, making it the 11th most common cancer, and the highest incidence and mortality rates due to pancreatic cancer are found in developed countries [2].

The causes of pancreatic cancer are still insufficiently known, but certain risk factors have been identified to have an impact in the development of pancreatic cancer. Risk factors implicated in pancreatic cancer are smoking, obesity, genetics, diabetes, diet, physical inactivity [81].

Diabetes mellitus is associated with an increased risk of pancreatic cancer; data in literature shown that both type I and type II diabetes have doubled the risk of pancreatic cancer [82]. Diabetes may be a risk factor for pancreatic cancer, but may also be the result of pancreatic cancer itself. Mechanism implicated is hyperinsulinemia, insulin has been shown to promote growth in pancreatic cell line and insulin resistance may enhance pancreatic carcinogenesis through enhanced proliferation of islet cells and increase cell turnover [83]. In type 2 diabetes exocrine pancreatic cells are exposed to high levels of insulin, and insulin act as mitogen leading to tumor growth. But this does not explain the increased risk of pancreatic cancer in type 1 diabetic patients and in patients treated with insulin therapy [84]. On the other hand, pancreatic cancer can be the cause of diabetes, through islet cell destruction and insulin resistance. It is not clear how pancreatic cancer can determine insulin resistance, but has been shown that diabetic patients with pancreatic cancer have increased plasma levels of islet amyloid polypeptide, a hormonal factor secreted by pancreatic cells that may cause insulin resistance [85].

Insulin resistance may appear early in pancreatic cancer, and patients may be diagnosed with diabetes long before developing sign or symptoms of pancreatic cancer. This concept was introduced by Gullo et al. [86]

In conclusion, further studies are necessary to explain this complicated association between diabetes and pancreatic cancer.

5.5. Diabetes and prostate cancer

Unlike others cancers that were discussed before, prostate cancer have been shown to have a decreased incidence among type 2 diabetic patients, studies show a decreased risk for prostate cancer in diabetic patients (9–16%) [87, 88].

High testosterone levels are associated with prostate cancer and type 2 diabetic patients commonly have low levels of testosterone, are obese and elderly and both are associated with low levels of testosterone, and this may be one of the reason that can explain the negative association with prostate cancer.

Some studies have suggested that the link between prostate cancer and diabetes is mediated by the effect of hyperinsulinemia on testosterone levels [89]. Other studies have shown a negative association between hyperglycemia, hyperinsulinemia and prostate cancer. For example, Stocks and colleagues [90] in their prospective study reported that increased insulin resistance and low glycemic control is associated with low risk for prostate cancer in diabetic patients.

Despite the fact that prostate cancer risk may be low in diabetic patients, they may have higher risk for cancer related mortality than non-diabetic patients.

Prostate cancer is an important example of the complexity of carcinogenesis associated with diabetes. On the one hand, an association between diabetes, IGF-1, hyperinsulinemia and insulin resistance appears plausible, but on the other, these features can be somewhat counterbalanced as well and can reduce the risk for the development of one of the leading cancer entities worldwide.

5.6. Diabetes and hepatic cancer

Hepatocellular carcinoma (HCC) represents the most common form of primary liver cancer. The association between HCC and type 2 diabetes was reported first 30 years ago, when Lawson documented that type 2 diabetes is more prevalent in patients with HCC, irrespective of viral hepatitis, alcoholic cirrhosis or hemochromatosis [91].

Since then, multiple studies have shown an association between type 2 diabetes and HCC, and documented the increased risk for HCC in diabetic patients, independent of age, sex, obesity, smoking, hypertension, presence of cirrhosis and hepatic steatosis [92–94].

The exact pathophysiological mechanisms linking type 2 diabetes and HCC are not completely understood, but the understanding of HCC pathophysiology has improved in recent years.

It is well known that type 2 diabetes is associated with increased hepatic and peripheral insulin resistance, lipotoxicity, increased oxidative stress and chronic low-grade inflammatory state, and several studies suggest that all these factors may contribute to the development of HCC by promoting hepatic cellular growth/proliferation and by inhibiting cellular apoptosis. In addition, in the presence of insulin resistance, insulin levels rise in blood, resulting in increased insulin-like growth factor-1 (IGF-1) production that is capable to stimulate hepatic cellular growth and proliferation and inhibit cellular apoptosis in the liver. Hyperinsulinemia also stimulates insulin receptor substrate-1 (IRS-1), which plays an important role in the activation of some intracellular cytokine signaling pathways implicated in hepatic carcinogenesis [95, 96].

There are ongoing studies trying to improve our knowledge about the pathophysiology of HCC. Recently, we have evidence that suggest that gut microbiota alteration may play a role in pathogenesis of type 2 diabetes [98], other studies reported some epigenetic alterations that might be also important for HCC development, for example, the hypermethylation of the E-cadherin-1 (*CDH-1*) gene has been related to increased incidence of NAFLD-related HCC [95–97].

6. Conclusions

Diabetes and cancer are common and serious global health problems, and incidence of both diseases is increasing all over the world. Many studies have suggested the relationship between diabetes and cancer and the fact that diabetes, may affect the risk of developing a variety of cancers, and this association is also biological plausible.

It is important as a clinician to take in consideration all aspects when treating a cancer patient who has diabetes. It is important to consider all complications, cardiac, neurologic and renal complications that are commonly associated with diabetes. Continued improvement of cancer outcomes may be dependent also by the control of diabetes. Taking in consideration the results of numerous epidemiologic and clinical studies involving diabetes and cancer, clinicians must also pay attention to the increased risk of new or longstanding diabetics for some tumor entities by regularly screening diabetic patients for early development of cancer.

The association between diabetes and cancer is complex and need further studies.

It is an important health problem worldwide, and scientists, clinicians and politicians have to develop national policies for early diagnosis and prevention of diabetes and cancer more effectively, otherwise both diseases with their biologic and sociologic relationships could overwhelm health systems.

Author details

Andra-Iulia Suceveanu[1*], Adrian-Paul Suceveanu[2], Andreea-Daniela Gheorghe[3] and Laura Mazilu[3]

*Address all correspondence to: andrasuceveanu@yahoo.com

1 Faculty of Medicine, Department of Gastroenterology, Emergency Hospital of Constanta, Ovidius University, Constanta, Romania

2 Faculty of Medicine, Department of Internal Medicine, Emergency Hospital of Constanta, Ovidius University, Constanta, Romania

3 Faculty of Medicine, Department of Oncology, Emergency Hospital of Constanta, Ovidius University, Constanta, Romania

References

[1] International Agency for Research on Cancer Section of Cancer Surveillance. CancerMondial [cited 12-01-2015]. Available from: http://www-dep.iarc.fr/

[2] Ferlay J, Soerjomataram I, Ervik M, Dikshit R, Eser S, Mathers C, et al. GLOBOCAN 2012 v1.0, Cancer Incidence and Mortality Worldwide: IARC CancerBase No. 11 [Internet]. [cited 30-07-2015]. Available from: http://globocan.iarc.fr

[3] Global report on diabetes, World Health Organization. 2016. http://apps.who.int/iris/bitstream/10665/204871/1/9789241565257_eng.pdf

[4] Lopez AD, Mathers CD, Ezzati M, Jamison DT, Murray CJ. Global and regional burden of disease and risk factors, 2001: Systematic analysis of population health data. Lancet. 2006; **367**:1747-1757. DOI: 10.1016/S0140-6736(06)68770-9

[5] Tuffier T. Diabete et neoplasmes. Archives Generales de Medecine. 1888;**7**:129-140

[6] Jiang Y, Ben Q, Shen H, Lu W, Zhang Y, Zhu J. Diabetes mellitus and incidence and mortality of colorectal cancer: A systematic review and meta-analysis of cohort studies. European Journal of Epidemiology. 2011;**26**:863-876 [PubMed]

[7] Larsson SC, Mantzoros CS, Wolk A. Diabetes mellitus and risk of breast cancer: A meta-analysis. International Journal of Cancer. 2007;**121**:856-862 [PubMed]

[8] Ben Q, Xu M, Ning X, Liu J, Hong S, Huang W, Zhang H, Li Z. Diabetes mellitus and risk of pancreatic cancer: A meta-analysis of cohort studies. European Journal of Cancer. 2011; **47**:1928-1937 [PubMed]

[9] Wang C, Wang X, Gong G, Ben Q, Qiu W, Chen Y, Li G, Wang L. Increased risk of hepatocellular carcinoma in patients with diabetes mellitus: A systematic review and meta-analysis of cohort studies. International Journal of Cancer. 2012;**130**:1639-1648 [PubMed]

[10] Friberg E, Orsini N, Mantzoros CS, Wolk A. Diabetes mellitus and risk of endometrial cancer: A meta-analysis. Diabetologia. 2007;**50**:1365-1374 [PubMed]

[11] Larsson SC, Orsini N, Brismar K, Wolk A. Diabetes mellitus and risk of bladder cancer: A meta-analysis. Diabetologia. 2006;**49**:2819-2823

[12] Mitri J, Castillo J, Pittas AG. Diabetes and risk of non-Hodgkin's lymphoma: A meta-analysis of observational studies. Diabetes Care. 2008;**31**:2391-2397. [PMC free article] [PubMed]

[13] Kasper JS, Giovannucci E. A meta-analysis of diabetes mellitus and the risk of prostate cancer. Cancer Epidemiology, Biomarkers & Prevention. 2006;**15**:2056-2062 [PubMed]

[14] Vigneri P, Frasca F, Sciacca L, Pandini G, Vigneri R. Diabetes and cancer. Endocrine-Related Cancer. 2009;**16**:1103-1123. Abstract/FREE Full TextGoogle Scholar

[15] Barone BB, Yeh HC, Snyder CF, Peairs KS, Stein KB, Derr RL, Wolff AC, Brancati FL. Long-term all-cause mortality in cancer patients with preexisting diabetes mellitus: A systematic review and meta-analysis. JAMA. 2008;**300**:2754-2764. [PMC free article] [PubMed]

[16] Zendehdel K, Nyrén O, Östenson C-G, Adami H-O, Ekbom A, Ye W. Cancer incidence in patients with type 1 diabetes mellitus: A population-based cohort study in Sweden. JNCI: Journal of the National Cancer Institute. December 2003;**95**(23):1797-1800. DOI: 10.1093/jnci/djg105

[17] Cannata D, Fierz Y, Vijayakumar A, LeRoith D. Type 2 diabetes and cancer: What is the connection? Mount Sinai Journal of Medicine. 2010;**77**:197-213. DOI: 10.1002/msj.20167

[18] Giovannucci E, Harlan DM, Archer MC, Bergenstal RM, Gapstur SM, Habel LA, Pollak M, Regensteiner JG, Yee D. Diabetes and cancer: A consensus report. CA: a Cancer Journal for Clinicians. 2010;**60**:207-221. DOI: 10.3322/caac.20078

[19] Aziz NM, Rowland JH. Trends and advances in cancer survivorship research: Challenge and opportunity. Seminars in Radiation Oncology. 2003;**13**:248-266. DOI: 10.1016/S1053-4296(03)00024-9

[20] CDC, Lance Armstrong Foundation. A National Action Plan for Cancer Survivorship: Advancing Public Health Strategies. Atlanta, Georgia: U.S. Department of Health and Human Services, CDC; 2004 Available at http://www.cdc.gov/cancer/survivorship/overview.htm

[21] Schienkiewitz A, Schulze MB, Hoffmann K, Kroke A, Boeing H. Body mass index history and risk of type 2 diabetes: Results from the European prospective investigation into cancer and nutrition (EPIC)-Potsdam study. The American Journal of Clinical Nutrition. 2006; **84**:427-433 PubMed

[22] Wei M, Gaskill SP, Haffner SM, Stern MP. Waist circumference as the best predictor of noninsulin dependent diabetes mellitus (NIDDM) compared to body mass index, waist/hip ratio and other anthropometric measurements in Mexican Americans–a 7-year prospective study. Obesity Research. 1997;**5**:16-23. DOI: 10.1002/j.1550-8528.1997.tb00278

[23] Ma J, Li H, Giovannucci E, et al. Prediagnostic body-mass index, plasma C-peptide concentration, and prostate cancer-specific mortality in men with prostate cancer: A long-term survival analysis. The Lancet Oncology. 2008;**9**:1039-1047. DOI: 10.1016/S1470-2045(08)70235-3

[24] Pischon T, Lahmann PH, Boeing H, et al. Body size and risk of colon and rectal cancer in the European prospective investigation into cancer and nutrition (EPIC). Journal of the National Cancer Institute. 2006;**98**:920-931. DOI: 10.1093/jnci/djj246

[25] Knowler WC, Barrett-Connor E, Fowler SE, et al. Diabetes prevention program research group. Reduction in the incidence of type 2 diabetes with lifestyle intervention or metformin. The New England Journal of Medicine. 2002;**346**:393-403. DOI: 10.1056/NEJMoa012512

[26] Eliassen AH, Colditz GA, Rosner B, Willett WC, Hankinson SE. Adult weight change and risk of postmenopausal breast cancer. JAMA. 2006;**296**(2):193-201. DOI: 10.1001/jama.296.2.193

[27] Eliassen AH, Colditz GA, Rosner B, Willett WC, Hankinson SE. Adult weight change and risk of postmenopausal breast cancer. JAMA. 2006;**296**:193-201

[28] Lee IM. Physical activity and cancer prevention–data from epidemiologic studies. Medicine and Science in Sports and Exercise. 2003;**35**:1823-1827. DOI: 10.1249/01.MSS.0000093620.27893.23

[29] Friedenreich CM, Orenstein MR. Physical activity and cancer prevention: Etiologic evidence and biological mechanisms. The Journal of Nutrition. 2002;**132**:3456S-3464S. PubMed

[30] Holmes MD, Chen WY, Feskanich D, Kroenke CH, Colditz GA. Physical activity and survival after breast cancer diagnosis. JAMA. 2005;**293**(20):2479-2486. DOI: 10.1001/jama.293.20.2479

[31] Meyerhardt JA, Giovannucci EL, Holmes MD, et al. Physical activity and survival after colorectal cancer diagnosis. Journal of Clinical Oncology. 2006;**24**:3527-3534. DOI: 10.1200/JCO.2006.06.0855

[32] Hamman RF, Wing RR, Edelstein SL, et al. Effect of weight loss with lifestyle intervention on risk of diabetes. Diabetes Care. 2006;**29**:2102-2107. DOI: 10.2337/dc06-0560

[33] Willi C, Bodenmann P, Ghali WA, Faris PD, Cornuz J. Active smoking and the risk of type 2 diabetes: A systematic review and meta-analysis. JAMA. 2007;**298**:2654-2664 [PubMed]

[34] Haire-Joshu D, Glasgow RE, Tibbs TL. Smoking and diabetes. Diabetes Care. 1999;**22**:1887-1898. DOI: 10.2337/diacare.22.11.1887

[35] Howard AA, Arnsten JH, Gourevitch MN. Effect of alcohol consumption on diabetes mellitus: A systematic review. Annals of Internal Medicine. 2004;**140**:211-219. DOI: 10.7326/0003-4819-140-6-200403160-00011

[36] Baliunas DO, Taylor BJ, Irving H, et al. Alcohol as a risk factor for type 2 diabetes: A systematic review and meta-analysis. Diabetes Care. 2009;**32**:2123-2213. DOI: 10.2337/dc09-0227

[37] Pollak M. Insulin and insulin-like growth factor signalling in neoplasia. Nature Reviews. Cancer. 2008;**8**:915-928. DOI: 10.1038/nrc2536

[38] Zhang H, Pelzer AM, Kiang DT, Yee D. Down-regulation of type I insulin-like growth factor receptor increases sensitivity of breast cancer cells to insulin. Cancer Research. 2007;**67**:391-397. DOI: 10.1158/0008-5472.CAN-06-1712

[39] Frasca F, Pandini G, Scalia P, Sciacca L, Mineo R, Costantino A, Goldfine ID, Belfiore A, Vigneri R. Insulin receptor isoform a, a newly recognized, high-affinity insulin-like growth factor II receptor in fetal and cancer cells. Molecular and Cellular Biology. 1999;**19**:3278-3288. [PMC free article] [PubMed]

[40] De Meyts P, Christoffersen CT, Urso B, Wallach B, Gronskov K, Yakushiji F, Shymko RM. Role of the time factor in signaling specificity: Application to mitogenic and metabolic signaling by the insulin and insulin-like growth factor-I receptor tyrosine kinases. Metabolism. 1995;**44**(10 Suppl 4):2-11 [PubMed]

[41] Papa V, Pezzino V, Costantino A, Belfiore A, Giuffrida D, Frittitta L, Vannelli GB, Brand R, Goldfine ID, Vigneri R. Elevated insulin receptor content in human breast cancer. The Journal of Clinical Investigation. 1990;**86**:1503-1510. DOI: 10.1172/JCI114868

[42] Chen W, Wang S, Tian T, et al. Phenotypes and genotypes of insulin-like growth factor 1, IGF-binding protein-3 and cancer risk: Evidence from 96 studies. European Journal of Human Genetics. 2009;**17**(12):1668-1675. DOI: 10.1038/ejhg.2009.86

[43] Major JM, Laughlin GA, Kritz-Silverstein D, Wingard DL, Barrett-Connor E. Insulin-like growth factor-I and cancer mortality in older men. The Journal of Clinical Endocrinology and Metabolism. 2010;**95**(3):1054-1059. DOI: 10.1210/jc.2009-1378

[44] Calle EE, Kaaks R. Overweight, obesity and cancer: Epidemiological evidence and proposed mechanisms. Nature Reviews. Cancer. 2004;**4**:579-591. DOI: 10.1038/nrc1408

[45] World Cancer Research Fund, American Institute for Cancer Research. Food, Nutrition, Physical Activity and the Prevention of Cancer: A Global Perspective. American Institute for Cancer Research: Washington, D.C.; 2007. DOI: 10.1126/science.1160809

[46] van Kruijsdijk RC, van der Wall E, Visseren FL. Obesity and cancer: The role of dysfunctional adipose tissue. Cancer Epidemiology, Biomarkers & Prevention. 2009;**18**:2569-2578. DOI: 10.1158/1055-9965.EPI-09-0372

[47] Wu Y, Antony S, Meitzler JL, Doroshow JH. Molecular mechanisms underlying chronic inflammation-associated cancers. Cancer Letters. 2014;**345**(2):164-173. DOI: 10.1016/j.canlet.2013.08.014

[48] Abbour S. Primary care physicians and insulin initiation: Multiple barriers, lack of knowledge or both? International Journal of Clinical Practice. 2008;**62**:845-847. DOI: 10.1111/j.1742-1241.2008.01757.x

[49] Richard M et al. Type 2 diabetes: Assessing the relative risks and benefits of glucose-lowering medications Bergenstal. The American Journal of Medicine. **123**(4):374. e9 - 374.e18. DOI: 10.1016/j.amjmed.2009.07.017

[50] Blin P, Lassalle R, Dureau-Pournin C, et al. Insulin glargine and risk of cancer: A cohort study in the French National Healthcare Insurance Database. Diabetologia. 2012;**55**(3):644-653. DOI: 10.1007/s00125-011-2429-5

[51] Hemkens LG, Grouven U, Bender R, et al. Risk of malignancies in patients with diabetes treated with human insulin or insulin analogues: A cohort study. Diabetologia. 2009;**52**(9):1732-1744. DOI: 10.1007/s00125-009-1418-4

[52] Chang C-H, Lin J-W, Wu L-C, Lai M-S, Chuang L-M. Oral insulin Secretagogues, insulin, and cancer risk in type 2 diabetes mellitus. The Journal of Clinical Endocrinology & Metabolism. July 2012;**97**(7):E1170-E1175. DOI: 10.1210/jc.2012-1162

[53] Bowker SL, Majumdar SR, Veugelers P, Johnson JA. Increased cancer-related mortality for patients with type 2 diabetes who use sulfonylureas or insulin. Diabetes Care. Feb 2006;**29**(2):254-258. DOI: 10.2337/diacare.29.02.06.dc05-1558

[54] Monami M, Colombi C, Balzi D, et al. Metformin and cancer occurrence in insulin-treated type 2 diabetic patients. Diabetes Care. 2011;**34**(1):129-131. DOI: 10.2337/dc10-1287

[55] Key TJ, Verkasalo PK, Bancks E. Epidemiology of breast cancer. The Lancet Oncology. **2**(3):133-140. DOI: 10.1016/S1470-2045(00)00254-0

[56] Xue F, Michels KB. Diabetes, metabolic syndrome, and breast cancer: A review of the current evidence. The American Journal of Clinical Nutrition. 2007 Sep;**86**(3):s823-35

[57] Larsson SC, Mantzoros CS, Wolk A. Diabetes mellitus and risk of breast cancer: A meta-analysis. International Journal of Cancer. 2007;**121**:856-862. DOI: 10.1002/ijc.22717

[58] Ish-Shalom D, Christoffersen C, Vorwerk P, et al. Mitogenic properties of insulin and insulin analogues mediated by the insulin receptor. Diabetologia. 1997;**40**(Suppl 2):S25. DOI: 10.1007/s001250051393

[59] Chappell J, Leitner JW, Solomon S. Effect of insulin on cell cycle progression in MCF-7 breast cancer cells. Direct and potentiating influence. The Journal of Biological Chemistry. 2001 Oct 12;**276**(41):38023-80. Epub 2001 Aug 10

[60] Brunet J, Vazquez-Martin A, Colomer R, Graña-Suarez B, Martin-Castillo B, Menendez JA. BRCA1 and acetyl-CoA carboxylase: The metabolic syndrome of breast cancer. Molecular Carcinogenesis. 2008;**47**:157-163. DOI: 10.1002/mc.20364

[61] Gunter MJ, Hoover DR, Yu H, Wassertheil-Smoller S, Rohan TE, Manson JE, Li J, Ho GY, Xue X, Anderson GL, Kaplan RC, Harris TG, Howard BV, Wylie-Rosett J, Burk RD, Strickler HD. Insulin, insulin-like growth factor-I, and risk of breast cancer in postmenopausal women. JNCI: Journal of the National Cancer Institute. January 2009;**101**(1):48-60. DOI: 10.1093/jnci/djn415

[62] Michels KB, Solomon CG, Hu FB, Rosner BA, Hankinson SE, Colditz GA, Manson JAE. Type 2 diabetes and subsequent incidence of breast cancer in the nurses' health. Study Diabetes Care. Jun 2003;**26**(6):1752-1758. DOI: 10.2337/diacare.26.6.1752

[63] Coughlin SS, Calle EE, Teras LR, Petrelli J, Thun MJ. Diabetes mellitus as a predictor of cancer mortality in a large cohort of US adults. American Journal of Epidemiology. June 2004;**159**(12):1160-1167. DOI: 10.1093/aje/kwh161

[64] DeCensi A, Gennari A. Insulin breast cancer connection: Confirmatory data set the stage for better care. Journal of Clinical Oncology. 2011;**29**(1):7-10

[65] Torre LA, Bray F, Siegel RL, et al. Global cancer statistics, 2012. CA: a Cancer Journal for Clinicians. 2015;**65**:87

[66] Siegel RL, Miller KD, Jemal A. Cancer statistics, 2016. CA: a Cancer Journal for Clinicians. 2016;**66**:7

[67] Joung KH, Jeong J-W, Ku BJ. The association between type 2 diabetes mellitus and women cancer: The epidemiological evidences and putative mechanisms. BioMed Research International. 2015;**2015**:920618. DOI: 10.1155/2015/920618

[68] Mu N, Zhu Y, Wang Y, Zhang H, Xue F. Insulin resistance: A significant risk factor of endometrial cancer. Gynecologic Oncology. 2012;**125**(3):751-757. DOI: 10.1016/j.ygyno.2012.03.032

[69] Bruchim I, Sarfstein R, Werner H. The IGF hormonal network in endometrial cancer: Functions, regulation, and targeting approaches. Frontiers in Endocrinology. 2014;**5**:76. DOI: 10.3389/fendo.2014.00076

[70] Syed V, Ulinski G, Mok SC, Ho S-M. Reproductive hormone-induced, STAT3-mediated interleukin 6 action in normal and malignant human ovarian surface epithelial cells.

JNCI: Journal of the National Cancer Institute. April 2002;**94**(8):617-629. DOI: 10.1093/jnci/94.8.617

[71] Wang T, Rohan TE, Gunter MJ, et al. A prospective study of inflammation markers and endometrial cancer risk in postmenopausal hormone nonusers. Cancer Epidemiology, Biomarkers and Prevention. 2011;**20**(5):971-977. DOI: 10.1158/1055-9965.EPI-10-1222

[72] Crosbie EJ, Zwahlen M, Kitchener HC, Egger M, Renehan AG. Body mass index, hormone replacement therapy, and endometrial cancer risk: A meta-analysis. Cancer Epidemiology, Biomarkers & Prevention. 2010;**19**(12):3119-3130. DOI: 10.1158/1055-9965.EPI-10-0832

[73] Friberg E, Mantzoros CS, Wolk A. Diabetes and risk of endometrial cancer: A population-based prospective cohort study. Cancer Epidemiology, Biomarkers & Prevention. 2007;**16**(2):276-280. DOI: 10.1158/1055-9965.EPI-06-0751

[74] Terry P, Baron JA, Weiderpass E, Yuen J, Lichtenstein P, Nyrén O. Lifestyle and endometrial cancer risk: A cohort study from the Swedish twin registry. International Journal of Cancer. 1999;**82**:38-42. DOI: 10.1002/(SICI)1097-0215(19990702)82:1<38::AID-IJC8>3.0.CO;2-Q

[75] Anderson KE, Anderson E, Mink PJ, Hong CP, Kushi LH, Sellers TA, Lazovich D, Folsom AR. Diabetes and endometrial cancer in the Iowa women's health study. Cancer Epidemiology, Biomarkers & Prevention. 2001;**10**(6):611-616. [PubMed]

[76] Friberg E, Orsini N, Mantzoros CS, Wolk A. Diabetes mellitus and risk of endometrial cancer: A metaanalysis. Diabetologia. 2007;**50**:1365-1374

[77] Larsson SC, Orsini N, Wolk A. Diabetes mellitus and risk of colorectal cancer: A meta-analysis. JNCI: Journal of the National Cancer Institute. November 2005;**97**(22):1679-1687. DOI: 10.1093/jnci/dji375

[78] Will JC, Galuska DA, Vinicor F, Calle EE. Colorectal cancer: Another complication of diabetes mellitus? American Journal of Epidemiology. May 1998;**147**(9):816-825. DOI: 10.1093/oxfordjournals.aje.a009534

[79] Yakar S, Nunez NP, Pennisi P, Brodt P, Sun H, Fallavollita L, Zhao H, Scavo L, Novosyadlyy R, Kurshan N, Stannard B, East-Palmer J, Smith NC, Perkins SN, Fuchs-Young R, Barrett JC, Hursting SD, Le Roith D. Increased tumor growth in mice with diet-induced obesity: Impact of ovarian hormones. Endocrinology. December 2006;**147**(12):5826-5834. DOI: 10.1210/en.2006-0311

[80] Yang YX, Hennessy S, Lewis JD. Insulin therapy and colorectal cancer risk among type 2 diabetes mellitus patients. Gastroenterology. 2004. DOI: 10.1053/j.gastro.2004.07.011

[81] Bosetti C, Bertuccio P, Negri E, La Vecchia C, Zeegers MP, Boffetta P. Pancreatic cancer: Overview of descriptive epidemiology. Molecular Carcinogenesis. 2012;**51**:3-13. DOI: 10.1002/mc.20785

[82] Batabyal P, Vander Hoorn S, Christophi C, Nikfarjam M. Association of diabetes mellitus and pancreatic adenocarcinoma: A meta-analysis of 88 studies. Annals of Surgical Oncology. 2014;**21**:2453-2462. DOI: 10.1245/s10434-014-3625-6

[83] Silverman DT, Schiffman M, Everhart J. Diabetes mellitus, other medical conditions and familial history of cancer as risk factors for pancreatic cancer. British Journal of Cancer. 1999;**80**:1830-1837. DOI: 10.1038/sj.bjc.6690607

[84] Stevens RJ, Roddam AW, Beral V. Pancreatic cancer in type 1 and young-onset diabetes: Systematic review and meta-analysis. British Journal of Cancer. 2007;**96**:507-509. DOI: 10.1038/sj.bjc.6603571

[85] Permert J, Larsson J, Westermark GT, Herrington MK, Christmanson L, Pour PM, Westermark P, Adrian TE. Islet amyloid polypeptide in patients with pancreatic cancer and diabetes. The New England Journal of Medicine. 1994, February 1994;**330**:313-318. DOI: 10.1056/NEJM199402033300503

[86] Gullo L, Pezzilli R, Morselli-Labate AM, the Italian Pancreatic Cancer Study Group. Diabetes and the risk of pancreatic cancer. The New England Journal of Medicine. 1994, July 1994;**331**:81-84. DOI: 10.1056/NEJM199407143310203

[87] Bonovas S, Filioussi K, Tsantes A. Diabetes mellitus and risk of prostate cancer: A meta-analysis. Diabetologia. 2004;**47**:1071. DOI: 10.1007/s00125-004-1415-6

[88] Kasper JS, Giovannucci E. A meta-analysis of diabetes mellitus and the risk of prostate cancer. Cancer Epidemiology, Biomarkers & Prevention. November 2006;**15**(11):2056-2062. DOI: 10.1158/1055-9965.EPI-06-0410

[89] Grossmann M, Thomas MC, Panagiotopoulos S, Sharpe K, MacIsaac RJ, Clarke S, Zajac JD, Jerums G. Low testosterone levels are common and associated with insulin resistance in men with diabetes. The Journal of Clinical Endocrinology & Metabolism. May 2008;**93**(5):1834-1840. DOI: 10.1210/jc.2007-2177

[90] Stocks T, Lukanova A, Rinaldi S, Biessy C, Dossus L, Lindahl B, Hallmans G, Kaaks R, Stattin P. Insulin resistance is inversely related to prostate cancer: A prospective study in northern Sweden. International Journal of Cancer. 2007;**120**:2678-2686. DOI: 10.1002/ijc.22587

[91] Lawson DH, Gray JM, McKillop C, et al. Diabetes mellitus and primary hepatocellular carcinoma. The Quarterly Journal of Medicine. 1986;**61**:945-955. [PubMed]

[92] Romeo S, Kozlitina J, Xing C, et al. Genetic variation in PNPLA3 confers susceptibility to nonalcoholic fatty liver disease. Nature Genetics. 2008;**40**(12):1461-1465. DOI: 10.1038/ng.257

[93] Falleti E, Fabris C, Cmet S, Cussigh A, Bitetto D, Fontanini E, Fornasiere E, Bignulin S, Fumolo E, Bignulin E, Pirisi M, Toniutto P. PNPLA3 rs738409C/G polymorphism in cirrhosis: Relationship with the aetiology of liver disease and hepatocellular carcinoma occurrence. Liver International. 2011;**31**:1137-1143. DOI: 10.1111/j.1478-3231.2011.02534.x

[94] Evans JMM, Donnelly LA, Emslie-Smith AM, Alessi DR, Morris AD. Metformin and reduced risk of cancer in diabetic patients. BMJ British Medical Journal. 2005;**330**(7503):1304-1305. DOI: 10.1136/bmj.38415.708634.F7

[95] Donadon V, Balbi M, Mas MD, Casarin P, Zanette G. Metformin and reduced risk of hepatocellular carcinoma in diabetic patients with chronic liver disease. Liver International. 2010;**30**:750-758. DOI: 10.1111/j.1478-3231.2010.02223.x

[96] Dapito DH, Mencin A, Gwak G-Y, et al. Promotion of hepatocellular carcinoma by the intestinal microbiota and TLR4. Cancer Cell. 2012;**21**(4):504-516. DOI: 10.1016/j.ccr.2012.02.007

[97] Liu YL, Patman GL, Leathart JB, et al. Carriage of the PNPLA3 rs738409 C>G polymorphism confers an increased risk of non-alcoholic fatty liver disease associated hepatocellular carcinoma. Journal of Hepatology. 2014;**61**:75-81. DOI: 10.1016/j.jhep.2014.02.030

4

Fine Particulate Matter ($PM_{2.5}$) Air Pollution and Type 2 Diabetes Mellitus (T2DM): When Experimental Data Explains Epidemiological Facts

Thiago Gomes Heck,
Pauline Brendler Goettems Fiorin,
Matias Nunes Frizzo and Mirna Stela Ludwig

Abstract

Epidemiologic and experimental studies suggest that environmental exposures to air pollutants can increase prevalence of metabolic and cardiorespiratory diseases. Among the risk factors, many studies have shown that air pollution, especially by fine particulate matter ($PM_{2.5}$), can lead to the development of type 2 diabetes mellitus (T2DM) or make diabetics more susceptible to other health complications. This chapter aimed to discuss the pathophysiologic mechanisms evolved in susceptibility to cardiorespiratory $PM_{2.5}$ effects in T2DM subjects, as well as the enhancing effect of $PM_{2.5}$ exposure on development of T2DM. We discussed the pathophysiologic mechanisms of $PM_{2.5}$ exposure and T2DM based on pro-/anti-inflammatory balance, metabolic regulation, redox status, and heat shock response, reinforcing the complex nature of T2DM etiology and highlighting the $PM_{2.5}$ air pollution as a critical health problem.

Keywords: fine particulate matter, type 2 diabetes mellitus, inflammation, oxidative stress, HSP70

1. Introduction: Epidemiology of sum of environmental and metabolic risk

In the last century, many epidemiological data demonstrated that the urbanization phenomenon corroborates to increasing prevalence of metabolic diseases and cardiorespiratory diseases. It is well known that high energy food offer and sedentarism are risk factors for metabolic diseases such as diabetes, while high levels of air pollutant emission represent a risk for cardio-respiratory diseases. Thus, almost all people living in great cities are exposed simultaneously to these two risk factors: food consumption in quantities above the necessary for health maintenance and exposure to environmental air pollution above the limits proposed by WHO.

Some numbers from WHO are really impressive. Data from Global report on diabetes (2016) show that at least 422 million people are diabetic in worldwide and that diabetes prevalence has been rising more rapidly in middle- and low-income countries [1]. In the same risk direction, Global Urban Ambient Air Pollution Database update 2016 [2] showed that 98% of these cities, with more than 100,000 inhabitants, do not meet WHO air quality guidelines. This data represents that 92% of the world population lives in places where air quality levels exceed WHO limits. Thus, we can hypothesize that probably a great amount of people are simultaneously exposed to urbanization risk factors to health.

Based on a biologically plausible hypothesis from 2004 [3], Brook et al. published data from respiratory clinics (n = 5228 patients) and conclude that traffic-related air pollutants were associated with type 2 diabetes mellitus (T2DM) prevalence among women [4]. Thus, in few years, at least eight studies corroborate with the first study and provide data from association between exposure to fine particulate matter (<2.5 μm, $PM_{2.5}$) and T2DM prevalence (for review, please see Rajagolapan and Brook, 2012).

Actually, the WHO air quality guidelines (WHO-AQG) [6] recommend that $PM_{2.5}$ levels not exceed annual mean concentration of 10 μg/m^3 and confirm that 92% of the world's population lives in places where air-quality levels exceed WHO limits. Interestingly, the information is presented via interactive maps, highlighting areas within countries that exceed WHO limits. Data obtained from "Most searched cities" and others in http://breathelife2030.org/ [7] and WHO ambient (outdoor) air pollution database 2016 are shown in **Figure 1**.

Just for hypothesize the population under $PM_{2.5}$ pollution risk, we listed in **Table 1** an estimate of habitants in each city listed in **Figure 1**. We may conclude that at least 140 millions of people are breathing an inadequate level of $PM_{2.5.}$ Additionally, according to WHO diabetes database, 1 person in each 11 is diabetic; thus, we can hypnotize that, only in these cities, more than 12 million of people are simultaneously under exposure of these 2 risk factors to health: diabetes and $PM_{2.5.}$

As can be observed in the data listed above, air pollution in middle- and low-income countries, in majority in Asia, Latin America, and Africa, is a significant public health burden. Here, we highlighted places that often present high concentrations of $PM_{2.5}$ and simultaneously a high population density suggesting an industrialized and modernized life style that corroborates to T2DM development. Accordingly, as was demonstrated more than 10 years ago, the sum of these conditions is critical for health. Diabetic patients are more susceptible to air pollution-induced cardiovascular morbidity and mortality [8, 9], and this susceptibility to $PM_{2.5}$ cardiovascular effects was associated with vasoconstrictive effects observed in episodes of high levels of pollution in T2DM [10].

In terms of "hard cardiovascular events," the recent review of Brook, et al. resume several meta-analyses assessing the impact of short-term exposures to $PM_{2.5}$. Accordingly, data extracted from 34 studies, each 10 μg/m^3 increase in $PM_{2.5}$ concentration (during few hours to

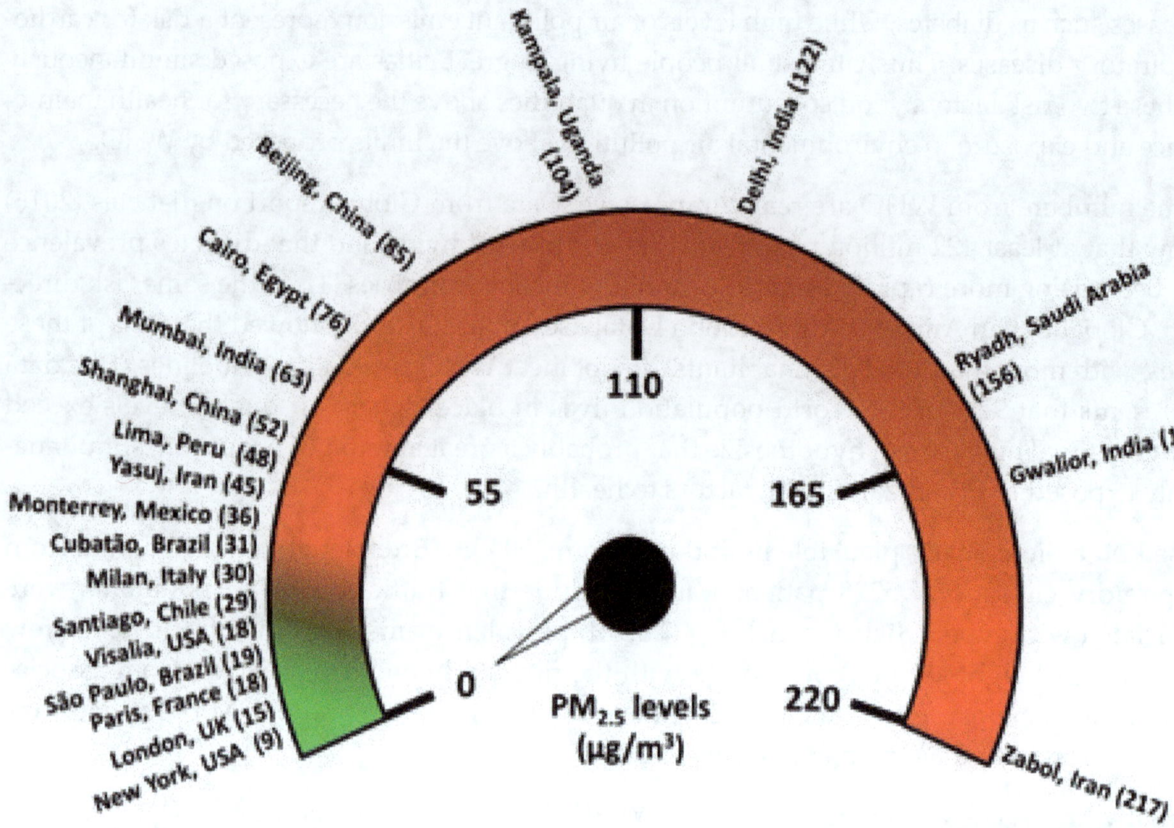

Figure 1. Fine particulate matter annual mean concentration in cities worldwide. Data obtained from WHO 2016 database [2] and published by breathlife2030.Org [7]. Data presented in terms of concentration of particles per air volume in µg/m^3.

City, Country	Population	City, Country	Population
Zurich, Switzerland	401,144	Shanghai, China	24,152,700
London, UK	8,787,892	Mumbai, India	12,442,373
Paris, France	2,229,621	Cairo, Egypt	9,500,000
Visalia, US	131,074	Beijing, China	21,700,000
São Paulo, Brazil	12,038,175	Kampala, Uganda	1,507,080
Santiago, Chile	7,314,176	Delhi, India	16,349,832
Milan, Italy	1,368,590	Bamenda, Cameroon	2,000,000
Cubatão, Brazil	127,006	Riyadh, Saudi Arabia	6,506,700
Monterrey, Mexico	1,130,960	Gwalior, India	1,953,505
Yasuj, Iran	108,505	Zabol, Iran	130,642
Lima, Peru	10,852,210	**Total**	**140,732,185**

Data extracted from wikipedia.com

Table 1. Estimate of population of cities listed in **Figure 1**.

days), increased the risk for acute myocardial infarction (by 2.5%), hospitalization or death from heart failure (2.1%), stroke (1.1%), and arrhythmia (1.5%). The risk increases for long-term exposure when people live in unhealthy urban area that exceeds $PM_{2.5}$ levels, reaching more than 10% increase in cardiovascular mortality. Also, if people live in polluted area, a peak of $PM_{2.5}$ levels increases 10–50 fold the risk for cardiovascular events [11]. Furthermore, elderly people and women are high susceptible profile to $PM_{2.5}$ effects and for T2DM development, mainly in menopause [11].

The pathophysiologic mechanisms evolved in susceptibility to cardiorespiratory $PM_{2.5}$ effects in T2DM subjects, as well as the enhancing effect of $PM_{2.5}$ exposure on development of T2DM, are discussed below. The number and the complexity of these mechanisms are positive correlated to the importance for life maintenance. In this chapter, we presented pathophysiologic mechanisms based on oxidative stress, inflammation, and heat shock response, with major contribution from experimental studies. These issues were selected considering as representative of the ability of an organism to respond physiologically (by adequate and quick ways) to the environmental challenges or internal changes in the metabolism as an essential characteristic that permits the life. As background of this discussion, there is the comprehension of the concept that homeostasis regulation of one variable is dependent on many cooperative or synergic mechanisms, that may be activated simultaneity or by steps, in terms of redox response, cell by cell signaling, and/or by molecular stress response. Since T2DM and $PM_{2.5}$ may be considered as stress situations that can promote damage to organism, and also are conditions that require adaptation/protection responses in the stressed cells, the comprehension of multi-integrative physiologic response can provide mechanistic explanation of epidemiological data listed above. Whereas high-intensity challenges to organism can overload the defensive response mechanisms, chronic and moderate intensity challenges can induce internal "recalibration" of many systems to survive [12]. Then, in the light of this "integrative" and "evolutionary" perspective is important to consider the expressive and complex effects of $PM_{2.5}$ exposure and T2DM on these variables discussed below: (a) the pro/anti-inflammatory balance; (b) the metabolic regulation (flux and consumption of energy sources); (c) the redox status (pro/antioxidant balance); and (d) heat shock response.

2. Pathophysiology of T2DM development: Role of inflammation, oxidative stress, and heat shock proteins

The plasma glucose level at any given time is determined by the balance between the amount of glucose entering the bloodstream and the amount leaving it. The principal determinants are therefore the dietary intake; the rate of entry into the cells of muscle, adipose tissue, and other organs; and the glucostatic activity of the liver. Thus, there are biochemical abnormalities as fundamental defects to T2DM development as reduced entry of glucose into various peripheral tissues and increased release of glucose into the circulation from the liver. The extracellular glucose excess (hyperglycemia) represents for many cells challenge to maintenance of intracellular glucose level [13, 14].

In animals, hyperglycemia state can be produced by pancreatectomy, by toxins administration that in appropriate doses cause selective destruction of the β cells of the pancreatic islets (as streptozocin or alloxan), by administration of drugs that inhibit insulin secretion, or by administration of anti-insulin antibodies. Also, strains of mice, rats, hamsters, guinea pigs, miniature swine, and monkeys that have a high incidence of spontaneous diabetes mellitus have also been described. However, due to high prevalence of T2DM related to lifestyle, several experimental data obtained from high fat diet (HFD) animal models have been used with success to induce the disruption of insulin signaling in liver, skeletal muscle, or adipose tissue causing hyperinsulinemia and thus, the development of T2DM [15, 16].

The HFD models help us to comprehension of the mechanisms described up to now for T2DM. As reviewed recently, it was proposed that the activation of transcription factor forkhead box protein O1 (FOXO1) in the liver and disruption of glucose-transporter translocation (GLUT4) to the surface membrane in skeletal muscle as the first steps of insulin resistance [17]. The resultant hyperglycemia and chronic hyperinsulinemia are hypothesized to disrupt insulin suppression of adipocyte lipolysis [17]. Additionaly, the active metabolism of adipose tissue may contribute to hyperinsulinemia since in HFD feeding, it occurs in the deregulation of hepatocyte gluconeogenesis (such as FOXO1), which causes increased hepatic glucose output, and deregulate the glucose transporter GLUT4 response to insulin in muscle, which results in decreased glucose uptake by muscle. In this case, the hypertrophy of adipose tissue can be interpreted as the first step of insulin resistance development that results in hyperglycemia and T2DM.

Persistent hyperglycemia causes tissue damage by different mechanism that involves oxidative stress. Increased uptake of glucose results in increased intracellular glucose concentration, that in turns, increased polyol pathway flux. This metabolic pathway uses dihydronicotinamide adenine dinucleotide phosphate (NADPH) that is required for maintaining the levels of the major intracellular nonenzymatic antioxidant defense, the glutathione. Nonenzymatic reaction of glucose and other glycation compounds formed advanced glycation products (AGEs) that modify intracellular proteins functions. Also, AGEs binding to specific receptors (RAGES) can induces reactive oxygen species (ROS) production. Finally, increased levels of AGEs and glucose (intracellularly and extracellularly) increased protein kinase C activation and hexosamine pathway flux. All these mechanisms listed above are involved in decrease nitric oxide (NO) production (vascular impaired function) and activation of factor nuclear kappa B (NF-kB), major pro-inflammatory transcript factor (for details, please see Giacco and Borwnlee, 2010).

Chronic hyperglycemia is strongly associated with enhanced oxidative stress with overproduction of ROS and nitrosative species (RNS), a reduction of the activity of antioxidant enzymes is known to cause endothelial dysfunction and insulin resistance [19]. Thus, oxidative stress constitutes as an important factor implicated not only in the T2DM development itself but also in the development of diabetic complications [18, 20]. T2DM is well known a cause of microangiopathies, observed at least by the three major diabetic complications, namely, diabetic retinopathy, nephropathy, and neuropathy. Also, T2DM constitutes a major risk factor for macroangiopathy, such as coronary artery disease and cerebrovascular disease.

Thus, oxidative stress in T2DM is associated with a wide array of complications associated with decreased quality of life of affected patients, thus contributing to the staggering increase in health-care expenditure.

Overweight and obesity is a risk factor for development of T2DM and is strongly related to chronic low grade inflammatory state. Adipose tissue metabolism is responsible for systemic oxidative stress and increase pro-inflammatory signaling, observed by increased plasma/serum cytokine levels. The development and the severity of the disease are related to immuno-inflammatory responses and thus, biomarkers. Inflammatory cells (monocytes/macrophage and Th1 lymphocytes) are stimulated to express high amounts of the inducible form of nitric oxide synthase (iNOS, that is, encode by NOS-2 gene) by activation of transcriptors factor of inflammation, as NF-kB [21]. Studies in human obesity and insulin resistance (as well as in animal models) have revealed a clear association between the chronic activation of pro-inflammatory signaling pathways and decreased insulin sensitivity.

Elevated levels of TNF-α, IL-6, and IL-8 have all been reported in various diabetic and insulin-resistant states. As part of the chronic inflammatory process, locally secreted chemokines attract pro-inflammatory macrophages to the adipose tissue, where they form crown-like structures around large dead or dying adipocytes. These "infiltrated" macrophages release cytokines that further activate the inflammatory response in neighboring adipocytes, exacerbating inflammation and insulin resistance. In addition, overnutrition and obesity are often accompanied by elevations in tissue and circulating free fat acids (FFA) concentrations, and saturated FFAs can directly activate pro-inflammatory responses in vascular endothelial cells, adipocytes, and myeloid-derived cells. Excess of free fatty acids accumulate (FFA), resulting in lipotoxicity and an increase in potentially harmful intracellular lipid products activating the NF-κB pathway and inflammation. Adipose tissue macrophages (ATMs) infiltrate adipose tissue to clear these excess lipids and produce pro-inflammatory cytokines, such as IL-1β, TNF-α and IL-6, which further propagate inflammation [22].

According Fontana et al., obesity is strongly associated with plasma IL-6 levels so that has been calculated that one third of total circulating concentrations of IL-6 originate from adipose tissue. A feed-forward paracrine inflammatory cycle involves co-cultured adipocyte release of FFA and macrophage FFA-induced TNF-α production, which blocks insulin-stimulated glucose uptake in adipocytes, and leads to increased release of FFA. TNF-α induces insulin resistance through several mechanisms including inhibition of insulin receptor signaling and increases in FFA. In addition, macrophages secrete a chemotactic pro-inflammatory lectin Galectin-3 that directly decreases insulin signaling and promotes adipose tissue inflammation. Thus, the overexpressed pro-inflammatory cytokines in obesity are considered the link between obesity and inflammation [23–25] and also, obesity and the concomitant development of inflammation are major components of insulin resistance [26].

Additionally with pro-inflammatory signaling and oxidative stress, hyperglycemia in T2DM is also associated with modifications in the cell stress response ability, with markedly undesirable effects in the metabolism. Cell stress response may be studied observing heat shock proteins (HSP) amount, synthesis, and release from cells and tissues. Since HSP are classified by their molecular weight, in this chapter, we use the term "HSP70" to describe all proteins from 70 kDa HSP family, including inducible 72 kDa and constitutive 73 kDa forms. Also we use the prefix "e" or "i" to identify protein location, as extracellular (eHSP70) or intracellular (iHSP70) located.

Pro-inflammatory signaling, oxidative stress, and hyperglycemia in T2DM is related to decreased iHSP70 levels. In obesity, it observed a reduction in iHSP70 levels and an increase in JNK activation in skeletal muscle. This effect may be a result of heat shock factor (HSF-1) inhibition. The levels of iHSP70 are correlated with the level of insulin resistance and negatively correlated with fast glucose levels [27]. Heat therapy, that increases iHSP70 levels and decreases JNK activation in muscle, protects against hyperglycemia, hyperinsulinemia, glucose intolerance, and insulin resistance [28].

Studies about cell stress response and oxidative stress using biopsies from T2DM patients showed that mRNA expression of HSP70 and heme-oxygenase-1 is reduced in this subjects. Furthermore, mRNA HSP70 levels were correlated with β-hidroxiacil-CoA dehydrogenase and citrate synthase enzymes activities, suggesting that insulin resistance is associated with poor heat shock and antioxidant defense of muscle [29]. In this way, mitochondrial dysfunction plays an essential role in T2DM development [30]. This organelle dysfunction may be a result of hyperglycemic state and/or oxidative state. The activation of key pathways that increases lipid oxidation and decreases lipid esterification reduces insulin resistance levels.

In a study with wild type and HSP70-knockout mice (HSP70-KO), it was demonstrated that HSP70 level is critical to maintenance of mitochondrial morphology and is a biomarker/sensor of mitochondrial stress levels and insulin signaling function in skeletal muscle. HSP70-KO mice showed impaired glucose homeostasis, insulin resistance, and increased adiposity levels. Also, muscles of HSP70 mice accumulated lipids probably as a result of reduction in fat acids oxidation, which in turns, promotes muscle inflammation. Moreover, muscle cells without HSP70 showed low levels of basal oxygen consumption and high levels of ROS mitochondrial production [31], whereas HSP72 overexpression mice are protected against insulin resistance by positive regulation of oxidative metabolism. Induction of HSP70 expression in skeletal muscle of these mice promoted an increase in mitochondrial number and oxidative capacity decreasing insulin resistance [32].

Intracellular HSP70 expression is associated with antiapoptotic and anti-inflammatory actions. Inhibition of NF-KB activation and translocation is a marked anti-inflammatory function of iHSP70 with great implications in immune system, inflammatory process and cell survival regulation [33]. Thus, HSP70 is well known by its molecular chaperon cytoprotective roles. However, this protein is also found in blood of health subjects [34] and a crescent number of studies have been demonstrated higher levels of HSP70 in blood in T2DM, T1DM, and gestational diabetes [35, 36]. The role of HSP70 in the extracellular space (eHSP70) involves immune regulatory actions, pro-inflammatory signaling, and alert/danger signal of cell damage [37].

In T2DM patients, it observed an increase in eHSP70 levels, and this increase is associated with diabetes duration, a biomarker of chronicity of the disease [36]. Also, chronic exposure of pancreatic β-cell *in vitro* to high levels of eHSP70 induces cell death and modifies cellular bioenergetics profile. Since T2DM and T1DM patients exhibit higher eHSP70 levels, the perpetuation of this pro-inflammatory signal may induce loss of cell integrity and consequently β-cell dysfunction [38].

In obese T2DM subjects, the eHSP70 level is higher than nonobese T2DM suggesting that adiposity, mainly visceral adiposity and its complications, may contribute to increasing eHSP70 levels. Actually, iHSP70 may be considered a cytoprotective proteins by anti-inflammatory functions associated with normal insulin sensitivity. On the other hand, increased levels of eHSP70 chronically may be a result of chronic low-grade inflammatory state of visceral obesity [39]. Therefore, the unbalance between eHSP70 and iHSP70 levels (eHSP70/iHSP70 ratio), known as H-index, can reveal the full context of inflammatory process and insulin resistance state [16, 40].

3. T2DM and $PM_{2.5}$: The mechanism of enhanced risk

Epidemiologic evidences have shown many effects of exposure to air pollution in the increase of hospital admissions in more susceptible individuals, as well as the increase of incidence of some diseases, from respiratory to cardiovascular diseases (Cote et al., 2008). In the last decade, the association between diabetes and air pollution was highlighted by some studies [10, 41–43].

Meo et al. reviewed studies that discuss insulin resistance, diabetes mellitus, and air pollution and conclude that in 10 studies, among 11 analyzed, the $PM_{2.5}$ exposure to is associated with abnormalities in glucose homeostasis and this effect is related with inflammation, insulin resistance mitochondrial alteration, cardio-metabolic disorders, and thus, related to T2DM development. The same work confirms a clear and strong association between T2DM and exposure to particulate material especially, the exposure to small particulate matter of 10 microns (PM_{10}) or less in diameter, such as $PM_{2.5}$ [15, 45].

The polluted air, mainly by $PM_{2,5}$, is related to inflammation, vascular dysfunction, and atherosclerosis by the toxicology mechanisms invocated by the $PM_{2,5}$ invasion into the bloodstream [42]. Beyond this, $PM_{2,5}$ is related to induction of insulin resistance and adiposity in high fat diet mice models [16, 43]. Chronic $PM_{2,5}$ exposure can induce glucose intolerance, oxidative stress, and mitochondrial alteration in Langerhans islet and adipose tissue. Thus, $PM_{2,5}$ inhalation represents a novel additional risk factor to T2DM [16, 43, 46].

Experimental studies attempt to explain the pathophysiological mechanisms that lead to metabolic outcomes described above. Xu et al. showed that $PM_{2.5}$ exposure for 12 weeks promoted significant liver damage, evidenced by elevated levels of hepatic stress biomarkers, such as transaminases (ALT and AST) and reduced glycogen levels, alterations involved in impaired glucose tolerance and insulin resistance in mice. Also, this work demonstrated that $PM_{2.5}$ exposure triggered Nrf2-mediated oxidative responses and activated the JNK-mediated inhibitory signaling pathway, resulting in hepatic dysfunction. Wherefore, hepatic insulin resistance can also be a potential mechanism of diabetes pathogenesis due to pollutants [45].

Oxidative stress is a common factor in both conditions, T2DM and $PM_{2,5}$. Furthermore, the oxidative stress induced by $PM_{2,5}$ also represents a pathogenic stimulus for pancreatic β-cell dysfunction [47], since it is responsible for debility on the antioxidant defenses [48].

The redox unbalance promoted by exposure to air pollution can stimulates an inflammatory processes, contributing to installation of a metabolic disorder. The role of inflammation in the toxicity mediated by $PM_{2,5}$ is associated to the increase in alveolar immunological response (increased phagocytic cell count) and to pro-inflammatory cytokines production by these cells in the alveolar surface [49], accompanied by increased lung oxidative damage [50–52], which generally evolute to systemic oxidative stress, a risk for diabetes complications.

Postulated mechanisms of action include oxidative stress and low-grade inflammation, endothelial dysfunction, visceral adipose tissue inflammation, endoplasmic reticulum stress, and mitochondrial dysfunction [5, 53]. Thus, both acute and chronic $PM_{2,5}$ exposures are associated to inflammatory and oxidative markers, as well as in T1DM and T2DM, but it is not clear the real effects of diabetes plus air pollution combination. However, the pathophysiology involved in this case increases the global risk of death by increasing the susceptibility to air pollution damage [10].

Cell stress response, observed by alteration in HSPs levels in different organs, is a defensive and cytoprotective response in both conditions, exposure to pollutants and metabolic diseases. However, there are few pieces of evidence about $PM_{2,5}$ exposure concomitant to T2DM development that explores heat shock response [16].

The HSPs naturally are very sensitive elements to any chemical attack to the cells and are extensive used as biomarker of environmental exposures. In this sense, the iHSP70 expression during cellular challenges indicates that these proteins can be candidate to monitoring air pollution aggression to the health organism [54]. One study showed increase in the iHSP70 in the lung and heart one day after course particle exposure [55], and the authors discussed the plausibility of oxidative stress and/or cytokines in HSPs-induced expression as cellular defense at molecular levels, inhibiting pro-inflammatory pathways. In this way, low doses (12.5 μg/ml) of $PM_{2,5}$ can increase eHSP70 in human bronquial epithelial culture [56]. Thus, the strong correlation among oxidative stress and inflammation induced by $PM_{2,5}$ inhalation promotes both increase in the iHSP70 and eHSP70 content, reinforcing the purpose of use these proteins as an important biomarker of homeostatic equilibrium in environmental challenges [16, 57, 58].

Simulating urbanized conditions (consumption of high fat diet and exposure to $PM_{2.5}$) [16] showed that subchronic exposure to $PM_{2.5}$, even at low doses (5 μg-day, intranasal administration), potentiates metabolic dysfunction in HFD-fed mice, which are T2DM-susceptible. The effects of $PM_{2.5}$ in T2DM mice presented a positive correlation between adiposity, increased body weight and glucose intolerance, and increased glucose and triacylglycerol plasma levels. Also, in this study, pancreas exhibited lower iHSP70 expression, accompanied by 3.7-fold increase in the plasma to pancreas [eHSP72]/[iHSP70] ratio (H-index). This study represents an experimental evidence that the combination of two relevant challenges to the organism, from different origins (environmental and dietary factors), promotes alterations in cell stress response (measurable by plasma/tissue H-index), reinforcing the chaperone balance [([eHSP72]/[iHSP70]) status] as a biomarker of T2DM risk.

If a short-term $PM_{2.5}$ exposure promotes innumerous damages, long-term exposure may evidence chronic effects on human health. Xu et al. showed in experimental mice model that long-term $PM_{2.5}$ exposure induces alterations on adipose tissue and leads to mitochondrial dysfunction. If $PM_{2.5}$ exposure is associated with other risk factors for T2DM, such as inadequate eating behavior, it observed an increase in adiposity, body weight, and glucose intolerance [16], as well as increase in glucose and triacylglycerol plasma levels. Exposure to $PM_{2.5}$ can markedly potentiate metabolic dysfunction in an already compromised organism, promoting relevant alteration in cell stress response.

The implications to health of a link between $PM_{2.5}$ pollutants exposure and T2DM are critical problems to public health since air pollution is a pervasive risk factor that affects many people worldwide. In this way, it is important to highlight that modest reduction of pollution exposure may provide substantial public health benefits [45]. The underlying mechanisms responsible for this adverse effect in response to ambient $PM_{2.5}$ air pollution need to be further investigated [43]. Both experimental and epidemiologic studies suggest that environmental exposures to air pollutants can increase the risk of insulin resistance, which lead to a link between air pollution and T2DM.

4. Conclusion

This chapter aimed to describe pathophysiological mechanisms of the association between exposure to atmospheric pollution by $PM_{2.5}$ and T2DM development, which are being highlighted in experimental studies connected to epidemiological data. The highlighted mechanisms involve inflammation, oxidative stress, and a clear participation of impaired cell stress response observed by alterations on HSP70 levels. Finally, epidemiological together with experimental studies reinforce the complex nature of T2DM etiology and highlights the $PM_{2.5}$ air pollution as a critical health problem.

It is known that type 2 diabetes results from the interaction between genetic susceptibility, environmental factors, and lifestyle choices, commonly accepted causes for the development of T2DM. However, it is argued that these factors alone cannot fully explain the rapid rise in the prevalence of diabetes [45]. If the high prevalence of T2DM is a result of an association between several risk factors, and air pollution is one, environmental protection represented by prioritization of steps to minimize the air pollution levels may be considered as health strategy to avoid T2DM [44]. Given the enormous number of people exposed to air pollution as shown in **Figure 1**, even conservative reduction of $PM_{2.5}$ emission would translate into a substantial decrease in the population attributable fraction of T2DM related to environmental factors [45]. In perspective, it is expected that future studies will describe molecular mechanisms involved, highlight the responsible pollutants and the role of combined exposures to mixtures, and susceptibility factors. These discoveries of metabolic effects of air pollution may help relevant public health guidelines discussion and government decision in this current context of global urbanization [59].

Appendices and nomenclatures (Optional)

AGEs: advanced glycation products.
ALT: alanine aminotransferase.
AST: aspartate aminotransferase.
ATMs: Adipose tissue macrophages.
eHSP70: 70 kDa extracellular heat shock proteins.
FFA: free fat acid.
FOXO1: forkhead box protein O1.
GLUT4: glucose-transporter type 4.
HFD: high fat diet.
HSF-1: heat shock factor.
HSP: heat shock proteins.
HSP70: 70 kDa heat shock proteins.
HSP70-KO: 70 kDa heat shock proteins knockout mice.
iHSP70: 70 kDa intracellular heat shock proteins.
IL-1β: interleukin-1beta.
IL-6: interleukin-6.
IL-8: interleukin-8.
iNOS: inducible nitric oxide synthase.
kDa: kilodalton.
mRNA: messenger RNA.
NADPH: dihydronicotinamide adenine dinucleotide phosphate;
NF-kB: factor nuclear kappa B.
NO: nitric oxide.
NOS-2: nitric oxide synthase-2.
$PM_{2,5}$: Fine Particulate Matter.
RAGES: advanced glycation products binding to specific receptors.
RNS: nitrosative species.
ROS: reactive oxygen species.
T2DM: type 2 diabetes mellitus.
TNF-α: tumor necrosis factor alpha.
WHO: world health organization.

Author details

Thiago Gomes Heck[1,2*], Pauline Brendler Goettems Fiorin[1,3], Matias Nunes Frizzo[1,2] and Mirna Stela Ludwig[1,2]

*Address all correspondence to: thiago.heck@unijui.edu.br

1 Department of Life Sciences, Research Group in Physiology, Regional University of Northwestern Rio Grande do Sul State (UNIJUI), Ijuí, RS, Brazil

2 Postgraduation Program in Integral Attention to Health (PPGAIS), Regional University of Northwestern Rio Grande do Sul State (UNIJUI), Ijuí, RS, Brazil

3 Postgraduation Program in Health Sciences, Federal University of Health Sciences of Porto Alegre, Porto Alegre, RS, Brazil

References

[1] World Health Organization. Global Report on Diabetes. Isbn [Internet]. 2016;**978**:88. Available from: http://www.who.int/about/licensing/%5Cnhttp://apps.who.int/iris/bitstream/10665/204871/1/9789241565257_eng.pdf

[2] World Health Organization. Global Urban Ambient Air Pollution Database (update 2016) Available from http://www.who.int/phe/health_topics/outdoorair/databases/cities/en/

[3] Brook RD, Franklin B, Cascio W, Hong Y, Howard G, Lipsett M, et al. Air Pollution and Cardiovascular Disease: A Statement for Healthcare Professionals from the Expert Panel on Population and Prevention Science of the American Heart Association. Circulation [Internet]. June 2004;**109**(21):2655-2671. Available from: http://www.ncbi.nlm.nih.gov/pubmed/15173049 [Accessed: 31 July 2017]

[4] Brook RD, Jerrett M, Brook JR, Bard RL, Finkelstein MM. The relationship between diabetes mellitus and traffic-related air pollution. Journal of Occupational and Environmental Medicine [Internet]. January 2008;**50**(1):32-38. Available from: http://www.ncbi.nlm.nih.gov/pubmed/18188079 [Accessed: 31 July 2017]

[5] Rajagopalan S, Brook RD. Air pollution and type 2 diabetes: Mechanistic insights. Diabetes. 2012;**61**(December):3037-3045

[6] World Health Organization. WHO Air Quality Guidelines for Particulate Matter, Ozone, Nitrogen Dioxide and Sulfur Dioxide: Global Update 2005: Summary of Risk Assessment. Geneva: World Health Organization [Internet]; 2006. p. 1-22 Available from: http://whqlibdoc.who.int/hq/2006/WHO_SDE_PHE_OEH_06.02_eng.pdf?ua=1

[7] BreatheLife [Internet]. Available from: http://breathelife2030.org/ [Accessed: 31 July 2017]

[8] Zanobetti A, Schwartz J. Cardiovascular damage by airborne particles: Are diabetics more susceptible? Epidemiology [Internet]. September 2002;**13**(5):588-592. Available from: http://www.ncbi.nlm.nih.gov/pubmed/12192230 [Accessed: 31 July 2017]

[9] Goldberg MS, Burnett RT, Yale J-F, Valois M-F, Brook JR. Associations between ambient air pollution and daily mortality among persons with diabetes and cardiovascular disease. Environmental Research. 2006;**100**:255-267

[10] O'Neill MS, Veves A, Zanobetti A, Sarnat JA, Gold DR, Economides PA, et al. Diabetes enhances vulnerability to particulate air pollution-associated impairment in vascular reactivity and endothelial function. Circulation [Internet]. 7 June 2005;**111**(22):2913-2920. Available from: http://circ.ahajournals.org/cgi/doi/10.1161/CIRCULATIONAHA.104.517110 [Accessed: 31 July 2017]

[11] Brook RD, Newby DE, Rajagopalan S. Air pollution and cardiometabolic disease: An update and call for clinical trials. American Journal of Hypertension [Internet]. June 2017; Available from: http://www.ncbi.nlm.nih.gov/pubmed/28655143; [Accessed: 31 July 2017]

[12] Hochachka PW, Somero GN. Biochemical Adaptation: Mechanism and Process in Physiological Evolution. Oxford: Oxford University Press; 2002. p. 480

[13] Barrett KE, Ganong WF. Ganong's review of medical physiology. McGraw-Hill Medical. 2012;752

[14] Heck TG, Ludwig MS, dos Santos AB, Goettems-Fiorin PB. Lifestyle and aging effects in the development of insulin resistance — Activating the muscle as strategy against insulin resistance by modulating cytokines and HSP70. In: Muscle Cell and Tissue [Internet]. InTech; 2015. Available from: http://www.intechopen.com/books/muscle-cell-and-tissue/lifestyle-and-aging-effects-in-the-development-of-insulin-resistance-activating-the-muscle-as-strate [Accessed: 17 August 2017]

[15] Xu J, Zhang W, Lu Z, Zhang F, Ding W. Airborne PM 2.5 -Induced Hepatic Insulin Resistance by Nrf2/JNK-Mediated Signaling Pathway. 2017

[16] Goettems-Fiorin PB, Grochanke BS, Baldissera FG, dos Santos AB, Homem de Bittencourt PI, Ludwig MS, et al. Fine particulate matter potentiates type 2 diabetes development in high-fat diet-treated mice: Stress response and extracellular to intracellular HSP70 ratio analysis. Journal of Physiology and Biochemistry. 2016;**72**(4):643-656

[17] Czech MP. Insulin action and resistance in obesity and type 2 diabetes. Nature Medicine [Internet]. July 2017;**23**(7):804-814. Available from: http://www.ncbi.nlm.nih.gov/pubmed/28697184 [Accessed: 31 July 2017]

[18] Giacco F, Brownlee M. Oxidative stress and diabetic complications. Circulation Research. 2010;**107**(9):1058-1070

[19] Roman-Pintos LM, Villegas-Rivera G, Rodriguez-Carrizalez AD, Miranda-Diaz AG, Cardona-Munoz EG. Diabetic polyneuropathy in type 2 diabetes mellitus: Inflammation, oxidative stress, and mitochondrial function. Journal of Diabetes Research. 2016; **2016**:3425617

[20] Kayama Y, Raaz U, Jagger A, Adam M, Schellinger I, Sakamoto M, et al. Diabetic cardiovascular disease induced by oxidative stress. International Journal of Molecular Sciences

[Internet]. October 2015;**16**(10):25234-25263. Available from: http://www.ncbi.nlm.nih.gov/pubmed/26512646 [Accessed: 31 July 2017]

[21] Newsholme P, de Bittencourt PIH. The fat cell senescence hypothesis: A mechanism responsible for abrogating the resolution of inflammation in chronic disease. Current Opinion in Clinical Nutrition and Metabolic Care [Internet]. July 2014;**17**(4):295-305. Available from: http://www.ncbi.nlm.nih.gov/pubmed/24878874 [Accessed: 10 June 2015]

[22] Fontana L, Eagon JC, Trujillo ME, Scherer PE, Klein S. Visceral fat adipokine secretion is associated with systemic inflammation in obese humans. Diabetes [Internet]. April 2007;**56**(4):1010-1013. Available from: http://diabetes.diabetesjournals.org/cgi/doi/10.2337/db06-1656 [Accessed: 31 July 2017]

[23] Kirwan AM, Lenighan YM, O'Reilly ME, McGillicuddy FC, Roche HM. Nutritional modulation of metabolic inflammation. Biochemical Society Transactions [Internet]. July 2017;**45**(4):979-985. Available from: http://biochemsoctrans.org/lookup/doi/10.1042/BST20160465 [Accessed: 31 July 2017]

[24] Ellulu MS, Patimah I, Khaza'ai H, Rahmat A, Abed Y. Obesity and inflammation: The linking mechanism and the complications. Archives of Medical Science [Internet]. 2017;**4**:851-863. Available from: https://www.termedia.pl/doi/10.5114/aoms.2016.58928 [Accessed: 31 July 2017]

[25] de Luca C, Olefsky JM. Inflammation and insulin resistance. FEBS Letters [Internet]. January 2008;**582**(1):97-105. Available from: http://doi.wiley.com/10.1016/j.febslet.2007.11.057 [Accessed: 31 July 2017]

[26] Thomas D, Apovian C. Macrophage functions in lean and obese adipose tissue. Metabolism [Internet]. July, 2017;**72**:120-143. Available from: http://linkinghub.elsevier.com/retrieve/pii/S0026049517301130 [Accessed: 31 July 2017]

[27] Hooper PL, Hooper JJ. Loss of defense against stress: Diabetes and heat shock proteins. Diabetes Technology & Therapeutics [Internet]. February 2005;**7**(1):204-208. Available from: http://online.liebertpub.com/doi/abs/10.1089/dia.2005.7.204 [Accessed: 31 July 2017]

[28] Chung J, Nguyen A-K, Henstridge DC, Holmes AG, Chan MHS, Mesa JL, et al. HSP72 protects against obesity-induced insulin resistance. Proceedings of the National Academy of Sciences of the United States of America. 2008;**105**(5):1739-1744

[29] Bruce CR, Carey AL, Hawley JA, Febbraio MA. Intramuscular heat shock protein 72 and heme oxygenase-1 mRNA are reduced in patients with type 2 diabetes: Evidence that insulin resistance is associated with a disturbed antioxidant defense mechanism. Diabetes [Internet]. September 2003;**52**(9):2338-2345. Available from: http://www.ncbi.nlm.nih.gov/pubmed/12941774 [Accessed: 31 July 2017]

[30] Morino K, Petersen KF, Shulman GI. Molecular mechanisms of insulin resistance in humans and their potential links with mitochondrial dysfunction. Diabetes [Internet].

December 2006;**55**(Suppl 2):S9-S15. Available from: http://diabetes.diabetesjournals.org/cgi/doi/10.2337/db06-S002 [Accessed: 31 July 2017]

[31] Drew BG, Ribas V, Le JA, Henstridge DC, Phun J, Zhou Z, et al. HSP72 is a mitochondrial stress sensor critical for parkin action, oxidative metabolism, and insulin sensitivity in skeletal muscle. Diabetes [Internet]. May 2014;**63**(5):1488-1505. Available from: http://diabetes.diabetesjournals.org/lookup/doi/10.2337/db13-0665 [Accessed: 31 July 2017]

[32] Henstridge DC, Bruce CR, Drew BG, Tory K, Kolonics A, Estevez E, et al. Activating HSP72 in rodent skeletal muscle increases mitochondrial number and oxidative capacity and decreases insulin resistance. Diabetes [Internet]. June 2014;**63**(6):1881-1894. Available from: http://diabetes.diabetesjournals.org/cgi/doi/10.2337/db13-0967 [Accessed: 31 July 2017]

[33] Ran R, Lu A, Zhang L, Tang Y, Zhu H, Xu H, et al. Hsp70 promotes TNF-mediated apoptosis by binding IKK gamma and impairing NF-kappa B survival signaling. Genes & Development [Internet]. June 2004;**18**(12):1466-1481. Available from: http://www.genesdev.org/cgi/doi/10.1101/gad.1188204 [Accessed: 31 July 2017]

[34] Pockley AG, Shepherd J, Corton JM. Detection of heat shock protein 70 (Hsp70) and anti-Hsp70 antibodies in the serum of normal individuals. Immunological Investigations [Internet]. December 1998;**27**(6):367-377. Available from: http://www.ncbi.nlm.nih.gov/pubmed/9845422 [Accessed: 31 July 2017]

[35] Garamvölgyi Z, Prohászka Z, Rigó J, Kecskeméti A, Molvarec A. Increased circulating heat shock protein 70 (HSPA1A) levels in gestational diabetes mellitus: A pilot study. Cell Stress Chaperones [Internet]. July 2015;**20**(4):575-581. Available from: http://link.springer.com/10.1007/s12192-015-0579-y [Accessed: 31 July 2017]

[36] Nakhjavani M, Morteza A, Khajeali L, Esteghamati A, Khalilzadeh O, Asgarani F, et al. Increased serum HSP70 levels are associated with the duration of diabetes. Cell Stress & Chaperones [Internet]. November 2010;**15**(6):959-964. Available from: http://link.springer.com/10.1007/s12192-010-0204-z [Accessed: 31 July 2017]

[37] Williams JHH, Hunter-Lavin C. Roles of extracellular heat shock proteins: A new sense of danger. In: . Heat Shock Proteins: Potent Mediators of Inflammation and Immunity. Netherlands. Springer. p. 39-57. Available from: http://linkspringer.com/10.1007/978-1-4020-5585-0_4 [Accessed: 31 July 2017]

[38] Krause M, Keane K, Rodrigues-Krause J, Crognale D, Egan B, De Vito G, et al. Elevated levels of extracellular heat-shock protein 72 (eHSP72) are positively correlated with insulin resistance in vivo and cause pancreatic β-cell dysfunction and death in vitro. Clin**ical** Scie**nce** (Lond) [Internet]. May, 2014;**126**(10):739-752. Available from: http://clinsci.org/lookup/doi/10.1042/CS20130678 [Accessed: 31 July 2017]

[39] Krause M, Heck TG, Bittencourt A, Scomazzon SP, Newsholme P, Curi R, et al. The chaperone balance hypothesis: The importance of the extracellular to intracellular HSP70 ratio to inflammation-driven type 2 diabetes, the effect of exercise, and the implications for

clinical management. Mediators of Inflammation [Internet]. January 2015;**2015**:249205: [Accessed: 1 April 2015]Available from: http://www.pubmedcentral.nih.gov/articlerender.fcgi?artid=4357135&tool=pmcentrez&rendertype=abstract

[40] Heck TG, Scomazzon SP, Nunes PR, Schöler CM, da Silva GS, Bittencourt A, et al. Acute exercise boosts cell proliferation and the heat shock response in lymphocytes: Correlation with cytokine production and extracellular-to-intracellular HSP70 ratio. Cell Stress & Chaperones. 2017;**22**(2):271-291

[41] Jacobs L, Emmerechts J, Mathieu C, Hoylaerts MF, Fierens F, Hoet PH, et al. Air pollution related prothrombotic changes in persons with diabetes. Environmental Health Perspectives [Internet]. February 2010;**118**(2):191-196. Available from: http://ehp.niehs.nih.gov/0900942 [Accessed: 31 July 2017]

[42] Pearson J, Bachireddy C, Shyamprasad S, Goldfine A, Brownstein J. Association between fine particulate matter and diabetes prevalence in the U.S. Diabetes Care. 2010; **33**(10):2196-2201

[43] Xu X, Liu C, Xu Z, Tzan K, Zhong M, Wang A, et al. Long-term exposure to ambient fine particulate pollution induces insulin resistance and mitochondrial alteration in adipose tissue. Toxicological Sciences. 2011;**124**(1):88-98

[44] Meo SA, Memon AN, Sheikh SA, Rouq FA, Usmani AM, Hassan A, et al. Effect of environmental air pollution on type 2 diabetes mellitus. European Review for Medical and Pharmacological Sciences [Internet]. January 2015;**19**(1):123-128. Available from: http://www.ncbi.nlm.nih.gov/pubmed/25635985 [Accessed: 31 July 2017]

[45] Esposito K, Petrizzo M, Maiorino MI, Bellastella G, Giugliano D. Particulate matter pollutants and risk of type 2 diabetes: A time for concern? Endocrine. 2016;**51**(1):32-37

[46] Liu C, Yang C, Zhao Y, Ma Z, Bi J, Liu Y, et al. Associations between long-term exposure to ambient particulate air pollution and type 2 diabetes prevalence, blood glucose and glycosylated hemoglobin levels in China. Environment International. 2016;**92**:416-421

[47] Zhang F, Li L, Krafft T, Lv J, Wang W, Pei D. Study on the association between ambient air pollution and daily cardiovascular and respiratory mortality in an urban district of Beijing. International Journal of Environmental Research and Public Health. 2011;**8**(6):2109-2123

[48] Domínguez C, Ruiz E, Gussinye M, Carrascosa A. Oxidative stress at onset and in early stages of type 1 diabetes in children and adolescents. Diabetes Care [Internet]. 1998;**21**(10):1736-1742. Available from http://www.ncbi.nlm.nih.gov/pubmed/9773740

[49] Dubowsky SD, Suh H, Schwartz J, Coull BA, Gold DR. Diabetes, obesity, and hypertension may enhance associations between air pollution and markers of systemic inflammation. Environmental Health Perspectives. 2006;**114**(7):992-998

[50] Rhoden CR, Lawrence J, Godleski JJ, González-Flecha B. N-acetylcysteine prevents lung inflammation after short-term inhalation exposure to concentrated ambient particles. Toxicological Sciences. 2004;**79**:296-303

[51] Rhoden CR, Wellenius GA, Ghelfi E, Lawrence J, González-Flecha B. PM-induced cardiac oxidative stress and dysfunction are mediated by autonomic stimulation. Biochimica et Biophysica Acta (BBA)-General Subjects. 2005;**1725**:305-313

[52] Rhoden CR, Ghelfi E, González-Flecha B. Pulmonary inflammation by ambient air particles is mediated by superoxide anion. Inhalation Toxicology. 2008;**20**:11-15

[53] Liu C, Xu X, Bai Y, Wang TY, Rao X, Wang A, et al. Air pollution-mediated susceptibility to inflammation and insulin resistance: Influence of CCR2 pathways in mice. Environmental Health Perspectives. 2014;**122**:17-26

[54] Mukhopadhyay I, Nazir A, Saxena DK, Kar CD. Heat shock response: Hsp70 in environmental monitoring. Journal of Biochemical and Molecular Toxicology. 2003;**17**(5):249-254

[55] Farina F, Sancini G, Battaglia C, Tinaglia V, Mantecca P, Camatini M, et al. Milano summer particulate matter (PM10) triggers lung inflammation and extra pulmonary adverse events in mice. PloS One. 2013;**8**(2):e56636

[56] Watterson TL, Hamilton B, Martin R, Coulombe RA. Urban particulate matter causes ER stress and the unfolded protein response in human lung cells. Toxicological Sciences. 2009;**112**(1):111-122

[57] El Golli-Bennour E, Bacha H. Hsp70 expression as biomarkers of oxidative stress: Mycotoxins' exploration. Toxicology [Internet]. 2011;**287**(1-3):1-7 Available from: http://dx.doi.org/10.1016/j.tox.2011.06.002

[58] Kido T, Bai N, Yatera K, Suzuki H, Meredith A, Mukae H, et al. Diesel exhaust inhalation induces heat shock protein 70 expression in vivo. Inhalation Toxicology. 2011; **23**(May):593-601

[59] Liu C, Ying Z, Harkema J, Sun Q, Rajagopalan S. Epidemiological and experimental links between air pollution and type 2 diabetes. Toxicologic Pathology. 2012; (October 2012)

5

Economic Evaluations in Health from the Perspective of the Costs Associated with Diabetes Mellitus Treatment

Maurílio de Souza Cazarim,
Ana Carolina de Oliveira Gonçalves,
Leonardo Régis Leira Pereira and
André de Oliveira Baldoni

Abstract

Diabetes mellitus (DM) is a morbidity that presents a wide range of difficulties for the patient to reach the control. This reality not only has impact on the clinical practice but also has serious financial and social consequences for both the patient and the health system. Health technologies that are capable of improving glycemic control have been tested in cost-effectiveness analysis to assess the efficiency of DM care. According to the Brazilian Society of Diabetes, patients with glycated hemoglobin (A1c) within the values considered adequate, less than 6.5%, present a relative risk of developing complications (neuropathy, retinopathy, diabetic foot, pressure ulcers, cardiovascular diseases and renal disease) equal to that of a nondiabetic patient. In highlight, health technologies health technologies have presented positive impact on reducing A1c and, consequently, on reducing diabetes complications. Thus, new health technologies have been capable saving of 72% of resources spent on DM care.

Keywords: diabetes mellitus, economics, pharmaceutical, technology assessment, biomedical

1. Economic evaluation in health

Historically, evaluation processes are part of the development of humanity as a society. After World War II, there was an increase in State activities in the control of services such as health and education in many countries. An economic current gained strength in the development of methodological processes to evaluate these State activities, assessing their costs and their advantages. These processes conformed themselves into economic health assessments [1].

In the course of time, economic evaluation in the area of health has been gaining more rigorous methodological contours, and nowadays, it is characterized as an important tool of public services, in the health economy sector. Health assessment has specific bodies in some developed countries such as the United States, Canada and France [1, 2]. In Latin America, Brazil is considered one of the pioneers in the implementation of economic health assessment methodologies, and countries such as Colombia, Mexico, Argentina and Chile have advanced a lot in the area's development [3].

The health area constantly goes through processes of technological innovation. Associated with the epidemiological changes of recent years, the incorporation of new health technologies has become a reality with which the management of health services has to deal constantly. This scenario has contributed to the increasing cost of maintaining health services and corroborated the increase in complexity in the administration and functioning of health services [2, 4]. It is noteworthy that health has limited and finite resources, which makes health evaluation a complex task, with criteria that go beyond the cost-related, ethical, safety and equity issues [2]. Given the complexity of the health scenario, economic evaluation in health aims to subsidize management in decision-making about the incorporation of new technologies, as well as its monitoring, with the standardization of criteria and practices that may facilitate the management of public health services [5, 6].

The researches of economic evaluation in the health area are constituted by some basic structural elements. Initially, it is necessary to define the costs that will be assessed during the study, which may be direct medical or nonmedical costs, which correspond to the costs directly applied to the provision of patient care, for example, the cost of medication (medical) or the cost of moving a patient to another municipality for care (nonmedical). There are also indirect costs that are related to the social losses of the individual or of society itself or of the State with the sick individual, such as, for example, days of work lost as a result of a disease. Another cost category is intangibles, which are considered difficult to measure monetarily, for example, pain. For any economic evaluation in health, it is necessary to define the perspective under which the costs will be analyzed, which will guide which costs will be included in the economic analysis, and how to carry out the costing. Costs can be assessed from the perspectives of the health system, the hospital service, the government or of the society as a service provider or buyer can be changed for payer [5, 7].

Another structural element of economic evaluation research is the identification of the outcome, that is, of the result that will be evaluated by the research. This outcome can be expressed as a monetary unit, a clinical outcome or quality of life. The use of primary outcomes (cure, eradication of infection, death) is preferable compared to intermediate outcomes (reduction of blood pressure or glucose levels). However, the measurement of primary resources is usually more difficult to perform and, consequently, little is used in research. According to the objective of the economic evaluation in health and the context in question, the type of economic evaluation to be performed must be defined [4, 7].

As evaluative surveys are still considered recent in the world scenario, it is important to highlight some concepts that may facilitate the understanding of terms that are given below, according to the Thematic Glossary – Health Economy [8]:

- Efficacy is the measurement of the results obtained from ideal or experimental situations.
- Effectiveness is the measurement of the results obtained in real situations, that is, as happens in the health service.
- Efficiency is the economic concept that relates the results obtained with the necessary financial resources to achieve these results.

In resume, economic evaluations in the health are structured through specifics scientific areas that produce analyses with specifics methods, which are preponderant for the rational process in decision-making; pharmacoeconomics is a science with multidisciplinary characteristics that has been standing out into this process [4].

2. Pharmacoeconomics

Pharmacoepidemiology is able to provide much information for routine health services. Pharmacoeconomics is one of the aspects of pharmacoepidemiology [9] and, following this logic of providing information for management, seeks to subsidize decisions regarding the economy and pharmaceutical services [10].

Currently, many medications are introduced into the market. The Ministry of Health and Regulatory Agencies (*ministério da saúde e as agências reguladoras*), the US Food and Drug Administration (FDA), the European Medicines Agency (EMA), and in Brazil, the National Agency of Sanitary Surveillance (*Agência Nacional de Vigilância Sanitária* – ANVISA), adopt measures with the aim of regulating this market. Among the strategies, we can mention the inclusion of medication in clinical protocols and the regulation of prices and public health financing. However, it can be seen that these measures are no longer sufficient to guide decision-making within public health services [11]. In this sense, pharmacoeconomic studies contribute to the degree of evidence subsidizing the discussion about the need to incorporate new pharmaceutical technologies [12].

Pharmacoeconomics is a component of the economic evaluation of health services, which assists decision-making and allocation of resources related to services, as well as products or health programs/strategies [13]. The products evaluated by pharmacoeconomics can be both tangibles such as medication and intangibles such as practices that promote the rational use of medication [14], in the case of pharmacotherapeutic empowerment and medication management treatment (MTM). **Figure 1** presents the interface between health and economy and how pharmacoeconomics fits into this scenario [15].

The analysis of the clinical-pharmacological viewpoint is usually limited to the binomial efficacy-safety; however, a discussion that considers other variables, such as secondary and final outcomes (death), adherence to treatment and social aspects, is necessary for the decisions to achieve broader aspects such as the social value attributed to a medicinal product. Social value is understood as all the positive effects produced by medication such as welfare promotion, satisfaction with treatment and social production capacity (family life, work) [11]. **Figure 2** shows how the complexity of pharmacoeconomic works evolves starting from the binomial efficacy-safety to more complex analyses that evaluate the quality of life of the patients [11].

Pharmacoeconomics uses specific methodologies for the construction of evaluation models that produce comparisons that adjust all the variables involved in this complex process [15]. **Figure 3** presents the scenario into which the pharmacoeconomic assessments are introduced. For this purpose, it needs different sources of information such as clinical trials, systematic reviews, meta-analyses and health service databases [15]. All these are important sources of information in the construction of pharmacoeconomic studies [11, 15].

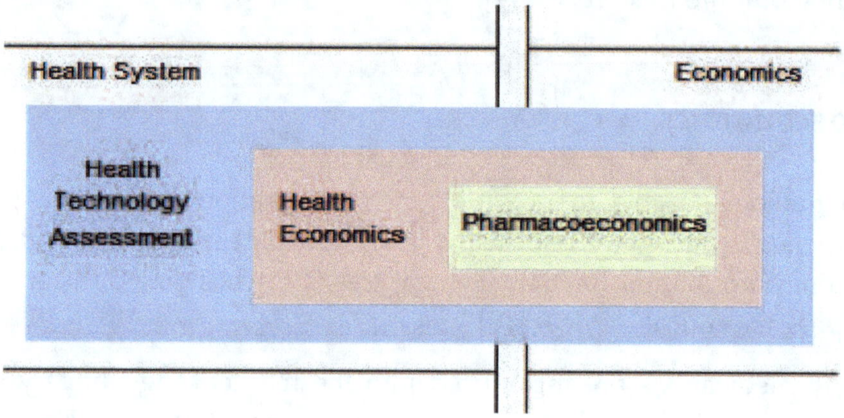

Figure 1. Pharmacoeconomics as one of the areas of evaluation of the technologies in health and its positioning within the health system scenario and economy. Source: Adapted from Bristol [15].

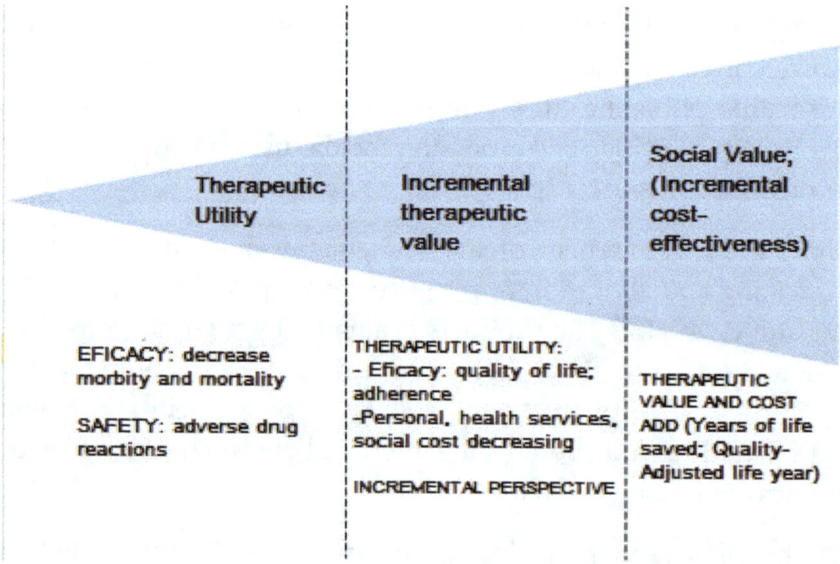

Figure 2. Evolution of pharmacoeconomic studies according to the complexity of the variables evaluated. Source: Adapted from Puig-Junoy et al. [11].

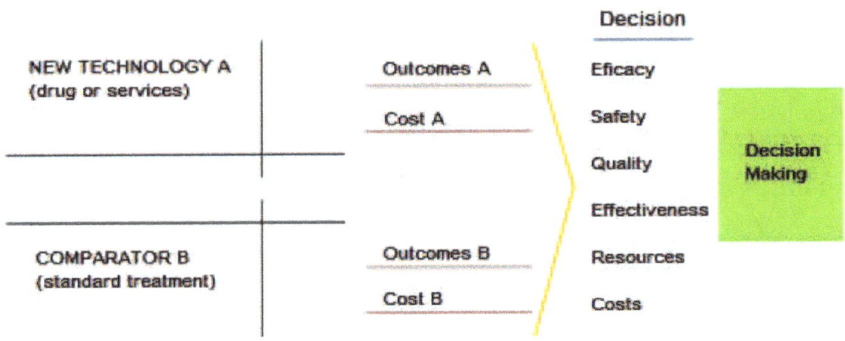

Figure 3. Scenario and variables involved in pharmacoeconomic studies. Source: Adapted from Bristol [15].

For a better understanding of the concepts worked in pharmacoeconomics, some definitions become relevant:

- Cost-minimization analysis: is performed by comparing two or more alternatives which assume the same safety profile and effectiveness; the comparison is between the costs of each alternative [7].
- Cost-benefit analysis: shows evidence of which alternative is most cost-effective, with benefits measured in monetary values [7].
- Cost-effectiveness analysis: allows comparison between alternatives as to their cost and their effect, measured in outcomes, and these outcomes are considered as a clinical parameter [7, 12].
- Cost-utility analysis: many authors defend this type of analysis as a variable of cost-effectiveness analysis. The great difference is in the measure of the outcome, which must measure quality of life and is usually a specific unit, quality-adjusted life year (QALY) or disability-adjusted life year (DALY), always comparing costs with these specific outcomes [7].
- Incremental cost-effectiveness ratio: predicts the cost increment for one more unit of outcome, and guides decision-making in relation to the threshold to be invested in health [7, 12].
- Markov modeling: a mathematical method that allows estimation of disease progression over the years, allocating patients a health status according to the probabilities, and predicting outcomes and costs [12].
- Sensitivity analysis: tests the oscillations of the variables involved in the study, improving the robustness of the study results [7].

3. Costs associated with the treatment of diabetes mellitus

Diabetes mellitus (DM) is a morbidity that is difficult for the patient to control, because it involves changes of habits with severe restrictions and a high demand of time for care. According to Stark et al. (2014), data between 2007 and 2010 from the National Health and Nutrition Examination Survey (2010) presented that 40% of Americans with DM failed to achieve adequate glycemic control [16]. This high prevalence of uncontrolled patients increases the occurrence of complications associated with diabetes [17, 18]. These complications can be summarized as acute and chronic, which give rise to more complex clinical conditions for the treatment of DM [19, 20]. This reality not only has impact on the clinical practice but also has serious financial and social consequences for both the patient and the health system [21].

Acute complications include hyperglycemia (casual glycemia >250 mg/dL), with or without ketoacidosis and hypoglycemia (casual glycemia <60 mg/dL). Acute complications require immediate intervention, so it is very important that patients and caregivers know how to identify the symptoms and manage care to prevent the situation from worsening. This stage of care is directed mainly to the direct costs. The glycemic value can be considered an intermediate outcome, and thus, health technologies capable of reducing glycemia have been tested in cost-effectiveness analysis to verify the efficiency of DM care [4, 5, 22].

Chronic complications can be divided into microvascular complications related to the natural evolution of DM and macrovascular complications, which are not necessarily related to DM, but are commonly more severe in patients with this clinical condition. Microvascular complications include retinopathy, nephropathy and neuropathy [6]. Retinopathy is the leading cause of blindness in adults, and after having DM for 20 years, approximately 60% of patients will already have some visual impairment. DM remains the leading cause of chronic kidney disease (CKD). About one in five patients with DM have a decreased glomerular filtration rate (GFR), that is, they have some degree of diabetic nephropathy. Neuropathy also has a high prevalence among DM patients. In DM, some degree of neuropathy may normally be verified at the time of diagnosis. Neuropathy stands out as a complication that directly impacts the patient's quality of life [23–24].

Macrovascular complications are represented by cardiovascular diseases; the major diseases associated with DM are as follows: ischemic heart disease, cerebrovascular disease and peripheral vascular disease [6]. In these cases, prevention of risk factors and pharmacotherapy are the main tools in the fight against the onset of these complications, which in patients with diabetes tend to occur earlier and be more severe than in the rest of the population [23]. Chronic complications can be considered in a cost-effectiveness analysis to measure costs against the years of life saved (YLS), cost-utility in the cost measurement by QALY or DALY and also in a cost-benefit analysis, when monetary values saved by reducing the chronic complications of DM by some health technology are compared to the cost of this technology. The best way to develop such an analysis would be to carry out Markov modeling for the projection of the patient's health status over time [7, 25].

Alfradique et al. [26] establishes DM as a condition sensitive to primary health care, that is, if managed correctly in basic care, it is possible to obtain positive results in reducing the complications and hospitalizations resulting from this clinical condition. The DM management is a complex process, which requires continuous clinical follow-up, preferably by a multidisciplinary team, and considers education for self-care as one of the pillars in preventing the occurrence of complications in both short- and long-term. In this sense, the primary care system and new health technologies play an important role for the systematized monitoring of diabetic [6, 19].

During the routine of the DM patient in primary care, their choices are able to impact more on their health condition, and consequently, on the results achieved, than the clinical decisions made by a health professional [27]. The health professionals involved in patient care play an important role in the search for glycemic control; however, this is only achieved with the active participation of the patient in their daily care [28].

Empowerment is a concept that was introduced by Anderson et al. in 1991 [29]. Subsequently, the WHO [30], defined empowerment as a strategy in which the patient gains control over decisions that interfere with their health conditions. Later, Kleba and Wendausen [31] added to this concept, the idea that empowerment drives people or groups of people to achieve a better quality of life by changing their daily practices.

In this sense, patient empowerment proves to be an effective strategy for glycemic control. It aims to promote a direct involvement of the patient in self-care, allowing them to know about their real situation and thereby make the best decisions about the care of their health. The health professional plays a supporting role in the process of empowerment, since the whole educational process is developed in a patient-centered way and provides information and contributes to the development of ability, so that the patient has control over their health [29].

Empowerment activities, when developed in an individual way, allow the patient's habits and routines to be understood, narrowing the patient-professional relationship and also allowing the creation of individualized goals and objectives, which consider the patient's psychosocial needs [32].

Studies have shown that empowerment is an efficient strategy for improving glycemic control as well as emotional control of the patient [32]. Kraemer et al., showed a 0.5% reduction in glycated hemoglobin (A1c) through individual pharmaceutical counseling for the empowerment of DM patients. In this sense, such training of the DM patient for their care has shown to be an important alternative in the search for the improvement of quality of life of the diabetic patient, being able to become an economically and clinically viable tool for primary health care [33].

It is worth noting that A1c is the clinical parameter, considered a gold standard for the clinical follow-up of DM, since it allows estimating the patient's glycemic profile for a period of approximately 90–120 days. In a clinical trial that considered diabetic patients on treatment or not, it showed mean values for A1c of 10.2% (3.9–19.1%) [34]. When only diabetic patients under treatment were considered, the mean A1c decreased to 7.7% [35]. According to the Brazilian Society of Diabetes, patients with A1c within the values considered adequate, that is, less than 6.5%, present a relative risk of developing complications (neuropathy, retinopathy, diabetic foot, pressure ulcers, cardiovascular diseases and renal disease) equal to that of a nondiabetic patient [23]. Whereas, values close to 8% for A1c presents a relative risk aproximately equal three. With an A1c value between 11 and 12%, type 2 diabetes mellitus (T2DM) patients are 20 times more likely to present these complications when compared to patients without diabetes. A reduction of 1% in A1c values reduces the risk of amputation by 43%, the risk of acute myocardial infarction by 14% and microvascular complications by 37% [23, 35].

The direct medical and nonmedical costs and indirect costs related to the diabetes patient increase over time, especially due to the consequences of the relative risk associated with A1c values, and consequently, to the presence of late complications [7, 36]. Thus, health services need to cope with rising costs in contrast to scarce resources [37]. This scenario becomes a challenge for the health system, considering the increase in the life expectancy of DM patients. Several studies are able to show that preventive measures have a positive benefit/cost ratio when considering the care of the diabetic individual [36, 38]. In addition, it is possible to have a 33% increase in expenses related to DM care in 2 years when glycemic levels are not at satisfactory levels and complications of the disease occur [39].

Expenditures on DM treatment consume up to 12% of the annual health expenditure in the world [40]. It is noteworthy that medications are responsible for 48.2% of the direct costs of a diabetic patient [41]. In a study performed by Marinho et al., in a medium-complexity institution for DM patients, direct costs related to type 2 diabetes mellitus (T2DM) totaled US $ 2,066,081 and 250,000 procedures were performed in the same period. Of this total, 36.3% was consumed by medication, 20.5% was third-party services (administrative, courses, rent, etc.) and 20.1% was spent by paying highly educated professionals in health care and management, high school educated supporting professionals and trainees involved in health care [42].

In Brazil, for example, the prevalence of T2DM patients is approximately 15% and annual expenditures are approximately 3.9 billion dollars. The Public Health System (PHS) spends an average of US$ 2108.00 per year for outpatient treatment with each diabetic patient. Of this, US$ 1335.00 is considered a cost directly related to diabetes [41]. In a Pharmaceutical Care program for diabetic patients, Obreli-Neto et al. showed a mean reduction of 0.7% in A1c values for patients who had empowerment, along with medication treatment management (MTM) in the program. In addition, US$ 660.80 of the total of US$ 916.30 spent per patient on DM care was saved [23, 35].

It is noteworthy that many patients become incapacitated as a result of the severity of DM complications, which leads to an increase in indirect costs for the health system [21, 43]. The WHO estimates that the costs of loss of productivity of DM patients can exceed up to five times the direct costs of this disease [20, 36]. It is seen that empowerment of the diabetic patient improves glycemic control and, consequently, reduces the incidence of DM complications over time, which is the main aspect to reduce costs with the treatment of the disease; empowerment of the diabetic patient can be considered an efficient health technology for health systems.

Many studies have presented the theme of economic evaluation focused on the care provided by the pharmacist, such as pharmaceutical care, which uses methods such as MTM and patient empowerment [22, 44]. Pharmaceutical care in a program for the elderly with T2DM and systemic arterial hypertension followed in primary health care in a municipality in the interior of the state of São Paulo, showed that the implementation of pharmaceutical care does not add significant costs to the health service when compared to the results of the best outcomes achieved in patient care [35]. In other words, care strategies such as pharmaceutical care may be more effective and efficient alternatives for health systems.

Acknowledgements

We thank the FAPESP funding agency for the scholarship support for the author Maurilio Souza Cazarim [grant number 2016/03584-1] from 07-01-2016 to 28-02-2019, URL (http://bvs.fapesp.br/en/pesquisador/673633/maurilio-de-souza-cazarim/). The funders had no role in study design, data collection and analysis, decision to publish or preparation of the manuscript. Opinions, assumptions and conclusions or recommendations expressed in this chapter are the authors' responsibility and do not necessarily reflect the viewpoint of FAPESP.

Conflict of interest

The authors declare no conflict of interest.

Author details

Maurílio de Souza Cazarim[1*], Ana Carolina de Oliveira Gonçalves[2], Leonardo Régis Leira Pereira[1] and André de Oliveira Baldoni[2]

*Address all correspondence to: mscazarim@usp.br

1 Faculty of Pharmaceutical Sciences of Ribeirão Preto, University of São Paulo (FCFRP-USP), Ribeirão Preto, SP, Brazil

2 Federal University of São João Del-Rei (UFSJ), Campus Centro-Oeste Dona Lindu (CCO), MG, Brazil

References

[1] Hartz ZMA. (Org). Avaliação em Saúde: dos modelos conceituais à prática na análise da implantação de programas [online]. Rio de Janeiro: Editora FIOCRUZ, 1997. 132 p. ISBN: 85-85676-36-1. Available from: SciELO Books. http://books.scielo.org

[2] Hartz ZM, Silva LM. Health Evaluation of the Theoretical Models to the Practice in the Evaluation of Health Programs and Systems. Salvador: EDUFBA. Rio de Janeiro: Fiocruz; 2005

[3] Augustovski F, Melendez G, Lemgruber A, Drummond M. Implementing pharmacoeconomic guidelines in Latin America: lessons learned. Value Health. 2011;**14**(suppl 1):3-7

[4] Drummond MF, Sculpher MJ, Claxton K, Stoddart GL, Torrance GW. Methods for the Economic Evaluation of Health Care Programmes. 3rd ed. Oxford: Oxford University Press; 2005. 379 p. ISBN: 10:0198529457

[5] Brazil Ministry of Health. Brazilian Network for Health Technology Assessment (BNHTA). Methodological Guidelines: Economic Evaluation Guideline. Series A. Standards and Technical Manuals. 2nd ed. Brasília: Ministry of Health Library; 2014. [Internet]. Available from: http://rebrats.saude.gov.br/diretrizes-metodologicas. ISBN: 978-85-334-2182-0

[6] Brazil Ministry of Health. Secretariat of Health Care. Department of Basic Attention. Strategies for care of the person with chronic disease: Diabetes mellitus. In: Cadernos de Atenção Básica. Vol. 36. 1st ed. Brasília-DF: Ministry of Health; 2013

[7] Rascati KL. Essentials of Pharmacoeconomics. 2nd ed. Baltimore, MD: Lippincott Williams & Wilkins; 2014. 289 p. ISBN: 978-1-4511-7593-6

[8] Brazil Ministry of Health. Health Economics Thematic Glossary. 3rd ed. Brasília-DF: Ministério da Saúde; 2013. 92 p. ISBN: 978-85-334-1917-9

[9] Strom BL. What is Pharmacoepidemiology? In: Strom BL, editor. Pharmacoepidemiology. 3rd ed. Chichester (UK): John Wiley & Sons Ltd.; 2005. pp. 3-15

[10] Baldoni AD, Guidoni CM, Pereira LR. A farmacoepidemiologia no Brasil: estado da arte da produção científica. Revista da Universidade Vale do Rio Verde. Jan 1, 2011;**9**(1):78-88

[11] Puig-Junoy J, Peiró S. De la utilidad de los medicamentos al valor terapéutico añadido ya la relación coste-efectividad incremental. Revista Española de Salud Pública. 2009 Feb;**83**(1): 59-70

[12] Ademi Z, Kim H, Zomer E, Reid CM, Hollingsworth B, Liew D. Overview of pharmacoeconomic modelling methods. British Journal of Clinical Pharmacology. Apr 1, 2013;**75**(4): 944-950

[13] Nita ME, Secoli SR, Nobre MRC, Ono-Nita SK, Capino ACC, Sarti FM, et al. Evaluation of Health Technologies: Clinical Evidence, Economic Analysis and Decision Analysis. 1st ed. Porto Alegre: Artmed; 2009. 600 p. ISBN: 9788536321059

[14] Marques Mota D, Gurgel Carlos da Silva M, Cazue Sudo E, Ortún V. Rational drug use: an economic approach to decision making. Ciência & Saúde Coletiva. 2008;**13**:589-601

[15] Bristol MS. Health Technology Assessment: A Practical Guide for Managers. 2010. Available from: http://www.bristol.com.br/Files/profissionais_saude/pdf_;Farmacoeconomia/Modulo1-Introducao.pdf

[16] Stark CS, Fradkin JE, Saydah SH, Rust KF, Cowie CC. The prevalence of meeting A1c, blood pressure, and LDL goals among people with diabetes, 1988–2010. Diabetes Care. 2014;**36**(8):2271-2279 Available from: http://care.diabetesjournals.org/content/36/8/2271.full.pdf+html

[17] Lachin JM, Orchard TJ, Nathan DM, DCCT/EDIC Research Group. Update on cardiovascular outcomes at 30 years of the diabetes control and complications trial/epidemiology of diabetes interventions and complications study. Diabetes Care. Jan 1, 2014;**37**(1):39-43

[18] Casagrande SS, Fradkin JE, Saydah SH, Rust KF, Cowie CC. The prevalence of meeting A1C, blood pressure, and LDL goals among people with diabetes, 1988–2010. Diabetes Care. Aug 1, 2013;**36**(8):2271-2279

[19] American Diabetes Association. Standards of Medical Care in Diabetes – 2016. Diabetes Care. Jan 2016;**39**:112

[20] World Health Organization. Definition and Diagnosis of Diabetes Mellitus and Intermediate Hyperglycemia: Report of a WHO/IDF Consultation. World Hearth Org. 2006. 1st ed. Geneva: WHO; [online] 2006. ISBN: 92 4 159493 4. Available from: http://www.who.int/diabetes/publications/Definition%20and%20diagnosis%20of%20diabetes_new.pdf>

[21] Silva I, Ribeiro JP, Cardoso H, Ramos H. Effects of social support on quality of life, metabolic control and development of chronic complications in individuals with diabetes. Psicologia, Saúde & Doenças. 2003;**4**(1):21-23

[22] Oliveira DM, Schoeller SD, Hammerschmidt KA, da Silva DM, Arruda C. Care challenges of diabetes mellitus acute complications in adult emergency services. Revista eletronica de enfermagem. 2016;**18**:e1163. Available from: http://dx.doi.org/10.5216/ree.v18.35523

[23] Brazilian Diabetes Society. Guidelines of the Brazilian Diabetes Society: 2014–2015. São Paulo: AC Pharmaceuticals; 2015

[24] Barrile SR, Ribeiro AA, da Costa AP, Viana AA, De Conti MH, Martinelli B. Sensitive-motor alteration of the lower limbs in diabetics type 2. Fisioterapia em Movimento. Sep 15, 2017;**26**(3):537-548

[25] Cazarim MS, Einarson TR. New prediction methods of indicators and costs capable of increasing the efficiency of pharmacoeconomic studies for health decision analysis. Pharmaceutica Analytica Acta. 2017;**8**:556. DOI: 10.4172/2153-2435.1000556

[26] Alfradique ME, Bonolo PD, Dourado MI, Costa MF, Macinko J, Mendonça CS, Oliveira VB, Sampaio LF, Simoni CD, Turci MA. Admissions due to conditions sensitive to primary care: The construction of the Brazilian list as a tool to measure the performance of the health system (Projeto ICSAP – Brasil). Cadernos de Saúde Pública. 2009;**25**(6):1337-1349

[27] Funnell MM, Anderson RM. Empowerment and self-management of diabetes. Clinical Diabetes. 2004;**22**(3):123-127

[28] Tol A, Baghbanian A, Mohebbi B, Shojaeizadeh D, Azam K, Shahmirzadi SE, Asfia A. Empowerment assessment and influential factors among patients with type 2 diabetes. Journal of Diabetes & Metabolic Disorders. 2013 Jan 19;**12**(1):6

[29] Anderson RM, Funnell MM, Barr PA, Dedrick RF, Davis WK. Learning to empower patients: Results of professional education program for diabetes educators. Diabetes Care. 1991 Jul 1;**14**(7):584-590

[30] World Health Organization. Division of Health Promotion, Education and Communications (HPR). Health Promotion Glossary. [online] Geneva: WHO; 1998. Available from: http://www.who.int/healthpromotion/about/HPR%20Glossary%201998.pdf

[31] Kleba ME, Wendausen A. Empowerment: strengthening process of subjects in spaces of social participation and political democratization. Saúde e Sociedade. 2009;**18**(4): 733-743

[32] Hermanns N, Kulzer B, Ehrmann D, Bergis-Jurgan N, Haak T. The effect of a diabetes education programme (PRIMAS) for people with type 1 diabetes: Results of a randomized trial. Diabetes Research and Clinical Practice. 2013 Dec 31;**102**(3):149-157

[33] Kraemer DF, Kradjan WA, Bianco TM, Low JA. A randomized study to assess the impact of pharmacist counseling of employer-based health plan beneficiaries with diabetes: The EMPOWER study. Journal of Pharmacy Practice. Apr 2012;**25**(2):169-179

[34] Velasquez PA, Agnes C, Svidzinsk TI. Hemoglobina Glicada como ferramenta na avaliação do controle glicêmico de pacientes. Revista Brasileira de Análises Clínicas. 2011;**43**(1):21-25

[35] Obreli-Neto PR, Marusic S, Guidoni CM, Baldoni AD, Renovato RD, Pilger D, Cuman RK, Pereira LR. Economic evaluation of a pharmaceutical care program for elderly diabetic and hypertensive patients in primary health care: A 36-month randomized controlled clinical trial. Journal of Managed Care & Specialty Pharmacy. Jan 2015;**21**(1):66-75

[36] Henriksson F, Agardh CD, Berne C, Bolinder J, Lönnqvist F, Stenström P, Östenson CG, Jönsson B. Direct medical costs for patients with type 2 diabetes in Sweden. Journal of Internal Medicine. Nov 1, 2000;**248**(5):387-396

[37] Guidoni CM, Olivera CM, Freitas OD, Pereira LR. Assistência ao diabetes no Sistema Único de Saúde: análise do modelo atual. Brazilian Journal of Pharmaceutical Sciences. Mar 2009;**45**(1):37-48

[38] Gross JL, Nehme M. Detecção e tratamento das complicações crônicas do diabetes melito: Consenso da Sociedade Brasileira de Diabetes e Conselho Brasileiro de Oftalmologia. Revista da Associação Médica Brasileira. Jul 1999;**45**(3):279-284

[39] Arredondo A, De Icaza E. Costos de la diabetes en Ameŕica Latina: evidencias del Caso Mexicano. Value in health. Aug 31, 2011;**14**(5):S85-S88

[40] International Diabetes Federation. Diabetes Atlas. 4th ed. Brussels: International Diabetes Federation; 2015. Available from: http://www.diabetesatlas.org/content/diabetes

[41] Bahia LR, Araujo DV, Schaan BD, Dib SA, Negrato CA, Leão MP, Ramos AJ, Forti AC, Gomes MB, Foss MC, Monteiro RA. The costs of type 2 diabetes mellitus outpatient care in the Brazilian public health system. Value in Health. Aug 31, 2011;**14**(5):S137-S140

[42] Marinho MGS, Cesse EÂ, Bezerra AF, Carvalho IM, de Sousa AF, de Carvalho EF. Cost analysis of health care for patients with diabetes mellitus and hypertension at a public health unit in Recife, Brazil. Arquivos Brasileiros de Endocrinologia e Metabologia 2011;**55**(6):406

[43] Santana Pereira D, Devidé Nogueira JA, da Silva CA. Quality of life and the health status of elderly persons: a population-based study in the central sertão of Ceará. Revista Brasileira de Geriatria e Gerontologia. 2015;**18**(4):893-908

[44] Cazarim MS, Freitas O, Penaforte TR, Achcar A, Pereira LRL. Impact assessment of Pharmaceutical Care in the Management of hypertension and coronary risk factors after discharge. PLoS One. 2016;**11**(6):e0155204. DOI: 10.1371/journal.pone.0155204

6

Amino Acid Plasma Concentrations and Urinary Excretion in Young Diabetics

Teodoro Durá-Travé, Fidel Gallinas-Victoriano, Ernesto Cortes-Castell and Manuel Moya-Benavent

Abstract

The aim of this study is to analyze amino acid plasma profile in a group of young diabetics and to evaluate its application as markers of metabolic control of the disease, as well as to analyze the urinary excretion of amino acids in these patients. A clinical assessment and metabolic study (amino acid serum concentrations and urinary excretion of amino acids) was accomplished in a group of 49 children diagnosed with diabetes, and a group of 48 healthy children (control group). The plasma levels of total amino acids as well as branchedchain, glucogenic and ketogenic amino acids were significantly higher ($p < 0.05$) in the diabetic group with respect to the control group. Total as well as branched-chain, glucogenic and ketogenic amino acids urinary levels were significantly lower ($p < 0.05$) in the diabetic group compared to the control group. The study of the amino acid plasma in the young diabetic reflect disturbances in protein/amino acid metabolism and, consequently, in metabolic control of the disease. The study of amino acid urinary excretion might have interest not only in the context of diabetic nephropathy, but also in the revealing of partial aspects of amino acid metabolism and, probably, in the metabolic control of the disease.

Keywords: amino acids, insulin-dependent diabetes mellitus, children, serum concentration, urinary excretion

1. Introduction

Most of the cells in our body are dependent on the anabolic effects of insulin, which enables the use and storage of different nutrients from the diet.

It has been experimentally proven that insulin deficiency involves a series of ultrastructural and/or functional changes at an intracellular level, within muscle as well as liver, which substantially inhibit protein synthesis and stimulate protein degradation. Therefore, being amino acidosis, the structural elements of proteins and its metabolism could be altered in diabetes mellitus [1, 2]. In fact, significant changes in amino acid plasma levels and urinary excretion have been described in diabetic ketoacidosis, as well as anomalies in postprandial plasma profile of such amino acids in diabetic patients, whose values will not even return to normal levels after intensive insulin therapy [3–6].

Diabetic nephropathy is one of the most frequent and severe late complications in infant-juvenile diabetes; its functional and structural pathology seems to be shaped from the early stages of the disease. Persistent microalbuminuria is a functional disruption that occurs in the emerging phases of diabetic nephropathy, whose early detection and monitoring is quite important due to its prognostic significance [7, 8].

An increased urinary excretion of low molecular weight proteins and lysosomal enzymes has been confirmed in diabetic patients in the absence of microalbuminuria, as a result of a disorder in renal tubular reabsorption; its significance in natural history of diabetic nephropathy would be interpreted as early markers of renal injury [9–11]. On the other hand, barely 2–3% of the total amount of amino acidosis filtered by the glomerulus is excreted in urine following a massive and active tubular reabsorption [12]. Hence, aminoaciduria in diabetic individuals might be conditioned by the degree of structural and/or functional integrity of the renal tubule.

The aim of this study is to analyze amino acid plasma profile in a group of young diabetic individuals and to evaluate its potential application as markers of metabolic control of the disease, as well as to analyze the urinary excretion of amino acids in the absence of microalbuminuria in these patients.

2. Material and methods

2.1. Participants

A clinical assessment and metabolic study was accomplished in 49 children diagnosed with insulin-dependent diabetes mellitus, aged 8.6–14.3 years, following conventional insulin therapy, and a group of 48 healthy children (control group) aged 7.4–14.8 years.

2.2. Clinical assessment

Information recorded from every patient/participant included age, weight and height, BMI, time and progress of the disease, and dosage of subcutaneous insulin.

Weight and height measurements were made in underwear while being barefoot. Weight was measured using the Año-Sayol scale (reading interval 0–120 kg and a precision of 100 g), and height was measured using the Holtain wall stadiometer (reading interval 60–210 cm, precision 0.1 cm). The Z-score values for the BMI were calculated using the epidemiologic data contained within the program Aplicación Nutricional, from the Spanish Society of pediatric gastroenterology, hepatology, and nutrition (Sociedad Española de Gastroenterología, Hepatología y Nutrición Pediátrica, available at http://www.gastroinf.es/nutritional/). The graphics from Ferrández et al. (Centro Andrea Prader, Zaragoza) (2002) were used as reference charts.

Blood pressure (BP) was measured in the right arm with the patient in the supine position using Visomat comfort 20/40 (Roche Diagnostics Inc.) digital blood pressure monitor, recording the lowest of three measurements.

2.3. Biochemical analysis

All participants (diabetic and control group) underwent blood testing after a 12-hour fast, in order to determine plasma glucose levels, glycosylated hemoglobin (Hb1Ac), creatinine and amino acid concentrations. In addition, a 24-hour urine sample was collected to determine albumin and amino acid concentrations and glomerular filtration rate (GFR).

The analyzed amino acids (in blood and urine) were the following: alanine (ALA), arginine (ARG), aspartic acid (ASP), cysteine (CYS), glutamine (GLN), glutamic acid (GLU), glycine (GLY), histidine (HIS), isolecucine (ILE), leucine (LEU), lisine (LYS), methionine (MET), phenylalanine (PHE), serine (SER), threonine (THR), tyrosine (TYR), valine (VAL), and taurine (TAU).

Measurements in plasma (glucose and creatinine) and urine (creatinine) were made using a Synchron CX5 (Beckman) analyzer. HbA1c was determined using Boehringer-Mannheim reagents.

The quantification of urinary albumin excretion (UAE) was made by nephelometry (Away Protein System-Beckman), and microalbuminuria was considered when values exceed 12 ug/min, being that a reason for exclusion. GFR was calculated using the endogenous creatinine clearance, and hyperfiltration was considered when values were over 145 ml/min/11.73 m^2.

The determination of urine and plasma amino acid concentrations was made by reversed-phase high pressure liquid chromatography (HPLC) with o-phthaldialdehyde precolumn derivatization.

2.4. Statistical analysis

Results are displayed as means (M) with corresponding standard deviations (SD). Statistical analysis (descriptive statistics, Student's *T* and Pearson's correlation) was done using the Statistical Packages for the Social Sciences version 20.0 (Chicago, IL, USA). Statistical significance was assumed when *p* value was lower than 0.05.

Parents and/or legal guardians were informed and provided verbal consent for the participation in this study in all cases. The study was approved by the Ethics Committee for Human Investigation at our institution (in accordance with the ethical standards laid down in the 1964 Declaration of Helsinki and later amendments).

3. Results

Table 1 shows the comparison of mean values for the clinical and biochemical characteristics (blood and urine) in the diabetic and control groups. Fasting glycaemia, Hb1Ac, and GFR were significantly higher ($p < 0.05$) within the diabetic group compared to the control group. There were not any significant differences in age, BMI Z-score, systolic and diastolic blood pressure, and urinary albumin excretion between both groups.

There was no correlation between glomerular filtration and Hb1Ac or urinary albumin excretion, not between blood pressure (systolic and diastolic blood pressure) and glomerular filtration or Hb1Ac. There was a positive correlation ($p < 0.05$) between diastolic blood pressure and the evolution of the disease (years) ($r = 0.515$).

Table 2 exposes and compares the mean values of amino acid plasma concentrations for the samples of the diabetic and control groups. Plasma concentrations of ARG, GLN, ILE, PHE, THR, TYR, VAL, and TAU were significantly higher ($p < 0.05$) within the diabetic group with respect to the control group.

Table 3 depicts and compares the mean values of plasma concentrations of different amino acids groups analyzed in the diabetic and control group. The plasma levels of total amino acids as well as branched-chain, glucogenic, and ketogenic amino acids were significantly higher ($p < 0.05$) in the diabetic group with respect to the control group.

There was no correlation between the single amino acid (or amino acid groups) plasma levels and the evolution of the disease (years) or Hb1Ac. There was a negative correlation ($p < 0.05$) among insulin dosage and amino acids THR ($r = -0.404$), MET ($r = -0.513$), PHE ($r = -0.456$), SER ($r = -0.442$), CYS ($r = -0.390$), GLY ($r = -0.451$), and TAU ($r = -0.479$), as well as a

Items	Diabetic group (n = 49)	Control group (n = 48)	p-Values
Age (years)	11.82 ± 1.78	12.05 ± 1.93	n.s.
BMI Z-score	0.05 ± 0.67	−0.01 ± 0.55	n.s.
Systolic BP	93.15 ± 8.85	89.0 ± 8.95	n.s.
Diastolic BP	55.0 ± 7.26	52.2 ± 8.36	n.s.
Evolution (years)	5.79 ± 2.67	—	—
Insulin (UI/kg/d)	0.82 ± 0.26	—	—
Glucose (mg(dl))	198.8 ± 55.5	89.57 ± 10.2	<0.01
Hb1Ac (%)	7.7 ± 1.68	4.56 ± 0.7	<0.05
GFR (ml/min/1.73 m^2)	135.65 ± 34.3	114.16 ± 9.13	<0.05
UAE (ug/min)	3.77 ± 1.8	3.42 ± 1.89	n.s.

GFR: glomerular filtration rate, UAE: urinary albumin excretion.

Table 1. Clinical and biochemical characteristics of the diabetic and control groups (M ± SD).

Amino acids	Diabetic group (n = 49)	Control group (n = 48)	p-Values
ALA	144.83 ± 36.32	134.84 ± 36.67	n.s.
ARG	49.01 ± 16.78	22.62 ± 6.94	<0.01
ASP	0.33 ± 0.95	1.34 ± 2.18	n.s.
CYS	34.77 ± 11.61	31.56 ± 10.90	n.s.
GLN	243.23 ± 59.42	187.84 ± 56.83	<0.01
GLU	18.28 ± 9.69	20.70 ± 10.22	n.s.
GLY	46.53 ± 22.3	35.34 ± 10.23	n.s.
HIS	133.62 ± 43.59	147.09 ± 53.89	n.s.
ILE	90.83 ± 19.37	66.54 ± 15.27	<0.001
LEU	74.74 ± 17.37	68.65 ± 14.65	n.s.
LYS	60.70 ± 27.32	57.15 ± 28.61	n.s.
MET	31.57 ± 10.68	29.18 ± 13.05	n.s.
PHE	81.84 ± 19.54	65.64 ± 16.45	<0.01
SER	53.93 ± 26.03	66.04 ± 22.04	n.s.
THR	73.26 ± 27.90	57.90 ± 18.07	<0.05
TYR	60.25 ± 27.18	38.25 ± 12.47	<0.05
VAL	190.46 ± 48.01	148.91 ± 35.31	<0.01
TAU	99.69 ± 36.82	75.66 ± 37.01	<0.05

ALA: alanine, ARG: arginine, ASP: aspartic acid, CYS: cysteine, GLN: glutamine, GLU: glutamic acid, GLY: glycine, HIS: histidine, ILE: isolecucine, LEU: leucine, LYS: lisine, MET: methionine, PHE: phenylalanine, SER serine, THR: threonine, TYR tyrosine, VAL: valine, TAU: taurine.

Table 2. Plasma concentrations of amino acids (nmol/ml) in the diabetic and control groups (M ± SD).

positive correlation ($p < 0.05$) among glycaemia and amino acids VAL ($r = 0.545$) and LEU ($r = 0.648$).

Table 4 displays and compares the mean values of urinary concentrations of different amino acids quantified in the diabetic and control group. The urinary level of amino acids, except for ASP, ILE, and PHE, was significantly lower ($p < 0.05$) in the diabetic group with respect to the control group.

Table 5 outlines and compares the mean values of urinary levels of the different amino acids groups in the diabetic and control group. Total as well as branched-chain, glucogenic and ketogenic amino acid urinary levels were significantly lower ($p < 0.05$) in the diabetic group compared to the control group. The mean values of the glucogenic/total amino acid ratio were significantly lower ($p < 0.05$) in the diabetic group with respect to the control group. There were no significant differences in the ketogenic/total amino acid ratio between both groups.

Amino acid groups	Diabetic group (n = 49)	Control group (n = 48)	p-Values
Total	1383.70 ± 353.67	1198.46 ± 261.16	<0.05
Branched-chain	347.65 ± 58.76	285.20 ± 45.20	<0.01
Glucogenic	1252.74 ± 236.82	1053.69 ± 211.19	<0.001
Ketogenic	441.62 ± 57.09	354.13 ± 53.45	<0.05

Table 3. Plasma concentrations of amino acids (nmol/ml) in the diabetic and control groups (M ± SD).

Amino acids	Diabetic group (n = 49)	Control group (n = 48)	p-Values
ALA	53.97 ± 36.68	118.07 ± 45.24	<0.001
ARG	2.45 ± 1.91	4.59 ± 2.97	<0.05
ASP	4.98 ± 3.23	8.84 ± 4.22	n.s.
CYS	19.25 ± 11.07	61.91 ± 29.17	<0.05
GLN	7.84 ± 4.52	95.02 ± 32.18	<0.001
GLU	16.62 ± 9.61	35.83 ± 15.77	<0.05
GLY	23.00 ± 15.05	192.41 ± 121.59	<0.001
HIS	74.12 ± 48.50	233.95 ± 89.36	<0.01
ILE	18.98 ± 10.31	29.83 ± 18.42	n.s.
LEU	12.46 ± 8.17	22.16 ± 9.13	<0.05
LYS	223.65 ± 150.75	525.32 ± 196.31	<0.05
MET	19.11 ± 8.01	86.04 ± 56.06	<0.05
PHE	40.64 ± 22.58	51.67 ± 13.71	n.s.
SER	10.64 ± 7.64	25.40 ± 13.65	<0.01
THR	14.47 ± 10.96	63.29 ± 19.36	<0.05
TYR	26.65 ± 16.28	79.08 ± 21.15	<0.001
VAL	25.61 ± 11.94	45.11 ± 13.67	<0.05
TAU	115.17 ± 56.70	172.31 ± 107.12	<0.01

ALA: alanine, ARG: arginine, ASP: aspartic acid, CYS: cysteine, GLN: glutamine, GLU: glutamic acid, GLY: glycine, HIS: histidine, ILE: isolecucine, LEU: leucine, LYS: lisine, MET: methionine, PHE: phenylalanine, SER serine, THR: threonine, TYR tyrosine, VAL: valine, TAU: taurine.

Table 4. Urinary levels of amino acids (μmol/m^2) in the diabetic and control groups (M ± SD).

Amino acid groups	Diabetic group (n = 49)	Control group (n = 48)	p-Values
Total	754.94 ± 427.16	1868.42 ± 662.36	<0.05
Branched-chain	54.58 ± 26.51	101.13 ± 36.76	<0.05
Glucogenic	252.51 ± 178.75	943.79 ± 370.50	<0.05
Ketogenic	236.40 ± 121.16	530.69 ± 215.78	<0.05
Ratio G/T	0.34 ± 0.09	0.50 ± 0.07	<0.05
Ratio K/T	0.33 ± 0.16	0.28 ± 0.12	n.s.

G/T: glucogenic/total, K/T: ketogenic/total.

Table 5. Urinary level of amino acid groups in the diabetic and control groups (M ± SD).

There was no correlation between the levels of each particular amino acid and/or group of amino acids in urine and the time of evolution, Hb1Ac, urinary albumin excretion, GFR, and blood pressure (systolic and diastolic blood pressure).

4. Discussion

4.1. Plasma concentrations

In diabetes mellitus, the deficiency in insulin, and in large part, the effects of the counter regulatory hormones would stimulate the synthesis of glucose—other than the glycogenolysis pathway—through the glyconeogenesis [1, 2, 13]. This might explain the differences found in the amino acid plasma levels within the diabetic and control group that, in general, would indicate that there is an increase in the bioavailability of glycogenic substrates in diabetic patients, even in basal conditions.

Insulin leads to a decrease in amino acid plasma levels through the stimulus of protein synthesis and the inhibition of proteolysis [2, 14]; this would largely explain the negative correlation found between insulin dosage and plasma level of the different amino acids. Therefore, the significantly high plasma concentrations of the different amino acids–particularly glucogenic amino acids–in the diabetic group with respect to the control group (probably as a consequence of the insulinopenia that characterizes diabetes), could be useful as plasma markers of a deficient metabolic control.

An increase in postprandial branched-chain amino acid (valine, leucine, and isoleucine) plasma concentrations has been described in diabetic patients, in relation to the metabolic control of the disease [4, 15]. This is probably due to a deficient peripheral metabolism of these amino acids (they undergo basically muscle metabolism). Since it has not been possible to prove an increase in the release of branched-chain amino acids from muscle and/or liver in diabetic patients during fasting [1, 2], and being conscious that biological effects of insulin are deficient in diabetes, it can be assumed that the increased branched-chain amino acid plasma levels in the diabetic group in comparison to the control group would be due to a low stimulation (by insulin) in amino acid transportation inside the cell. Even though no correlation has been found between branched-chain amino acids and metabolic control or time of evolution of diabetes, a positive correlation has been detected between valine and leucine and fasting glycaemia, a fact that would support the hypothesis of a more intense relationship among basal plasma concentration of these amino acids and single determination glycaemia rather than with mediumterm metabolic control.

Even though amino acids are appropriate substrates for hepatic and/or renal synthesis of glucose (gluconeogenesis), glutamine and especially alanine are the most important glucogenic amino acids in quantitative terms [16]. However, while glutamine plasma levels in basal conditions were significantly higher in the diabetic group in comparison to control group, alanine plasma levels did not differ in those groups.

During fasting, alanine release does not exclusively correspond to a mechanism of proteolysis and posits muscle synthesis of new molecules of alanine from the glucose captured by the muscle or glucose alanine cycle [2, 16]. Nevertheless, since glucose uptake by the muscle is lowered due to insulinopenia in the diabetic patient, the conversion of glucose into alanine would be decreased, and consequently, this would explain why alanine plasma levels in the diabetic group do not differ from the control group.

Amino acid metabolism in insulin-dependent diabetes mellitus appears to be intrinsically disrupted, since insulin deficiency and to a great extent, the effects of the counter regulatory hormones imply an increase in hepatic gluconeogenesis and muscle proteolysis, as well as a deficient peripheral use and/or disturbance in hepatic amino acid metabolism; this would result in a plasma profile characterized by an increase of total amino acids, at the expense mainly of branched-chain and glucogenic amino acids. In this way, the study of the amino acid plasma profile in diabetic patients would be worthwhile, since it would reflect disturbances in protein and/or amino acid metabolism and consequently, in metabolic control of the disease.

4.2. Urinary excretion

Diabetic nephropathy is preceded by a window period, which might show different renal functional and/or structural disturbances, even in the early stages of the disease [7, 8]. In fact, the results obtained, in line with other researchers [17, 18], reveal significantly higher glomerular filtration in the diabetic group in comparison to the control group, and especially in those patients with a shorter period of disease and regardless of metabolic control of the disease. In addition, even when the whole diabetic group had normal blood pressure measurements, the existing correlation between diastolic blood pressure and the time of evolution of the disease suggests a situation of window period in diabetic nephropathy in this group of young diabetics, and highlights the importance of periodic blood pressure measurements in diabetics from the early stages of the disease. This allows for the beginning of a dietary and/or medical treatment earlier than was recommended until now [19]. However, it can be concluded that the structural integrity of the glomerulus in these diabetic patients would be relatively well preserved, since the urinary excretion of albumin was similar in both groups.

On another note, several researchers have noted a higher beta 2 microglobulin and lysosomal enzyme urinary excretion in diabetic patients in the absence of microalbuminuria, as a sign of functional disorder in the proximal tubule with no glomerular lesion, from the early stages of the disease [10, 11]. In this context, the study of amino acid urinary excretion in the diabetic could be of great interest, since different mechanisms of specific tubular reabsorption for different amino acids have been described on an experimental basis [20]. Hence, any tubular malfunction might condition significant qualitative and/or quantitative aminoaciduria, and therefore, it could have a potential clinical application in the early detection of tubular lesion and/or silent diabetic nephropathy.

All the same, and according to the results obtained, urinary excretion of each single amino acid (except for isoleucine, aspartic acid, and taurine), as well as each amino acid groups analyzed were significantly lower in the diabetic group with respect to the control group. This may seem paradoxical; however, the difference observed in the relation glucogenic and total amino acid (G/T ratio) between both groups reveals that the lower amino acid urinary excretion in the diabetic would greatly be at the expense of glucogenic amino acids, probably because the glomerular filtration is also lower, as a consequence of a greater organic use of these amino acids in the endogenous synthesis of glucose. No correlation has been found between aminoaciduria and time of evolution, glomerular filtration, blood pressure, and metabolic control.

In sum, the study of amino acid urinary excretion in the young diabetic might have interest not only in the context of diabetic nephropathy, but also in the revealing of partial aspects of amino acid metabolism, and probably, in the metabolic control of the disease.

Author details

Teodoro Durá-Travé[1,2]*, Fidel Gallinas-Victoriano[2], Ernesto Cortes-Castell[3] and Manuel Moya-Benavent[3]

*Address all correspondence to: tduratra@cfnavarra.es

1 Department of Pediatrics, School of Medicine, University of Navarre, Pamplona, Spain

2 Department of Pediatrics, Navarre Hospital Complex, Pamplona, Spain

3 Department of Pediatrics, School of Medicine, University of "Miguel Hernández", Elche, Spain

References

[1] Kimball SR, Flaim KE, Peavy DE, Jefferson LS. Protein metabolism. In: Rifkin H, Porte D, editors. Diabetes Mellitus. Theory and practice. New York: Elsevier SP; 1990. pp: 41-50

[2] Liu Z, Barret EJ. Protein metabolism in health and diabetes. In: Defronzo RA, Ferrannini E, Keen H, Zimmet P, editors. International Textbook of Diabetes Mellitus. Chichester, England: Wiley; 2004. pp. 319-334

[3] Trevisan R, Marescotti C, Avogaro A, Tessari P, del Prato S, Tiengo A. Effects of different insulin administrations on plasma amino acid profile in insulin-dependent diabetic patients. Diabetes Research 1989;**12**:57-62

[4] Szabó A, Kenesei E, Körner A, Miltényi M, Szücs L, Nagy I. Changes in plasma and urinary amino acid levels during diabetic ketoacidosis in children. Diabetes Research and Clinical Practice. 1991;**12**:91-97

[5] Ohtsuka Y, Agishi Y. Abnormal amino acid metabolism in diabetes mellitus. Nihon Rinsho. 1992;**50**:1631-1636

[6] Adeva MM, Calviño J, Souto G, Donapetry C. Insulin resistance and the metabolism of branched-chain amino acids in humans. Amino Acids. 2012;**43**:171-181

[7] Drummond K, Mauer M, International Diabetic Nephropathy Study Group. The early natural history of nephropathy in type 1 diabetes: II. Early renal structural changes in type 1 diabetes. Diabetes. 2002;**51**:1580-1587

[8] Mauer M, Drummond K. The early natural history of nephropathy in type 1 diabetes: I. Study design and baseline characteristics of the study participants. Diabetes. 2002;**51**: 1572-1579

[9] Hsiao PH, Tsai WS, Tsai WY, Lee JS, Tsau YK, Chen CH. Urinary N-acetyl-beta-D-glucosaminidase activity in children with insulin-dependent diabetes mellitus. American Journal of Nephrology. 1996;**16**:300-303

[10] Holmquist P, Torffvit O. Tubular function in diabetic children assessed by Tamm-Horsfall protein and glutathione S-transferase. Pediatric Nephrology. 2008;**23**:1079-1083

[11] Saif A, Soliman N. Urinary alfa1-microglobulin and albumin excretion in children and adolescents with type 1 diabetes. Journal of Diabetes. 2017;**9**:61-64

[12] Mitch WE, Chesney RW. Amino acid metabolism by the kidney. Mineral and Electrolyte Metabolism. 1983;**9**:190-202

[13] Newgard CB. Regulation of glucose metabolism in the liver. In: Defronzo RA, Ferrannini E, Keen H, Zimmet P, editors. International Textbook of Diabetes Mellitus. Chichester, England: Wiley. 2004. pp. 253-275

[14] Grill V, Björkman O, Gutniak M, Lindqvist M. Brain uptake and release of amino acids in nondiabetic and insulin-dependent diabetic subjects: Important role of glutamine release for nitrogen balance. Metabolism. 1992;**41**:28-32

[15] Hagenfeldt L, Dahlquist G, Persson B. Plasma amino acids in relation to metabolic control in insulin-dependent diabetic children. Acta Paediatrica Scandinavica. 1989;**78**:278-282

[16] Nelson AL, Cox MM. Glucolisis, gluconeogénesis y ruta de las pentosas fosfato. In: Principios de Bioquímica. Omega. Barcelona. 2006. pp. 521-559

[17] Bjornstad P, Roncal C, Milagres T, Pyle L, Lanaspa MA, Bishop FK, Snell-Bergeon JK, Johnson RJ, Wadwa RP, Maahs DM. Hyperfiltration and uricosuria in adolescents with type 1 diabetes. Pediatric Nephrology. 2016;**31**:787-793

[18] Tonneijck L, Muskiet MH, Smits MM, van Bommel EJ, Heerspink HJ, van Raalte DH, Joles JA. Glomerular hyperfiltration in diabetes: Mechanisms, clinical significance, and treatment. Journal of the American Society of Nephrology 2017;**28**:1023-1039

[19] Warady BA, Abraham AG, Schwartz GJ, Wong CS, Muñoz A, Betoko A, Mitsnefes M, Kaskel F, Greenbaum LA, Mak RH, Flynn J, Moxey-Mims MM, Furth S. Predictors of rapid progression of glomerular and nonglomerular kidney disease in children and adolescents. The chronic kidney disease in children (CkiD) cohort. American Journal of Kidney Diseases. 2015;**65**:878-888

[20] Rossi R, Danzebrink S, Linnenbürger K, Hillebrand D, Grüneberg M, Sablitzky V, Deufel T, Ullrich K, Harms E. Assessment of tubular reabsorption of sodium, glucosa, phosphate and amino acids based on spot urine samples. Acta Paediatrica. 1994;**83**:1282-1286

7

DPP-4 Inhibitors and Fat Metabolism in Patients with Type 2 Diabetes

Alexander S. Ametov and Dinara G. Gusenbekova

Abstract

Objective. To evaluate the influence of combined therapy of Sitagliptin and metformin on fat metabolism in patients with T2 DM.

Methods. The study included 82 patients with obesity. The following were evaluated at base line and after 6 months of therapy: fasting glucose, postprandial glucose, glycated hemoglobin, weight, waist circumference, lipid profile, proinsulin, leptin,adiponectin, HOMA-β,HOMA-IR, MRI of visceral fat.

Results. After 6 months, HbA1c decreased by 18.52% ($p < 0.001$) in-group 1 and by 8.17% ($p < 0.001$) in-group 2. HOMA-β increased by 33% in group 1 ($p < 0.001$) and by 11% in group 2 ($p > 0.05$). Adiponectin levels increased by 27.06% ($p < 0.001$) in group 1 and by 7.16% in group 2 26 ($p < 0.001$). Leptin levels were reduced by 30.47% ($p < 0.001$) in group 1 and by 5.41% in group 2 ($p < 0.001$). MRI showed a 7.52% reduction in visceral fat for group 1 ($p < 0.001$) and a 1.76% reduction for group 2 ($p < 0.01$).

Conclusion. Sitagliptin and metformin combination therapy had a prominent effect on nonglycemic parameters, with more marked decreases in visceral fat and leptin and increases in adiponectin levels.

Keywords: Sitagliptin, visceral fat, fat metabolism, type 2 diabetes, adiponectin, leptin

1. Introduction

Diabetes mellitus (DM) occupies a prominent place among chronic diseases due to the rapid spread, tendency to increase in the number of patients, high disability due to numerous macro- and microvascular complications and the leading position among the main causes of death [1]. The relationship between epidemics of type 2 diabetes and obesity initiated conducting research studying the adipose tissue as an endocrine organ that plays a crucial role in the development of metabolic disorders in patients suffering from obesity. Due to excessive accretion of visceral adipose tissue, there is an imbalance of adipokines, lipid metabolism, hyperinsulinemia, which lead to the development and progression of insulin resistance (IR), DM 2. According to modern concepts, in the pathogenesis of DM 2, in addition to IR and impaired insulin secretion, an important role is played by abnormalities related to the "incretin effect," which led to the creation of a class of inhibitors of dipeptidyl peptidase-4 (iDPP-4). The advantage of this class is the restoration of the physiological concentration of glucagon-like peptide-1 (GLP-1). Due to the physiological mechanism of action, the use of drugs of this class is associated with a low risk of hypoglycemia. It should be noted that therapy with DPP-4 inhibitors, along with glycemic ones, also has favorable nonglycemic effects, among which, a positive effect on body weight (BW), lipid profile and blood pressure (BP) [2–5]. One of the first approved representatives of iDPP-4 (registered by the FDA in 2007) is Sitagliptin. According to the literature, the use of Sitagliptin has been studied both in the form of monotherapy, and in double, triple combinations of hypoglycemic drugs combined with insulin [6–12]. Particular attention is drawn to the possibility of the combination of iDPP-4 with a first line drug-metformin. It is important to note that metformin can lead to an increase in total GLP-1 and potentially enhance the effects of the inhibitor DPP-4 [13]. The combination of metformin and iDPP-4 suggests an impact on all the major pathogenetic mechanisms of development of type 2 diabetes type [14]. A number of studies [15, 16] reported the identification of DPP-4 as a new adipokine, which can be a link between an increase in adipose tissue mass and obesity-associated diseases. The excessive content of DPP-4 in visceral adipose tissue may be a marker of inflammation of adipose tissue, which is associated with insulin resistance. Conversely, animal studies have shown that suppression of DPP-4 prevents the development of inflammation and impaired glucose tolerance, which develops on the background of obesity, in adipose tissue.

Thus, due to poor knowledge, a comprehensive study of lipid metabolism, with the visualization of fat dynamics, the evaluation of adipocytokine-adiponectin and leptin secretion, and the possibility of disease management by changing the parameters of lipid metabolism, on the background of iDPP-4 therapy in combination with metformin, the best variant of physiological intervention mobilizing the body's own resources, is of the scientific and practical interest, which determined the relevance of the study. The solution of this problem will allow us to expand our understanding of the nonglycemic effects of iDPP-4, to improve the effectiveness of therapy in patients with type 2 diabetes and obesity. The study was conducted at the Department of Endocrinology of the Russian Medical Academy of Postgraduate Education.

The aim of our study was to evaluate the effect of combined therapy with Sitagliptin and metformin on the parameters of fat metabolism in patients with type 2 diabetes and obesity.

The study protocol was approved by the expert commission of therapeutic faculty of the State-Funded Educational Institution "Russian Medical Academy of Postgraduate Education" of the Ministry of Health of Russia on issues of medical ethics 14.11.2013 (Minutes № 8 of 14.11.2013).

Materials and methods. The study included 82 patients with type 2 diabetes with excessive body weight of varying severity, dyslipidemia, not taking lipid-lowering therapy, who did not reach the target levels of HbA1c on metformin monotherapy and dietary treatment. The average age of the patients was 55.3 ± 9.1 years. Group I included 42 patients with type 2 diabetes and obesity on combination therapy with metformin 2000 mg/day + Sitagliptin 100 mg/day. Before entering the study, patients in this group received monotherapy with metformin at a dose of 1500–2000 mg/day. Group II included 40 patients on metformin alone at a dose of 2000 mg/day. Before entering the study, patients were on dietary treatment. All patients were overweight and obese. A brief description of the groups by main parameters is presented in **Table 1**.

After the formation of comparable clinical groups, all patients underwent clinical, instrumental and laboratory tests. Methods of examination included the collection of anamnesis, measurement of anthropometric parameters (height, body weight (BW), waist circumference (WC), hip circumference (HC) and their ratio).

To evaluate the carbohydrate metabolism, the levels of fasting plasma glycemia (GH), postprandial glycemia (PPG) and glycated hemoglobin (HbA1c) were determined.

For the study of fat and lipid metabolism, the concentrations of leptin, adiponectin, total cholesterol (OX), triglycerides (TG), high-density lipoprotein (HDL) cholesterol, low-density lipoprotein (LDL) cholesterol and apolipoprotein β (apo β protein) were determined.

The quantity and nature of the distribution of adipose tissue were assessed by MRI of visceral fat at L4 level. The area of visceral fat (VFA) ≥ 130 cm^2 and the ratio of VFA/SFA > 0.4 were interpreted as visceral obesity.

Insulin resistance and functional activity of β-cells were determined using the HOMA IR and HOMA β indices. The calculation was carried out according to the following formulas:

HOMA IR = Fasting insulin (μE/ml) X Fasting plasma glucose (mmol/L)/22.5.

Index of HOMA-IR <2.77 was considered normal. IRI-immunoreactive insulin.

HOMA β = 20X IRI (μU/ml)/fasting glycemia (mmol/L) −3.5.

A biochemical blood test was performed on Advia 1800 automatic analyzers from Bayer (Germany) and Olympus AU 2700 from Beckman Coulter (USA). The level of HbA1c was determined by capillary electrophoresis on a Capillaris 2 device from Sebia (France). The study of the content of adiponectin was carried out by ELISA (immunoenzyme method) with Bio Vendor test systems (Germany). The levels of leptin and proinsulin were evaluated using DRG kits for enzyme immunoassay on the Multiscan Labsystems analyzer (Finland). Insulin level in serum of venous blood was evaluated by the method of chemiluminescent immunoassay on the automatic device Architect i2000 (Abbot, USA). The level of C-peptide was determined in the serum of venous

Group characteristics by main parameters			
Parameters	**Group 1**	**Group 2**	**P**
Total number of patients, abs%	42 (100)	40 (100)	–
Men's, abs. (%)	10 (23.8)	8 (20)	–
Women, abs. (%)	32 (76.1)	32 (80)	–
Average age, years	55.3 ± 9.1	56.1 ± 5.4	>0.05
Duration of DM type 2, years	2.4 ± 2.0	2.4 ± 1.5	>0.05
Fasting glycemia, mmol/l	9.7 ± 279	9.6 ± 2.1	>0.05
Postprandial glycemia, mmol/l	11.01 ± 3.19	9.45 ± 1.96	<0.05
HbA1c, %	8.3 ± 1.66	8.35 ± 1.7	>0.05
Total cholesterol, mmol/l	6.85 ± 0.95	7.11 ± 6.39	>0.05
Adiponectin, μkg/ml	7.63 ± 2.56	7.41 ± 2.43	>0.05
Leptin, ng/ml	23.87 ± 13.43	23.84 ± 9.61	>0.05
BMI, kg/m^2	34.78 ± 4.87	35.45 ± 4.3	>0.05
Visceral fat area (VFA, L4), sm^2	300.73 ± 80.88	334.62 ± 70.55	>0.05
Subcutaneous fat area (SFA, L4), sm^2	375.88 ± 91.55	431.25 ± 54.13	>0.05
Proinsulin, pmol/l	9.66 ± 10.49	10.02 ± 12.65	>0.05
Insulin, μU/ml	14.24 ± 9.3	14.72 ± 8.51	>0.05
C-peptide, ng/ml	3.3 ± 1.6	3.2 ± 1.7	>0.05
HOMA-β	40.63 ± 25.99	57.05 ± 35.43	>0.05
HOMA-IR	5.85 ± 4.15	6.32 ± 5.0	>0.05

Table 1. Characteristics of groups by main parameters.

blood by the method of chemiluminescent immunoassay on the Immulite 2000 automatic analyzer (Siemens, USA). To assess the lipid profile, the levels of OX, HDL cholesterol, LDL cholesterol and TG in serum were determined after 12 h of fasting by enzymatic colorimetry on automatic Advia 1800 analyzers. Apolipoprotein β (apo-β-protein) was determined by immunoturbidimetry using an Olympus AU 400 automatic analyzer, manufactured by Beckman Coulter (USA).

Before entering the study, patients provided written informed consent, were trained in the school of diabetes, were secured by means of self-control and self-monitoring diaries.

The statistical analysis of the data was carried out using the Statistica 8 software package. The Wilcoxon test was used to assess the difference in the parameters before and after treatment. The difference in dynamics between the groups was determined by the Mann–Whitney U test. The pair relationships of the indicators were determined by the Spearman rank correlation coefficient.

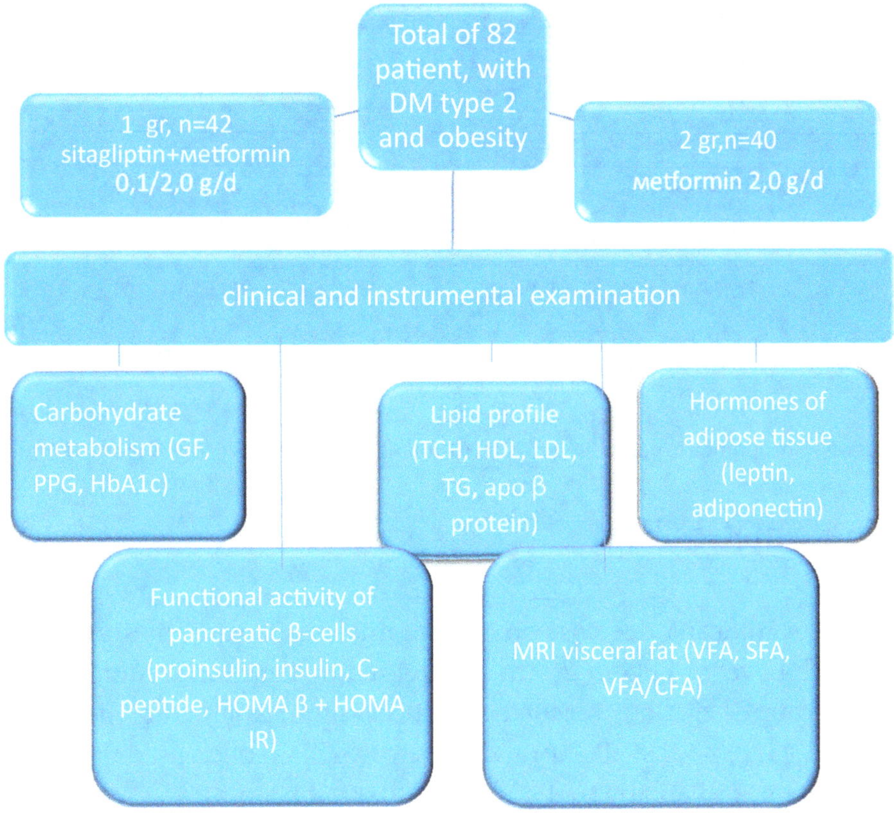

Figure 1. Study design.

To test the statistical hypotheses on the type of distribution, the Shapiro-Wilks criterion was applied. The significance level of p was set at 0.05.

The design of the study is shown in **Figure 1**.

2. Anthropometric measures

After 24 weeks of therapy, a significant decrease in all anthropometric measures was observed in both groups, but more statistically significant differences were observed in group I. BMI decreased on average by 1.81 ± 1.33 (5.29%), $p < 0.001$ in group I, and by 0.68 ± 0.35 (1.96%), $p < 0.001$ in group II. Body weight (BW) decreased by 4.97 ± 3.22 kg (5.2%), $p < 0.001$ in group I, and by 2 ± 0.94 kg (2.07%), $p < 0.001$ in group II. Waist circumference (WC) decreased by 6.52 ± 4.71 cm (5.88%), $p < 0.001$ in group I and by 2.42 ± 1.06 (2.18%), $p < 0.001$ in group II. Accordingly, WC/HC ratio decreased from 0.95 ± 0.06 to 0.91 ± 0.05 (3.28%), $p < 0.001$ in group I, and from 0.94 ± 0.03 to 0.93 ± 0.03 (0.98%), $p < 0.001$ in group II (**Figure 2**). The decrease in WC as well as in the WC/HC ratio indicates a decrease in the amount of visceral fat, which means a decrease in insulin resistance and hyperinsulinemia, the underlying basis of the metabolic syndrome.

The decrease of body weight on Sitagliptin and metformin combined therapy is likely associated with an integrated effect from caloric restriction of the diet, a synergistic effect of iDPP-4 and metformin on GLP-1, which has an anorectic effect.

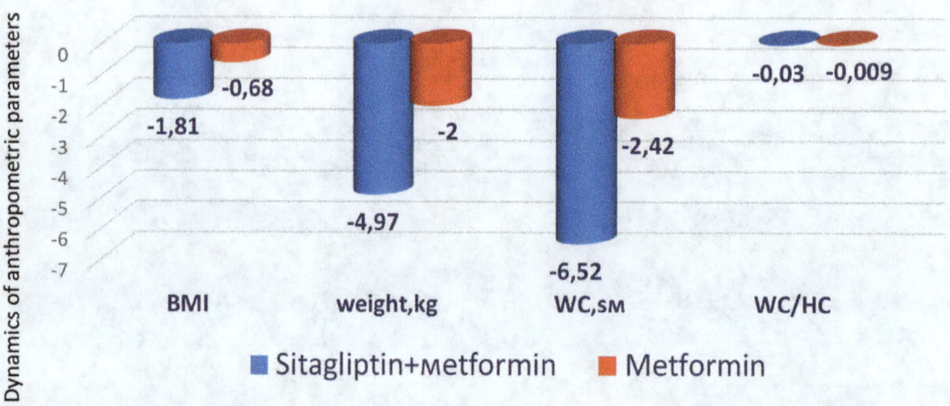

Figure 2. Dynamics of anthropometric parameters. P < 0.001 for all values; P between groups <0.001 for all value.

3. Carbohydrate metabolism

After 24 weeks, a significant decrease in all parameters of carbohydrate metabolism was observed in group I. Level of FPG in group I decreased by 2.67 ± 2.37 mmol/L (21%), p <0.001, FPG decrease in group II has not reached statistical significance with the mean decrease of 0.33 ± 1.6 mmol/L (1.45%), p > 0.05. Postprandial glucose (PPG) decreased by 3.26 ± 2.54 mmol/L (26.35%), p <0.001 in group I and by 0.64 ± 1.2 mmol/L (5.31%), p < 0.05 in group II. HbA1c level decreased by 1.63 ± 1.31% (18.52%), p <0.001 in group I, and by 0.72 ± 0.47% (8.17%) in group II (**Figure 3**).

The largest success in achieving glycemic control in patients on combined treatment is associated with complimentary action of the therapy components. Metformin lowers insulin resistance and hepatic glucose production, while Sitagliptin delays inactivation of GLP-1, thus enhancing glucose-dependent insulin secretion and decreasing glucagon secretion [17]. In addition, it was demonstrated that metformin leads to increase in overall GLP-1 and can

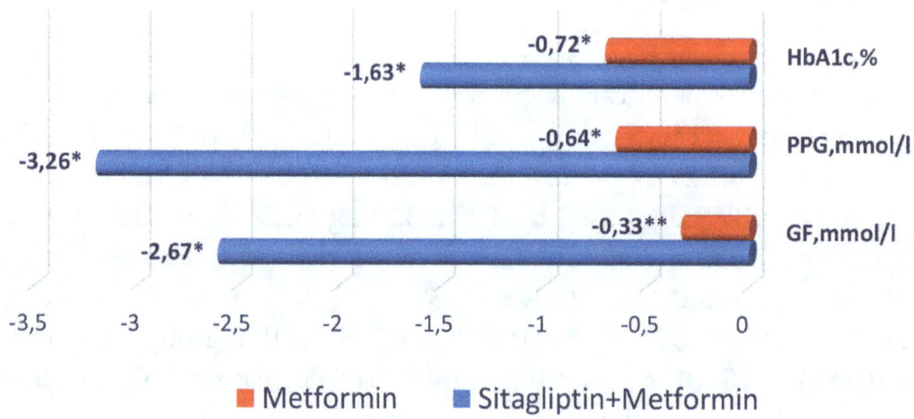

Figure 3. Dynamics of carbohydrate metabolism in the groups. GF-glucose fasting, PPG-postprandial glycemia; *P < 0.05; ** P > 0.05.

potentially enhance the effects of DPP-4 inhibitor. It is notable that the study achieved a significant PPG decrease in metformin monotherapy group, which is potentially associated with metformin ability to increase GLP-1 level and to slow down carbohydrate absorption in the intestine.

4. Lipid profile

Lipid profile parameters belong to the improvement indices of the metabolic health.

The analysis of the lipid profile showed significant positive dynamics of TC, HDL and Apo B in both groups. The only difference between groups was in HDL and TG dynamics. HDL level decreased by 0.78 ± 0.5 mmol/L (17.43%), p < 0.001 in group I, and by 0.37 ± 0.17 mmol/L (9.63%), p <0.001 in group II; TG decreased by 1.33 ± 1.16 mmol/L (28.15%), p < 0.001 in group I, and by 0.63 ± 0.39 mmol/L (15.19%), p <0.001 in group II. **Figure 4** displays parameter dynamics in both groups.

Possible mechanisms partaking in the positive effect on lipid profile from therapy by DPP-4 inhibitor in combination with metformin could be weight loss, lowering of glucose level, decrease in visceral fat (VF), which is accompanied by improvement in metabolic status.

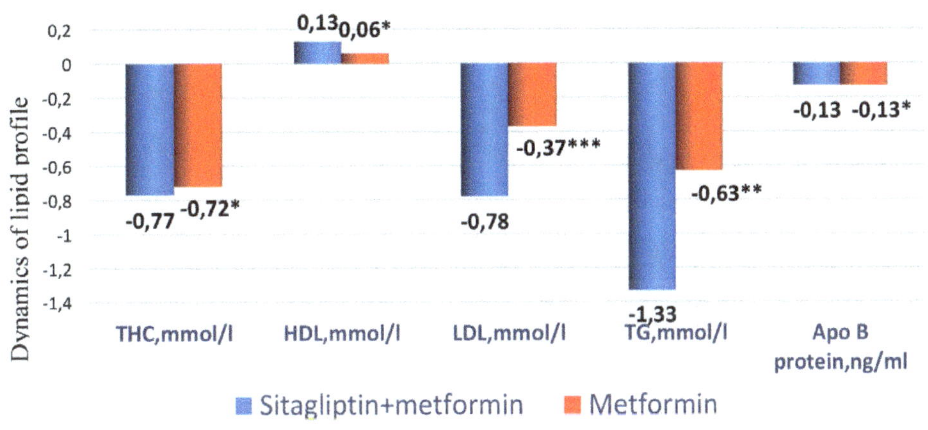

Figure 4. Dynamics of lipid profile. *** P < 0.001; **P < 0.05; *P > 0. 05 between groups.

5. Subcutaneous and visceral fat

MRI visualization of visceral fat dynamics demonstrated positive fat redistribution by lowering VFA in group I by 20.62 ± 13.54 cm^2 (7.52%), p <0.001. In group II of metformin monotherapy, VFA decreased by 5.77 ± 3.75 cm^2 (1.76%), p <0.001. SFA decreased by 4.51 ± 14.43 cm^2 (1.69%), p < 0.05 in group I, and by 1.95 ± 1.05 cm^2 (0.46%), p < 0.05 in group II. Significant improvement in SFA dynamic was observed in both groups; however, we have not detected

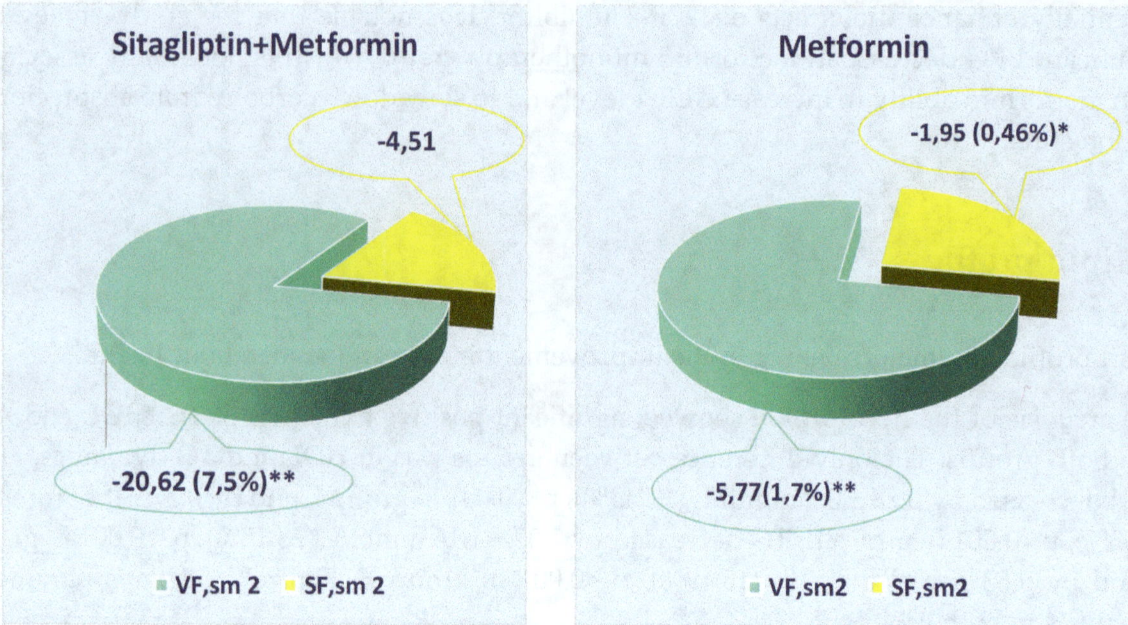

Figure 5. Dynamics of visceral and subcutaneous fat by results MRI. VF-visceral fat, SF- subcutaneous fat; *P between groups >0.05; **P between groups <0.05.

statistically significant difference between the groups (**Figure 5**). VFA/SFA ratio significantly lowered by 0.18 ± 0.24 (15.26%), $p < 0.001$ in group I; and by 0.008 ± 0.008 (1.14%), $p < 0.001$ in group II, which is also indicative of more marked lowering of visceral fat in group I.

6. Adipose tissue hormones

Of note, decrease in VFA and improvement in anthropometric measures were associated to change in secretion of adipose tissue hormones. On Sitagliptin and metformin therapy, a more marked decrease in leptin level by 7.37 ± 5.69 ng/ml (30.47%), $p < 0.001$ was registered, while on metformin monotherapy, leptin level decreased by 1.21 ± 1.34 ng/ml (5.41%), $p < 0.001$.

The study also indicates dynamics of another adipokine-adiponectin that plays a significant role in glucose and lipid metabolism. The initial adiponectin levels in both groups were lower than reference values. After 6 months of therapy, a more marked adiponectin level increase by 1.95 ± 1.53 μg/mL (27.06%), $p < 0.001$ was observed in group I compared to group II, where it is increased by 0.49 ± 0.26 μg/mL, (7.16%), $p < 0.001$. It is known that this hormone secretion is diminished at T2D. The recovery of secretion is accompanied by the improvement in carbohydrate metabolism indicators, lowering of atherogenesis and slowing down of the progression of diabetes vascular events [18].

Adipose tissue hormones dynamics is displayed in **Figure 6**.

Thus, visceral fat area increased on the background of increasing concentration of adiponectin and decreasing leptin content.

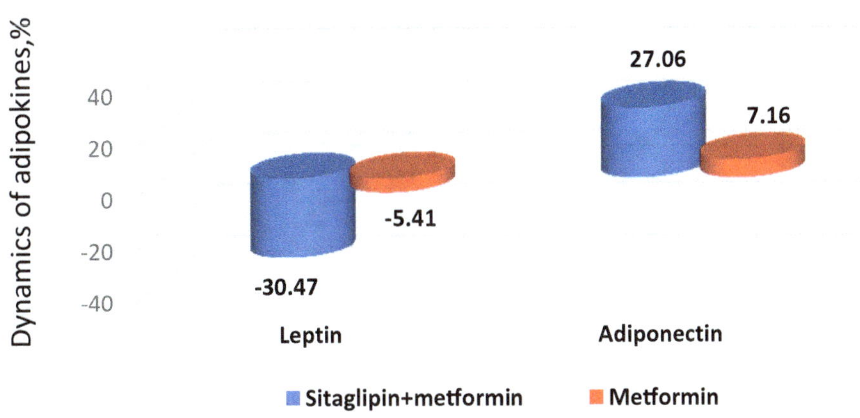

Figure 6. Dynamics of adipokines.

7. Functional activity of β-cells and HOMA-IR

Data from the analysis of pancreatic β-cell function condition have certain scientific and practical interest. For instance, in the Sitagliptin and metformin combined therapy group, a significant increase in HOMA-β index by 23.4 ± 22.6 relative units (33.06%), $p < 0.0001$ was observed compared to the group that receiving metformin monotherapy, where increase in this index has not reached a statistical significance and equaled 4.86 ± 1.63 relative units (11.08%), $p > 0.05$.

Furthermore, the work has obtained statistically significant insulin level lowering in both groups. For instance, on a background of Sitagliptin therapy in combination with metformin therapy, insulin level decreased by 15.68%, ($p < 0.001$), and on metformin monotherapy, insulin level decreased by 7.57%, ($p < 0.001$).

Before treatment, both groups showed increase in proinsulin level, after 6 months of therapy, we achieved significant decrease in the proinsulin level in group I (Sitagliptin + metformin) by 29.17%, ($p < 0.001$), and in group II (metformin) by 13.79%, ($p < 0.001$). Proinsulin/insulin ratio is increased when the functional activity of β-cells is decreased and is an indication of more marked apoptosis in pancreatic β-cells. We established that on Sitagliptin therapy in combination with metformin, a significant decrease by 10.38%, ($p < 0.05$) was observed in proinsulin/insulin ratio, while in metformin monotherapy group, a decrease in this ratio was insignificant, by 2.84%, ($p > 0.05$) (**Figure 7**). This should be considered as a long-term positive effect of Sitagliptin on the function of pancreatic β-cells.

It is important to note that on combined therapy C-peptide level increased by 55.83%, ($p < 0.0001$); and by 6.3%, ($p < 0.05$) in metformin monotherapy group. HOMA-IR significantly lowered in both groups. However, we have not detected statistically significant difference between the groups' dynamics. It decreased by 32% ($p < 0.0001$) in group I, and by 11.05% ($p < 0.0001$) in group II. The decrease in homeostasis model assessment of insulin resistance is the evidence of improvement in peripheral glucose disposal. Positive effect on β-cell function is associated with lowering of glucotoxicity, weight loss, insulin resistance, and improvement

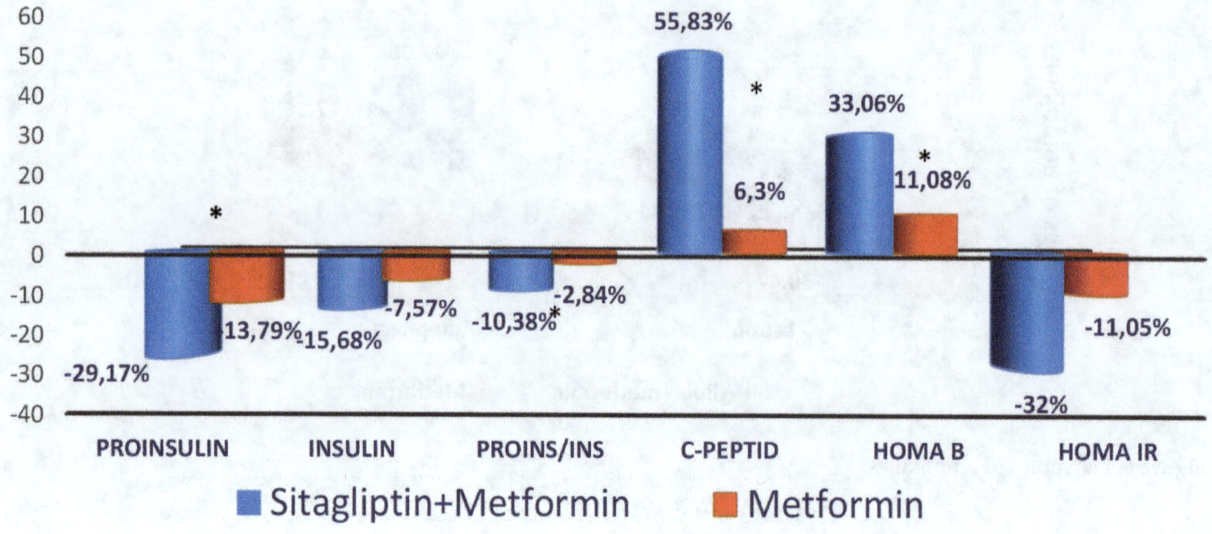

Figure 7. Function of β-cells of the pancreas and HOMA IR in dynamics. *P between groups <0.05.

in metabolic health, which promoted lowering of the "stress" on the insular apparatus of the pancreas. β-cell function improvement is promising in stabilization of T2D progression.

The results of the correlation analysis are displayed in **Table 2** and in **Figure 8**.

Thus, as can be seen from the correlation analysis, an additional therapeutic effect on glycemic control in patients with T2D and obesity is associated with a decrease in the amount of visceral fat and a change in the secretion of adipose tissue hormones. **Table 3** presents a comparative analysis of the main parameters, depending on the type of therapy.

Показатели, динамика	Адипонектин	Лептин
HbA1c	r = −0.39*	r = 0.32*
VF	r = −0.54*	r = 0.33*
body mass	r = −0.75**	r = 0.45**
BMI	r = −0.74**	r = 0.45**
WC	r = −0.62**	r = 0.43**
LDL	r = −0.29**	r = 0.3**
TG	r = −0.33**	r = 0.16
HOMA IR	r = −0.53**	r = 0.37**
HOMA β	r = 0.29**	r = −0.33**
Leptin	r = −0.63*	—

*p < 0.01 significance of correlation coefficient at p < 0.01.
**p < 0.05 significance of correlation coefficient at p < 0.05.

Table 2. Correlation analysis.

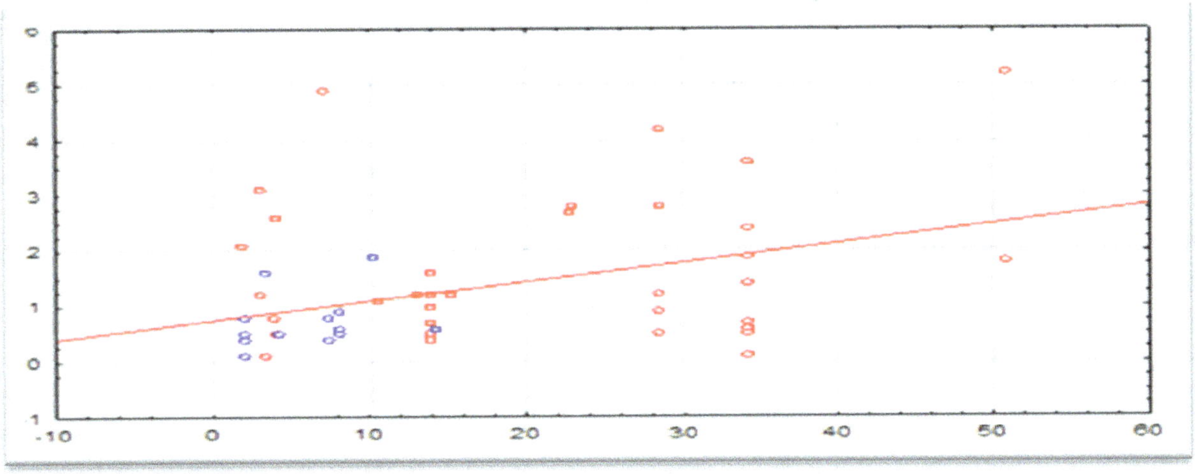

Figure 8. Correlation between the dynamics of the VF and HbA1c.

Parameters	Group 1, Sitagliptin + metformin		Group 2, Metformin		P between groups
	Before treatment	After treatment	Before treatment	After treatment	
HbA1c	8.3 ± 1.66	6.66 ± 1.24	8.35 ± 1.75	7.62 ± 1.39	<0.001
BMI, kg/m^2	34.78 ± 4.87	32.96 ± 5.04	35.45 ± 4.3	34.76 ± 4.33	<0.001
Adiponectin, mkg/ml	7.63 ± 2.56	9.59 ± 3.03	7.41 ± 2.43	7.9 ± 2.44	<0.001
Leptin, ng/ml	23.87 ± 13.43	16.49 ± 9.63	23.87 ± 9.61	22.66 ± 9.61	<0.001
VF, sm^2	300.73 ± 80.88	280.11 ± 84.16	334.62 ± 70.55	328.85 ± 70.4	<0.001
SF, sm2	375.88 ± 91.55	371.37 ± 98.04	431.25 ± 54.13	429.3 ± 54.52	>0.05
LDL, mmol/l	4.31 ± 0.73	3.53 ± 0.58	3.89 ± 0.61	3.51 ± 0.61	<0.001
TG, mmol/l	4.28 ± 2.4	2.95 ± 1.73	4.31 ± 2.04	3.68 ± 1.86	<0.05
HOMA-IR	5.85 ± 4.15	3.49 ± 2.44	6.32 ± 5.0	4.32 ± 2.77	>0.05
HOMA-β	40.63 ± 25.99	64.04 ± 29.01	57.05 ± 35.43	61.91 ± 30.82	<0.005

Table 3. Comparative characteristics of the main parameters depending on the type of therapy.

8. Discussion

The study investigates the effect of Sitagliptin in combination with metformin as well as of metformin monotherapy on carbohydrate and fat metabolism in patients who required their therapy to be intensified. According to the data received, after 24 weeks, the positive dynamics of HbA1c was followed by a significant decrease in mean fasting glycemia and postprandial glycemia in group I, while in group II (on metformin monotherapy), the decrease in glycemia did not reach statistical significance. An important advantage in our study was that, despite the common belief about neutral effect that DPP-4 inhibitors have on weight, we demonstrated that with the addition of Sitagliptin to metformin, there was a more marked weight loss and decrease of BMI and visceral fat depot, compared to the group of patients on metformin monotherapy. What was a "pure" contribution of DPP-4 inhibitor + metformin combination, and what was due to lifestyle changes in both groups could not be determined in this work, therefore, further prospective studies including quantitative calculation of energy inputs are required. The study of adipokine status, specifically leptin and adiponectin, was of particular interest. The main function of leptin is forming a communication pathway link between adipocytes and the brain [19]. Leptin secretion positively correlates with the amount of adipose tissue, which we also demonstrated in our work. In addition to the anorectic effect in the adjustment of eating behavior, leptin also stimulates energy intake. During increased energy intake exceeding the body's requirements, the leptin level increases, which prevents further food consumption and increases energy expenditure, and that leads to negative energy balance and rebalancing of energy. Most obese patients have high leptin levels, but this does not lead to weight loss, which confirms the fact that obese patients may develop resistance to leptin. Leptin's effect disorder in obesity can be a leading factor in the development of insulin resistance and fat and glucose metabolism disorder. In our work, on a background of combined Sitagliptin and metformin therapy, the leptin level was reduced by 30.47% and in the metformin monotherapy group by 5.41%. We associate decrease in leptin level with weight loss and a decrease in the amount of fat.

In both study groups, the initial adiponectin levels were lower than reference values. After 24 weeks of therapy, adiponectin content in blood increased by 27.06% in the group receiving Sitagliptin and metformin combination, and by 7.16% in the group receiving metformin monotherapy. Adiponectin with its effect on the reduction of insulin resistance, which is characteristic of patients with T2D and obesity, and also its anti-inflammatory, antidiabetic and antisclerotic effects make it an additional therapeutic target. In our study, an increase of adiponectin is most likely associated with a decrease of body weight and VFA, according to the data of the correlation analysis. However, there are publications which make it known that GLP-1 promotes an increase in adiponectin level [20, 21], the Sitagliptin therapy was followed by increase in adiponectin level [22, 23].

Correlational analysis demonstrated correlation of glycemic control in T2D obese patients with reducing visceral fat amount and with recovery of secretion of adipose tissue hormones.

In addition, the study showed a significant improvement in the functional activity of pancreatic β-cells against combined Sitagliptin and metformin therapy, which was confirmed by an increase in the HOMA-β index, a decrease in the ratio of proinsulin/insulin, in contrast to metformin monotherapy, where the change in these indices did not reach statistical significance. A possible mechanism for improving the function of β-cells can be a decrease in lipotoxicity, against a background of a decrease in the level of TG inhibiting β-cell function.

9. Conclusion

Our study demonstrated the important role of correction of fat metabolism disorders in improving glycemic control in patients with diabetes and obesity. Regression of visceral fat according to the MRI results was accompanied by the recovery of levels of adipokine hormones, which led to an improvement in the parameters of carbohydrate and fat metabolism. Contrary to common belief, we consider Sitagliptin as a drug that promotes weight loss. The chapter demonstrates that ultimately it is the reduction of the visceral depot that plays a key role in the correction of carbohydrate metabolism disorders. The parameters of the lipid profile and glycemic control are significantly improved as the pathogenetic effect on patient's body weight as well as on the structure of its adipose tissue. Recovery of such indicators as HOMA-IR and HOMA-β proves the possibility of disease management by correcting disorders of fat metabolism in patients with T2D and obesity in the early stages.

Information regarding funding and conflict of interest

The study has been performed at the personal expense of the authors. The authors claim that there is no conflict of interest regarding data disclosed in the article.

List of abbreviations

DM	diabetes mellitus
IR	insulin resistance
DPP-4	dipeptidyl peptidase type 4
GLP	glucagon-like peptide
BM	body mass
BMI	body mass index
HbA1c	glycated hemoglobin
GF	glucose fasting
PPG	postprandial glycemia
VF	visceral fat
VFA	visceral fat area
SFA	subcutaneous fat area
MRI-MPT	

WC	waist circumference
HC	hip circumference
TCH	total cholesterol
LDL	low-density lipoproteins
HDL	high-density lipoproteins
TG	triglycerides

Author details

Alexander S. Ametov and Dinara G. Gusenbekova*

*Address all correspondence to: drdinara@yandex.ru

Russian Medical Academy of Postgraduate Education, Moscow, Russian Federation

References

[1] Dedov II. Novel technologies for the treatment and prevention of diabetes mellitus and its complications. Diabetes mellitus. 2013;**3**:4-10

[2] Van Genugten R. Moller-Goede D, van Raatle D, et al. Extra-pancreatic effects of incretin-based therapies: Potential benefit for cardiovascular-risk management in type 2 diabetes. Diabetes, Obesity and Metabolism. 2013;**7**:593-606

[3] Jose T, Inzucchi S. Cardiovascular effects of the DPP-4 inhibitors. Diabetes and Vascular Disease Research. 2012;**2**:109-116

[4] Satoh-Asahara N, Sasaki Y, Wada H, et al. A dipeptidyl peptidase-4 inhibitor, sitagliptin, exerts anti-inflammatory effects in type 2 diabetic patients. Metabolism. 2013;**3**:347-351

[5] Derosa G, Ragonesi P, Fogaria E, et al. Sitagliptin added to previously taken anti-diabetic agents on insulin resistance and lipid profile: a two years study evaluation. Fundamental & Clinical Pharmacology. 2012;**2**:221-229

[6] Aschner P, Kipnes M, Lunceford J, et al. Effect of the dipeptidyl peptidase-4 inhibitor sitagliptin as monotherapy on glycemic control in patients with type 2 diabetes. Diabetes Care. 2006;**12**:2632-2637

[7] Aschner P, Katzeff H, Guo H, et al. Efficacy and safety of monotherapy of sitagliptin compared with metformin in patients with type2 diabetes. Diabetes Obesity and Metabolism. 2010;**3**:252-261

[8] Aschner P et al. Insulin glargine versus sitagliptin in insulin-naïve patients with type 2 diabetes mellitus uncontrolled on metformin (EASIE): A multicenter randomized open-label trial. The Lancet. 2012;**9833**:2262-2269

[9] Derosa G, Carbone A, Franzetti I. Effects of a combination of sitagliptin plus metformin vs metformin monotherapy on glycemic control, β-cell function and insulin resistance in type 2 diabetic patients. Diabetes Research and Clinical Practice. 2012;**1**:51-60

[10] Hong E, Khang A, Yoon J, et al. Comparison between sitagliptin as add-on therapy to insulin and insulin dose-increase therapy in uncontrolled Korean type 2 diabetes: CSI study. Diabetes, Obesity, Metabolism. 2012;**9**:795-802

[11] Vilsbøll T, Rosenstock J, Yki-Järvinen H, et al. Efficacy and safety of sitagliptin when added to insulin therapy in patients with type 2 diabetes. Diabetes Obesity Metabolism. 2010;**2**:167-177

[12] Xu L, Man C, Charbonnel B, et al. Effect of sitagliptin, a dipeptidyl peptidase-4 inhibitor, on beta-cell function in patients with type 2 diabetes: a model-based approach. Diabetes Obesity Metabolism. 2008;**12**:1212-1220

[13] Migoya E, Bergeron R, Miller J, et al. Dipeptidyl peptidase-4 inhibitors administered in combination with metformin result in an additive increase in the plasma concentration of active GLP-1. Clinical Pharmacology & Therapeutics. 2010;**6**:801-808

[14] Ametov AS, Pakus EN. Efficacy and safety of metformin-sitagliptin combination for the treatment of patients with diabetes mellitus and obesity. Diabetes Mellitus. 2010;**3**:62-64

[15] Lamers D, Famulla S, Wronkowitz N, et al. Dipeptidyl peptidase 4 is a novel adipokine potentially linking obesity to the metabolic syndrome. Diabetes. 2011;**7**:1917-1925

[16] Sell H, Matthias B. Kloting N, et al. Adipose dipeptidyl peptidase-4 and obesity: Correlation with insulin resistance and depot-specific release from adipose tissue in vivo and in vitro. Diabetes Care. 2013;**12**:4083-4090

[17] Seck T, Nauck M, Sheng D. Safety and efficacy of treatment with sitagliptin or glipizide in patients with type 2 diabetes inadequately controlled on metformin: A 2-year study. International Journal of Clinical Practice. 2010;**5**:562-576

[18] Klebanova EM, Balabolkin MI. Hormones of adipose tissue and their role in the pathogenesis of diabetes mellitus type 2. Lechashchii vrach. 2010;**11**:27

[19] Ametov AS. Diabetes type 2: Problems and solutions. Vol. 2. 3rd ed. Moscow. p. 37-41. 2015

[20] Pocai A, Carrington P, Adams J, et al. Glucagon-like peptide 1/glucagon receptor dual agonism reverses obesity in mice. Diabetes. 10-2009:2258-2266

[21] Kim Ch, Hosaka T, Yoshida M, et al. Exendin-4, a GLP-1 receptor agonist, directly induces adiponectin expression through protein kinase A pathway and prevents inflammatory adipokine expression. Biochemical and Biophysical Research Communications. 2009;**3**:613-618

[22] Nomura S, Omoto S, Taniura T, et al. Anti-atherosclerotic effects of sitagliptin in patients with type 2 diabetes mellitus. Diabetes, Metabolic Syndrome and Obesity: Targets and Therapy. 2015;**339**

[23] Nagao H, Kashine S, Nishizawa H, et al. Vascular complications and changes in body mass index in Japanese type 2 diabetic patients with abdominal obesity. Cardiovascular Diabetology. 2013;**1**:88

8

Molecular Signal Integration of Aging and Diabetes Mellitus

Irina Sarvilina

Abstract

DM is considered as the cause of accelerated aging. Numerous biomedical studies have proved the key role of neuroimmune-endocrine interactions in the human body, which trigger the universal molecular pathways in the development of aging and DM (GH/IGF-1, Ras-MAPK, FOXO3A, sirtuin, mTOR, CETP, Timeless gene, TZAP pathways). Modern methods of proteomic and bioinformatic analysis allow us to investigate key genomic-proteomic interactions that underlie diabetic nephropathy (DN) in patients with type 2 DM. The study of the formation and development of DN can become the model for studying molecular pathways of aging of kidney tissue. Future biomedical research based on methods of high-throughput screening (HTS) of a pool of target molecules will lead to great advances in the diagnosis of aging stages and DM, as well as the development of methods for the prevention and therapy of accelerated aging of the human body and various violations of carbohydrate metabolism (1D-2D/MALDI-TOF-MS, HTS, biochips, biosensors).

Keywords: aging, diabetes mellitus, pathway, gene expression, proteomics

1. Introduction

The latest data show that the prevalence of diabetes mellitus (DM) in the world has increased more than in two times, peaking at 415 million by the end of 2015 [1]. In accordance with the current evaluation of the International Diabetes Federation, 642 million patients will be with DM by 2040 [2]. Increased incidence of DM caused the adoption of the United Nations (UN) resolution 61/225 dated 20 December 2006 about DM. In the 2011, political declaration was adopted by the UN to the national healthcare systems to create a multidisciplinary strategy in the area of prevention and control of noninfectious diseases, where particular attention is drawn to the problem of DM as one of the leading causes of disability and mortality [3].

There is significant increase of the prevalence of DM in the Russian Federation. According to the Federal Register of Diabetes Mellitus, at the end of 2016, 4.35 million outpatients with DM (3% of the total population) were registered in Russia, of whom 92% (4 million people) had type 2 DM, 6% (255,000 people) - type 1 DM and 2% (75,000 people) -other types of DM. Actual number of patients with DM remains underestimated, since only identified and reported cases are considered. The results of the large-scale Russian epidemiological study NATION confirmed that only 50% of type 2 DM cases are diagnosed. Actual number of patients with DM can be at least 8-9 million people (about 6% of the population) in Russia [4]. Because of the lack of timely diagnostics of DM, some patients do not receive necessary therapy and have higher risk of the developing of such complications of DM as retinopathy, nephropathy, ischemic heart disease, cerebral ischemia, peripheral angiopathy. These complications are responsible for most cases of disability and mortality of DM.

Today, DM is considered as the cause of accelerated aging [5]. Twenty percent of middle-aged people and 35% of the population of older persons are characterized by varying degrees of impaired glucose tolerance (IGT) and symptoms of insulin resistance. An increase in the frequency of obesity and sedentary lifestyle and the major risk factors for type 2 DM suggests that the prevalence of DM in the world will increase. The management of this disease becomes difficult for persons aged 60, 70 and 80 years. The risk of complications, such as ischemic heart disease, increases with age, as well as damage with age of organs of vision, hearing and physical activity, can amplify in the presence of DM.

The modern stage of the development of researches in the field of DM and aging is interrelated and involves the use of unified technological platforms for molecular diagnostics and pharmacology of stages of aging and DM. Unified technological platforms presuppose the performing of comparative genomic and proteomic studies, the results of which allow to study interrelated pathogenesis of aging and DM. Also new technological platforms are necessary for the development of new prophylaxis and treatment of these interconnected pathological states. The analysis of data from comparative genomic and proteomic studies allows the formation of unified molecular pathological pathways of DM and aging. The chapter presents new technological platforms for the early identification and the development of anti-aging and anti-diabetic agents.

2. Neuroimmune and neuroendocrine communications: aging, metabolic syndrome and diabetes mellitus

Aging is a universal factor for metabolic and immune disorders in humans and related diseases, including DM [6]. So, analysis of the reciprocal effect of neuroendocrine factors and immunological processes at the system level, human organs and tissues is very important. It is the basis for the development of processes of aging and the emergence of DM formation of mechanisms at cellular and molecular levels.

The maintenance of the homeostasis of nervous and immune systems is carried out by comparable number of cellular elements. The integration of nervous and immune systems is due

of DM development. Lipostatic theory postulates the existence of a feedback mechanism between the amount of fat stored by the body, nutritional behavior and fat burning.

The theory predicts the presence of chemical signal produced in adipose tissue, which controls food behavior, physical and metabolic activity [31]. In 1994, leptin was discovered, that is, produced by adipocytes, moves with blood to the brain and acts on the hypothalamic receptors, suppressing the appetite [32]. Decreased leptin concentration leads to the development of obesity and is considered as one of the factors of the pathogenesis of type 2 DM. There is an increased level of cortisol, heat release, the restriction of growth, the lack of reproductive function, unlimited appetite and insulin resistance in mice with the ob/ob genotype. Leptin receptors belong to the family of cytokine receptors of class 1 and are present in the hypothalamus, fatty tissue, liver, skeletal muscles, pancreas, ovaries, prostate, placenta, kidneys and lungs. Leptin reaches the arcuate nuclei of the hypothalamus, interacts with its receptors in centers of hunger and satiety and reduces appetite. The binding of leptin activates the release of adrenaline, which increases the level of cAMP and the activity of protein kinase A through the adrenergic α-3 receptors, and triggers the synthesis of thermogenin, which converts mitochondria of adipocytes into unconjugated state [33].

In the arcuate nuclei of the hypothalamus, energy consumption is controlled by two types of neurons: orexigenic neurons stimulate the appetite by producing and releasing neuropeptide Y (NPY), which acts on the next neuron sending the brain a signal to eat. The concentration of NPY in the blood rises during fasting. It is the high level of peptide NPY that causes obesity in mice od/od and db/db [34]. Anorexigenic neurons of arcuate nuclei of the hypothalamus produce α-melanocyte-stimulating hormone (α-MSH). The release of α-MSH results in the next neuron sending a signal to the brain to stop eating. Mutations in the melanocortin receptor, which is expressed in the brain cells and plays a role in the regulation of appetite, lead to the appearance of obesity and type 2 DM [35]. Insulin acts on the hypothalamic receptors, suppressing appetite by inhibiting the release of NPY by the orexigenic neurons and also stimulating the production of MCH by anorexigenic receptors, reducing food intake and increasing thermogenesis. Leptin makes the liver and muscle cells more sensitive to insulin.

Adiponectin—a protein, consisting of 224 amino acids, is encoded by the ADIPOQ gene and secreted by adipocytes under the action of insulin. Adiponectin regulates energy homeostasis, has anti-inflammatory and anti-atherogenic effects. Its level decreases with obesity and is associated with glucose metabolism. Adiponectin increases the absorption of fatty acids by myocytes and the rate of β-oxidation of fatty acids in muscles, blocks the synthesis of fatty acids and gluconeogenesis in hepatocytes and stimulates the absorption and metabolism of glucose in muscles and the liver. These effects of adiponectin are provided by increasing the level of cAMP and activating cAMP-dependent protein kinase. A low level of adiponectin is characteristic for obesity, DM and cardiovascular diseases [36]. The similarity of adiponectin to TNF-α was found.

TNF-α is one of the key pro-inflammatory cytokines, secreted by macrophages and released by adipose tissue cells. One of the main targets of TNF-α is the adipocytes themselves, where it blocks the transcription of several genes and activates the expression of others. These effects can lead to insulin resistance, chronic inflammation with systemic consequences for the body. Many genes transcribed by TNF-α are activated by the transcription factor in NF-κB adipose tissue cells.

The peroxisome proliferator-activated receptors (PPARs) alter gene expression, affecting the metabolism of fats and carbohydrates in response to changes in lipid levels in food. Ligands of these transcription factors are fatty acids and their derivatives. PRAPs act on the nucleus of the cell by forming heterodimers with another nuclear receptor—retinoid X receptor (RXR) that binds to regulatory regions of DNA. PPARs include genes necessary for β-oxidation of fatty acids and the formation of ketone bodies during fasting and stimulate the expression of genes encoding proteins that provide β-oxidation and dissipation of energy due to the formation of mismatched mitochondria. In mice with non-functioning receptor, leptin-activated PPAR-γ prevents the development of obesity by stimulating the synthesis of proteins involved in the cleavage of fatty acids and thermogenesis [37].

Ghrelin is a peptide hormone consisting of 28 amino acids produced by P/D1 cells of mucous membrane of the fundus of the stomach. Ghrelin receptors are expressed by neurons in the arcuate nucleus and ventromedial hypothalamus, here the processes associated with the action of ghrelin are mediated: stimulation of the production of releasing hormones, increased appetite, changes in the level of glucose and lipid metabolism, regulation of secretion and contractions of walls of the gastrointestinal tract [38]. It stimulates the release of GH. The concentration of ghrelin in the blood increases before eating and falls immediately after its intake. The concentration of ghrelin in the blood plasma increases with age, which contributes to weight gain in people as they age [39].

Consequently, numerous biomedical studies have proved the key role of neuroimmune-endocrine interactions in the human body, which trigger the universal molecular pathological pathways in the development of aging and DM.

3. The complex role of molecular pathways in the aging process and DM

Human body cells constantly receive signals from the body and the environment, causing processes such as damage, infection and stress. The modern field of research, called "epigenetics," explores how the environment and time affect the functioning of genes and the development, health and aging of humans. Some epigenetic changes are serious triggers for the development of DM or conditions that increase the risk of developing related DM to age. The response to internal and external signals from cells and the production of these signals occurs through biological pathways that are important for the development of aging and DM, including oxidative stress and/or cellular metabolism. Everyday millions of destructive events occur in the DNA structure, but in cells there are powerful mechanisms that protect DNA from damage, and these mechanisms remain active in old age.

Today, the goal is to sequester 100 genes in 1000 healthy elderly people, which can shed light on the inherited variability that underlies the protection of some people from aging diseases, including DM, enabling them to live a healthy life at their age. Sequencing allows researchers to determine whether the presence of mutation carrier makes the elderly more secure or more vulnerable to the effects of damaging factors. Topol et al. perform study compared genetic sequencing in healthy volunteers, aged 80 years, and persons whose death has been linked to diseases associated with aging, including type 2 DM [40]. Scientists are finding that healthy people have an extremely low probability of genetic variations associated with the development of the disease. This fact proves the idea that protective genes play major role in the successful aging people. Therefore, the identification of molecular bases of protective effect would develop similar medicines, including effective means of preventing type 2 DM. Barzilai et al. sequenced several candidate genes of centenarians, including a variant gene that modifies the mechanism of cholesterol metabolism [41]. Scientists have sequenced genes of IGF1, its receptor and have identified mutations that are unique to women aged 100 years [42]. Calorie restriction increases life span and reduces age-related deterioration of work systems and physiological responses of age-related diseases, including with the development of DM. Restriction of caloric intake in animals in the experiment leads to a decrease in the level of glucose and insulin in the blood plasma and reduces inflammatory responses and the intensity of oxidative stress.

Genetic analysis identified several genes that affect life span and associated with damage to the pituitary development, the decrease of the secretion of GH, food intake and apoptosis. The work of these genes converges in the region of the IGF-1 receptor pathway and reproduces many effects of limiting calorie intake. Although *dwarf* mice having the defect in the synthesis of GH or the IGF-1 signaling pathway are also characterized by an increase of life expectancy, people with signaling defects associated with GH are prone to the development of diseases associated with aging. One of the targets of IGF-1, the signal pathway within the cell, is the repression of proteins responsible for stress resistance, including SOD and heat shock proteins, as well as a decrease in IGF signaling can increase life expectancy by increasing the expression of genes responsible for stress resistance. The mutation of the receptor to IGF-1, a phosphorylation target (p66 Shc), also increases the life span without affecting other organs and systems. When Shc is activated, the levels of intracellular oxygen radicals increase, suppressing the factor FKHRL1, which is involved in apoptosis (**Figure 1**).

Let us consider the scheme of molecular pathological pathway insulin/IGF-1 in humans, where mechanisms of aging and the appearance of type 2 DM are converging.

IGF-1 and IGF-1R provide the activity of proliferative signaling system that stimulates growth in many cell types and blocks apoptosis. In vivo, IGF-1 acts as an immediate response to effects of many growth factors and GH. One of the components of IGF-1, mitogenic signaling, is associated with the tyrosine kinase receptor via Shc, Grb2 and Sos-1, activating the RAS and MAP kinase cascade (raf, Mek, Erk). The end point of the MAP kinase pathway is the modification of the activity of transcription factors, such as the activation of ELK transcription factors. The serum response factor (SRF) and AP-1 provide mitogenic activity of many growth factors. IGF-1R signals for cellular survival and growth in response to IGF-1 and IGF-2. IGF-1R activates three signaling pathways that converge on the phosphorylation process of the BAD protein and block apoptosis. The first pathological pathway is activated by the

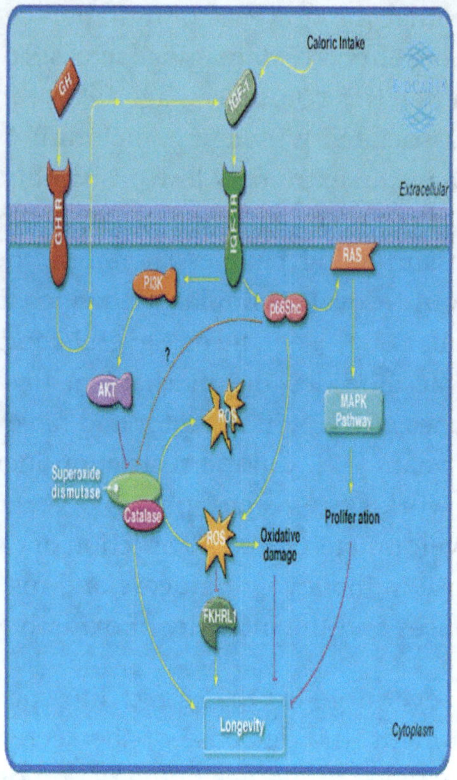

Figure 1. Scheme of participation of IGF-1-signaling in the regulation of life expectancy (database of pathways of BioCarta).

IGF-1R PI3 kinase, and the AKT signaling pathway phosphorylates BAD and blocks apoptosis. The second pathological pathway is activated by IGF-1R involving the Ras-Map-kinase pathway with the blockade of apoptosis. The third pathological pathway involves the interaction of Raf with mitochondria in the response to the activation of IGF-1R. The similarity of these pathological ways blocks apoptosis and increases the response to IGF-1R stimulation. The function of proapoptotic BAD molecule is regulated by the phosphorylation of three sites (ser 112, 136 and 155), which reduces the possibility of BAD heterodimerization by survival proteins of BCL-XL or BCL-2 cells. Phosphorylated BAA binds to 14-3-3 and is sequestered in the cytoplasm. Phosphorylation of ser-136 is associated with activation of Akt and phosphorylation of Ser-112 is due to the activation of the Ras-MAPK pathway. BAD Ser 155 is a large phosphorylation site that induces the formation of growth factors and is protected by inhibitors of protein kinase A.

It is known that FOXO3A gene prevails among long livers and probably determines longer life span, being one of the members of the family of transcription factors that mediate insulin action and resistance to stress. The relationship between polymorphisms of the FOXO3A gene and human life expectancy is presented in eight independent cohorts of centenarians [43]. Cell resistance to stress and cell survival in aging and DM may increase with high expression of the protein of the FOXO3A gene due to its effect on the activation of several members of the family of serum glucocorticoid-regulated kinases.

Genome-wide association studies (GWAS) have identified genes associated with DM and aging [44]. Most of the detected longevity genes have distant effect on one of the three molecular pathways in the cell: insulin/IGF-1, sirtuins and mTOR. In the 1980s, scientists discovered the first gene that limited the lifespan of *Caenorhabditis elegans* and called it *Age-1*. The effects of the gene *Age-1* are realized through the molecular pathway of insulin/IGF-1: when the activity of the gene *Age-1* decreases, the molecular pathway of insulin/IGF-1 decreases and the life of *C. elegans* lengthens. Recent studies have shown that in people with mutations in the pathway of insulin/IGF-1, the risk of developing DM may be reduced.

The sirtuin pathological pathway in the cell regulates the metabolism of the cell. In the 1990s, scientists from the Massachusetts Institute of Technology discovered an extrocopy of the equivalent of sirtuin, sirtuin 2, which increases the life span of yeast. mTOR pathway (mammalian target of rapamycin) plays a role in the aging processes of various organisms, controlling the rate of protein synthesis, which is important for the functioning of the cell. The inhibition of this pathway in rapamycin mice leads to an increase in life expectancy [45].

The development of DM is associated with hyperlipidemia III and IV types. An example of a gene associated with healthy aging and long life expectancy is the cholesteryl ester transfer protein gene. The homozygous variant 405VV of the *CETP* gene is associated with low concentrations of the CETP protein in the blood, high concentrations of HDL cholesterol and large HDL particles, which determines the protection of the human body from the development of DM, cardiovascular diseases and Alzheimer's disease [46].

The work of biological clock is determined by oscillatory genes and genes responsible for unidirectional movement of time (telomere activity). Oscillatory genes synchronize behavioral and biochemical processes with a day/night cycle. Telomeres, which are repetitive series of DNA sequences that form terminal regions of chromosomes, are shortened during each subsequent division of the cell. The shortened telomeres are registered in various pathological conditions associated with aging. The activity of all processes in human cells is supported by NADH and ATP, synthesized from nutrients. Limiting the intake of calories increases the level of AMP and NAD and healthy life span of animals. Silent Information Controller T1 (SIRT1), NAD-dependent deacetylase, reduces the telomere reduction process, whereas the 1α receptor activator γ, activated by the peroxisome proliferator-activated receptor γ coactivator 1α (PGC-1α), is phosphorylated by kinase AMP and deacetylated SIRT1. Thus, PGC-1α is a key component of circadian oscillator that combines human biological clock and energy metabolism. Reactive forms of oxygen, formed in conditions of genetic mutation of biological clocks, lead to an accelerated reduction of telomeres. The above-mentioned processes are described in patients with DM.

The *Timeless* gene (Tim) was found in Drosophila and encodes a protein that regulates the circadian rhythm [47]. Oscillations of mRNA and protein rhythmically occur in time as part of the work of negative coupling in the transcription-translation system involved in the work of the period (per) gene of the periodic oscillatory protein [48–50].

The timeless protein connects the cell cycle with the circadian rhythm in humans. In the model of "direct coupling," two cycles are separated by key protein, the expression of which is determined by the circadian pattern [51]. The special role of the Tim gene in creating circadian rhythm is realized with the help of the *Cry* gene in humans. The transcription of the *Cry* and *Per* genes is activated by the *CLOCK/BMAL1* complex and suppressed by the PER/CRY complex.

Timeless protein in humans (hTIM) is responsible for the production of electrical oscillations emanating from the suprachiasmatic nucleus of the hypothalamus (SCN) and determining for all circadian rhythms in the human body. This protein interacts with the key products of the activity of the oscillation genes *CLOCK, BMAL, PER1, PER2* and *PER3*. Sancar et al. investigated the role of hTIM in the work of cell cycle in humans [52]. It plays integral role in phases of G2/M and the intra-S cell cycle. In the G2/M phase of the cell cycle, hTIM binds the ATRIP subunit to the ATR protein kinase responsible for DNA damage. Binding of hTIM and ATR subsequently leads to phosphorylation of Chk1, resulting in cell cycle arrest or apoptosis. The *Timeless* gene influences to the development of human diseases. DNA damage associated with telomeres is increased in cells with reduced replication of the *Timeless* gene, along with disruption of telomere replication. Swi1 is a protein associated with the Timeless protein, which is responsible for DNA replication in the telomere region [53]. Single nucleotide polymorphism in the *Timeless* gene, which leads to the replacement of glutamine by arginine in the amino acid sequence of the protein, has not demonstrated an association with changes in morning or evening diurnal rhythms in humans [54]. The Timeless protein can be responsible for circadian rhythms in pancreatic β-cells [55]. It is believed that the Timeless protein can be identified as a kinase suppressor with Ras-1-like activity [56].

The telomeric zinc finger-associated protein (TZAP) associated with long telomeres that have low concentration of protective complex competing with TRF1 and TRF2 factors linking telomeric repeats. In telomeres, TZAP causes a purification process that leads to rapid removal of telomere repeats. The regulation of the length of telomeres in human cells has been proposed: reduced concentration of protective complex in long telomeres leads to binding of TZAP protein and initiation of telomeres purification and sets an upper limit of telomere length [57]. Telomere shortening was previously associated with the development of DM in several pilot studies and in two large studies. Zee et al. showed that telomere length was less in the study group of patients with type 2 DM than in the control group (adjusted odds ratio = 1.748) [58].

Salpea et al. performed a study in which it was found that telomere length was less in type 2 DM and this fact corresponded to a high level of oxidative stress in these patients. Short telomeres are an independent predictor of the progression of diabetic nephropathy (DN) in patients with type 1 DM in the early onset of the disease [59, 60]. Astrup et al. showed that short telomere length is the predictor of all causes of death in type 1 DM [61]. Short telomeres were detected in arterial wall cells in patients with type 1 and type 2 DM [62]. Patients with IGT demonstrated shorter telomere length compared to healthy controls, and patients with DM and severe atherosclerosis showed the presence of shorter telomeres compared with patients with DM without atherosclerosis. The presence of obesity and insulin resistance was associated with the length of telomere leukocytes in the adult population [63]. The study found direct causal relationship between telomerase activity and insulin secretion, as well as glucose tolerance: the TERC-/- mutation showed ITG, which was caused by impaired glucose-stimulated insulin secretion from pancreatic islet cells due to a decrease in pancreatic cell size and replication damage of producing insulin β-cells [64].

Klass showed that the life expectancy of *C. elegans* could vary with the presence of the mutation of the *Age-1* gene, and this effect is associated with caloric restriction [65]. Later,

Johnson showed that life expectancy increased to 65% due to the mutation of the *Age-1* gene to greater extent than caloric restriction [66]. The *Age-1* gene encodes catalytic subunit of class I phosphatidylinositol 3-kinase (PI3K). Ten years after Johnson's research, the analysis of the *daf-2* gene was performed, and Cynthia Kenyon demonstrated an increase in the half-life of *C. elegans* [67].

Despite the fact that long livers can be characterized by unique set of genes, future biomedical research based on methods of high-performance screening of a pool of target molecules will lead to great advances in the diagnosis of aging stages and DM, as well as the development of methods for the prevention and therapy of accelerated aging of the human body and various violations of carbohydrate metabolism.

4. New technological platform for diagnostic and predictive pharmacology of aging stages and diabetes mellitus

Research in the field of aging and diabetology is related to recent discoveries in genomics and proteomics, new analytical equipment allows identifying biomarkers of aging and DM, the development of new drugs occurs through high-throughput screening of target molecules in human body [68].

At present, we have created unified technology platform for diagnostics and predictive pharmacology of aging and DM, taking into account interdisciplinary approach, including complex solution of problems of genomics, proteomics and metabolomics in the range of universal molecular pathways [69].

The technological platform for diagnostics and predictive pharmacology of DM includes three components taking into account a unique instrument base:

- *Scientific component*: Search for target biomarkers (α-β-subunit of insulin receptor, tyrosine kinase, MEK1/2-MAPK-cascade, Shc-Grb2-SOS-Ras–Raf mitogen, atypical isoforms of protein kinases, molecular cascade of GH/IGF-1, etc.) with aging and DM as the basis for a new level of diagnosis; the development of cellular technologies in the treatment of DM in combination with the development of new drugs based on targeted biomarkers; *in vitro* and *in vivo* studies of individual PK processes of drugs for the prevention of aging and treatment of DM; combining information on phenotypic manifestations of drug effects on the basis of pharmacoproteomic profile with the results of PK studies; PK/PD modeling; personalization of therapy for stages of aging and each type of DM.
- *Technological component*: New methods of genomic, proteomic, pharmacokinetic, pharmacoprotein, pharmacogenomic studies; biomodeling; software on bioinformatics and for the registration of ADR; methods of visualization of molecular PD effects of drugs in biological fluids and body tissues; creation of bank of biosamples.
- *Medical component*: The introduction of technological platform for molecular diagnostics and drug monitoring in aging and DM, diagnostic of ADR, new biomolecular methods

of control and prevention of aging and complications of DM in the clinic; clinical trials of drugs; economic evaluation of the platform.

Methods of genomic and proteomic analysis of human biosamples at various stages of aging and aging-related DM are used most widely in biomedical research (**Figure 2**).

Modern systems for high-throughput screening (HTS) of molecules in cellular structures (for Image-Based High Content Screening, High Content Analysis and High Content Imaging) allow to investigate the proliferation and cytotoxicity, cell viability, cell cycles, the expression of nuclear, cytoplasmic proteins and plasma membrane proteins, mitochondrial mass, phospholipidosis, signaling pathways, the increase and the decrease of nuclear sizes, apoptosis and fragmentation of nuclei. These systems allow performing complex analysis of cellular structures in real time, obtaining universal biological information about the development of aging processes and related diseases at the molecular level in the cell. Model of diabetic cardiomyopathy has been developed with the help of Operetta High Content Screening (Perkin Elmer, UK)—the system of high-performance screening of cell structures. The ways of pharmacological influence on the key targets of the development of this complication of DM have been developed. The model of this state in vitro was developed taking into account reproduced environmental conditions and genetic factors from human pluripotent stem cells of cardiomyocytes.

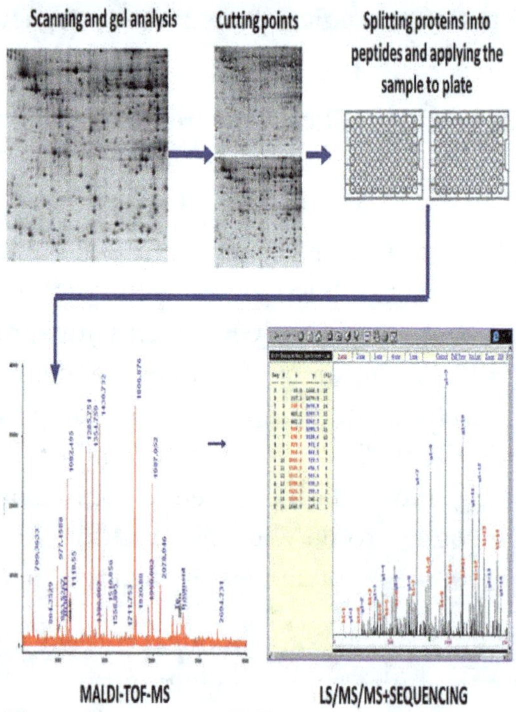

Figure 2. Molecular pattern of patient's biosample, obtained by methods of proteomic analysis (two-dimensional polyacrylamide gel electrophoresis, MALDI-TOF-MS, HPLC / MS / MS).

Biochemistry of DM was obtained, which stimulates the development of the phenotype of cardiomyopathy and which allowed us to analyze structural and functional changes in cardiomyocytes. The cardiomyopathic phenotype was reproduced definitively in specific cells of patients and determined by the initial clinical status. *In vitro* model was included in the stages of screening platform that identifies drugs that prevent the development of the phenotype of cardiomyopathy [70].

Thus, the current stage in the development of biomedical research in the field of aging and DM is associated with the introduction of new technology platform for HTS of molecules in human cells and the pharmacology of the aging stages and all types of DM.

The newest biomedical tools of the twenty-first century are biological microchips (biochips, DNA microarrays). Developed biological microchips make it possible to realize in an accessible form very complex integrative approaches of genomics, proteomics and selomics. An important medical application of biochips is the early diagnosis of DM and the development of new therapy, as well as the correlation of diagnostic markers of DM with diagnostic markers of stages of aging of the human body. Researchers conduct on-chip simultaneous analysis of tens of thousands of genes and compare the expression of these genes in healthy and diseased cells. Biochips are also an indispensable tool for biomedical research, which can in one experiment recognize the influence of various factors (drugs, proteins, nutrition) on the work of tens of thousands of genes. The effectiveness of biochips is due to the possibility of parallel carrying out a huge number of specific reactions and interactions of molecules of biopolymers, such as DNA, proteins and polysaccharides, with each other and low molecular ligands. The task is to quickly and effectively determine the concentration of the desired compound, for example, glucose for people with DM.

The use of protein chips for search of markers of aging and DM is promising direction. The following two tasks are of particular interest: simultaneous qualitative and quantitative determination of large number of proteins in cells of various tissues or in various functional states; study of interactions of cellular proteins with each other and other cellular ligands (DNA, low molecular compounds).

Bioelectronic devices are able to raise the quality of medical analyzes to new level, they will contribute to a one-stage definition of stages of aging and early diagnosis of DM.

Highly sensitive oligonucleotide microarrays were used to evaluate mRNA levels and identify transcriptional profiles of fibroblast cultures obtained from donors of different ages. The mRNA levels were measured in actively dividing fibroblasts isolated from young, middle-aged and elderly patients, as well as patients with progeria. The study identified genes, the expression of which is associated with phenotypes of different age groups and diseases. The aging process is based on a mechanism that includes an increasing number of errors in the mitosis of dividing cells at the post-productive stage of human life [71].

The progress and development of biosensors used in the clinic was related to the development of glucose biosensor in the 1960s and obtained on the basis of early integration of the redox enzyme glucose oxidase with an oxygen electrode [72]. New materials, sensory configurations and technical innovations have been proposed for the determination of glucose [73–75]. Currently, glycemic control is based on the study of blood glucose, which still requires frequent blood sampling with a certain degree of inconvenience. Despite the intensive application of the existing method of blood glucose testing, precise monitoring of glucose fluctuations during the day cannot yet be performed. Therefore, today, subcutaneous biosensors are used, which measure glucose periodically during the day [76, 77]. However, the creation of an accurate implantable biosensor for glucose, acceptable for patients with DM, is an open question. Today, the most promising results were obtained on biosensors, which are based on amperometric detection of hydrogen peroxide formed by enzymes immobilized on electrodes. Updike et al. created a biosensor for glucose, implanted subcutaneously, with maximum duration of up to 5 months [78].

Interstitial levels of lactate should reflect its systemic level when hypoxia appears in the tissues. There is an opportunity to control lactate *in vivo* in the interstitium; however, it is difficult to introduce monitoring methods into the clinic because of their unreliability due to the influence on the level of lactate of a lot of endogenous factors. Several types of biosensors for the determination of lactate are presented in the literature. A microfluidic biochip was developed, which is integrated with a highly sensitive fiber-optic biosensor of glucose. Experimental results showed that the biochip determines an ultra-low glucose concentration (1 nM) [79]. Due to the fact that DM as an aging-related disease progresses and due to complex and stepwise processes of malfunctioning of the pancreatic β-cells at the molecular level that can be registered in the blood, early detection of DM requires the use of supersensitive systems for detecting molecular changes. To this end, a protein microchip was developed, including the use of polyfluorophor technology. The innovative system is characterized by high sensitivity: the possibility of the determining of biomarkers at the level of femtograms in 10 μl of the biosample is 92% within 10 minutes [80].

It is believed that the stages of aging and related diseases, including DM, are characterized by their bar code—a change in the level of transcription of a set of genes specific for this disease. It is assumed that in the future, according to the barcode, changes in the expression in particular set of genes can be diagnosed with specific diseases and the stages of their development and, consequently, develop targeted treatment regimen.

At present, bioinformatics is ready to provide data about tens of thousands of new drug targets, predicting the function of genes and deciphering the sequence of proteins. Promising bioinformatic developments are presented in such sections of medicine as gerontology and diabetology. The main directions of bioinformatics are distinguished, depending on the objects of study: sequence bioinformatics, structural bioinformatics and computer genomics. The main task of bioinformatics in the development of new drugs is to provide technologies that allow the formation of target targets for directed action of drug having specific structure for this target.

Today, an extended analysis is available, including the molecular pathways presented in most databases; so, large array of information about altered proteins can be obtained, including their expression and/or post-translational modifications in molecular pathways. Comparative analysis of two web products for the analysis of pathways and intermolecular interactions—Ingenuity Pathway Analysis (IPA) and STRING—is published. Data about key proteins, participating in molecular pathological pathways (Wnt, APP, insulin signaling, mitochondrial apoptosis, tau-phosphorylation), were obtained on the basis of medical literature and data of proteomic analysis of the HEK293 cell line.

Information about protein interactions in complexes is found in databases such as MINT, BioGRID, IntAct or HRPD. It is possible to provide high percentage of predicted protein-protein interactions and interactions based on literature data (PubMed database). Widely used web resource for the analysis of inter-protein interactions STRING is not only a database but also linked to several other resources with large volume of literature sources [81]. The Cytoscape graphical tool allows us to create network interactions of high degree of complexity. Recently, web platform has been launched that integrates data on molecular pathways for the development of pathological processes and the analysis of intermolecular interactions, including six different databases (KeGG, Bio-Carta, Gene Ontology, Reactome, Wiki, NCI pathways) and interacts functionally with database on molecular activity of proteins (Interpro) and database of complex information about proteins (Corum).

Identification of the protein in the study of the biosample should be accompanied by a detailed analysis of its primary, secondary and tertiary structure, as well as its post-translational modifications and intermolecular interactions (BLAST search engine). The amino acid sequence of the protein can be analyzed in software products such as Pfam, Interpro, SMART or DAVID [82], whereas sequence analysis of post-translational protein modifications can be performed using algorithms such as MotifX or PhosphoMotif [83].

Modern methods of proteomic and bioinformatic analysis allow us to investigate key genomic-proteomic interactions that underlie DN in patients with type 2 DM. The study of the formation and development of DN can become the model for studying molecular pathways of aging of kidney tissue [84].

We carried out prospective comparative cohort study with parallel design for the search of molecular prognostic markers of DN of different stages using methods of proteomics and bioinformatic analysis on the basis of the Department of Nephrology of the Dagestan State Medical University (Makhachkala, Dagestan, Russia) and the Department of Nephrology of the Rostov State Medical University (Rostov-on-Don, Russia), MC "Novomeditsina" (Rostov-on-Don, Russia) [85]. It included 205 patients with T2DM and DN (stages 1–4). Patients corresponded to the criteria for the DN classification proposed by the Committee on Diabetic Nephropathy [86]. The duration of DN was 10.5 years. Molecular phenotyping of biosamples (urine) was processed with methods of proteomics: the prefractionation, the separation of proteins with standard sets (MB-HIC C8 Kit, MB-IMAC Cu, MB-Wax Kit, «Bruker», USA) and matrix-assisted laser desorption-ionization time-of-flight mass spectrometry (MALDI-TOF-MS/MS, Ultraflex II, «Bruker», USA). The partially identified sequences were then submitted to "BLAST protein-protein" and screened against the *Homo sapiens* Swissprot database to check if this identification matched the MASCOT-identification (Matrix Science). The data of the molecular interactions and functional features of proteins were received with STRING 10.0 database.

Protein name	Group 1 (n = 42)	Group 2 (n = 48)	Group 3 (n = 65)	Group 4 (n = 50)	Control group (n = 30)	MW (Da)	Functional process (sources: InterPro, Entrez, SWISS-PROT, NRDB, PDB, KEGG
TGF-β1	18 *PCG*-1 = 0.001	27 *PCG*-2 = 0.000	52 *PCG*-3 = 0.000	48 *PCG*-4 = 0.000	2	44,341	Pro-fibrotic and anti-inflammatory activities, the regulation of tubular EMT
E-cadherin	22 *PCG*-1 = 0.000	38 *PCG*-2 = 0.000	62 *PCG*-3 = 0.000	49 *PCG*-4 = 0.000	1	97,456	The regulation of tubular EMT; the maintenance of epithelial integrity, cell phenotype; the progression of renal fibrosis
Cystatin C	15 *PCG*-1 = 0.001	40 *PCG*-2 = 0.000	60 *PCG*-3 = 0.000	45 *PCG*-4 = 0.000	1	15,799	Cysteine proteinase inhibitor, tubular damage marker
Collagen IV	4 *PCG*-1 > 0.05	32 *PCG*-2 = 0.000	48 *PCG*-3 = 0.000	42 *PCG*-4 = 0.000	1	164,038	Constituent of mesangial matrix, marker of the phase of compromised renal filtration function
MMP 9	8 *PCG*-1 > 0.05	32 *PCG*-2 = 0.000	60 *PCG*-3 = 0.000	49 *PCG*-4 = 0.000	1	78,458	Potent modulator of ECM turnover and also of shedding of syndecans
Fibronectin	4 *PCG*-1 > 0.05	35 *PCG*-2 = 0.000	52 *PCG*-3 = 0.000	43 *PCG*-4 = 0.000	1	262,625	Adhesive glycoprotein, locally stimulated mesangial and epithelial cell production
NGAL	10 *PCG*-1 = 0.043	42 *PCG*-2 = 0.000	62 *PCG*-3 = 0.000	48 *PCG*-4 = 0.000	1	22,588	Kidney development; it loses through the damaged glomerulus, injured tubular cells produce NGAL as a compensatory mechanism against intracellular oxidative stress and complement- induced apoptosis.
Ceruloplasmin	12 *PCG*-1 = 0.006	37 *PCG*-2 = 0.000	42 *PCG*-3 = 0.000	35 *PCG*-4 = 0.000	1	122,205	Marker of damaged glomerulus

Protein name	Group 1 (n = 42)	Group 2 (n = 48)	Group 3 (n = 65)	Group 4 (n = 50)	Control group (n = 30)	MW (Da)	Functional process (sources: InterPro, Entrez, SWISS-PROT, NRDB, PDB, KEGG
β2-microglobulin	6 *PCG-1* > 0.05	37 *PCG-2* = 0.000	62 *PCG-3* = 0.000	49 *PCG-4* = 0.000	1	11,774	The indicator of incipient DN; detecting injured epithelial cells in the proximal tubules
Podocin	23 *PCG-1* = 0.000	45 *PCG-2* = 0.000	63 *PCG-3* = 0.000	49 *PCG-4* = 0.000	1	42,201	Podocyte-specific protein, interact with the PI3K/AKT-signaling pathway for maintenance of functional integrity
MCP-1	11 *PCG-1* = 0.011	39 *PCG-2* = 0.000	48 *PCG-3* = 0.000	46 *PCG-4* = 0.000	1	2583	Chemotactic factor for monocytes; regulates the memory T lymphocytes, NK cells; increases with TNFα and IL-6 in damaged kidneys

Table 1. Qualitative profile of urine proteins in T2DM patients with DN.

All changes in patients with DN are associated with a higher expression of urine proteins in the progression of epithelial-to-mesenchymal transition (EMT) and changes in the extracellular matrix (ECM) in kidneys in T2DM patients with DN (**Table 1**). Proteomic analysis helps in the detection of differences in the component composition of the urine proteins in patients with DN of varying stages compared with the control group. Molecules interact among themselves and with other molecules as participants in universal pathways in T2DM patients with DN, which are the key elements for EMT formation and changes in ECM: Smad, p38 MAPK, TLRs, Wnt, mTOR, Notch, small GTPase and Hedgehog and PI3K/AKT-signaling pathways.

Each protein molecule in the functional group interacts with other protein molecules. For example, the molecular interactions of NGAL are presented in **Figure 3**. The concentration of NGAL increases in the urine of T2DM patients with DN. The study identified the biomarkers of tubular damage that have a key role in the development and progression of DN. The research into signaling pathways and molecules that are involved in ECM formation may help in developing strategies to prevent DN. Molecular pathways for the development of DN constitute a model for the study of molecular pathways in the development of aging of kidney tissue.

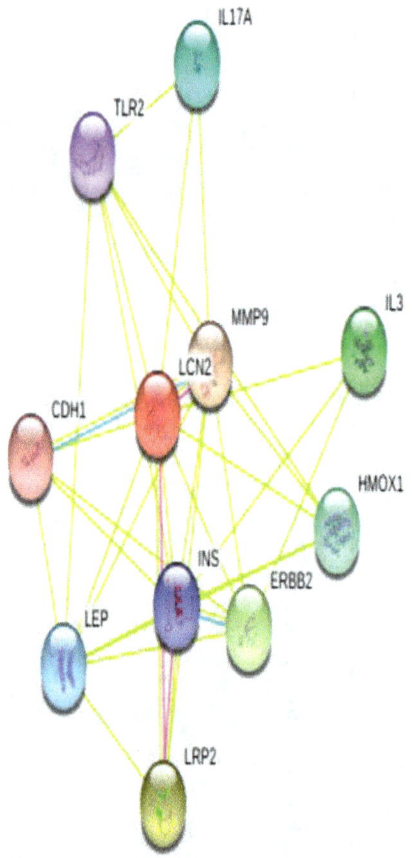

Figure 3. Molecular interactions of NGAL (STRING 10.0 database). LCN2, lipocalin-2; MMP-9, matrix metallopeptidase 9; LRP2, low density lipoprotein-related protein 2; ERBB2, erythroblastic leukemia viral oncogene homolog 2 (neuro/glioblastoma derived oncogene homolog); IL3, interleukin 3 (colony-stimulating factor, multiple); HMOX1, heme oxygenase (decycling) 1; IL-17A, interleukin 17A; LEP, leptin; INS, insulin; TLR2, toll-like receptor 2 and CDH1, cadherin 1, type 1, E-cadherin (epithelial cadherin).

Thus, the future progress in biomedical research of the aging stages of the human body and DM is associated with the development of experimental genomics, transcriptomics, proteomics and selomics and with the development of typical human development scenario, starting from the postnatal period on the basis of modern technological platforms. The development of methods for the systematic analysis of molecular interactions in cell and the subsequent study of their functional activity makes it possible to discover new pathways for the development of human pathology associated with aging.

Author details

Irina Sarvilina

Address all correspondence to: isarvilina@mail.ru

Medical Centre "Novomeditsina,"Rostov State Medical University, Rostov-on-Don, Russia

References

[1] American Diabetes Association. Standards of medical care in diabetes. Diabetes Care. 2017;**40**(Supplement 1):S4-S5. DOI: https://doi.org/10.2337/dc17-S003

[2] International Diabetes Federation. IDF Diabetes Atlas – 7th edition. Available at: https://www.idf.org/sites/default/files/EN_6E_Atlas_Full_0.pdf [Accesed: 1 Feb 2016]

[3] Silink M. UN Resolution 61/225: 'World Diabetes Day'; A United Nations Resolution on Diabetes—The Result of a Joint Effort. US Endocrinology. 2007;**12**(1):12-14. DOI: 10.17925/USE.2007.00.1.12

[4] Dedov I, Shestakova M, Mayorov A. Standards of specialized diabetes care. Diabetes Mellitus. 2017;**20**(1S):1-112. DOI: 10.14341/DM20171S8

[5] Morley J. Diabetes and aging: Epidemiologic overview. Clinics in Geriatric Medicine. 2008;**24**(3):395-405. DOI: 10.1016/j.cger.2008.03.005. Review

[6] Ford E, Giles W, Dietz W. Prevalence of the metabolic syndrome among US adults: Findings from the third National Health and nutrition examination survey. JAMA. 2002;**287**:356-359. DOI: https://doi:10.1001/jama.287.3.356

[7] Smirnov V, Freidlin I. Immunodeficiency Conditions. St. Petersburg: Foliant; 2000. p. 568p. DOI: https://doi:10.1016/j.ijantimicag.2015.03.001

[8] Zatz M, Goldstein A. Thymosins, lymphokines, and the immunology of aging. Gerontology. 1985;**31**(4):263-277. DOI: https://doi.org/10.1159/000212709

[9] Poveshchenko A, Orlov N, Kazakov O, Poveshchenko O, Kim I, et al. Age and gender differences in cytokine profile of lymph and blood serum. Advances in Aging Research. 2014;**3**:216-221. DOI: 10.4236/aar.2014.33030

[10] Banerjee M, Saxena M. Interleukin-1 (IL-1) family of cytokines: Role in type 2 diabetes. Clinica Chimica Acta. 2012;**413**(15-16):1163-1170. DOI: 10.1016/j.cca.2012.03.021

[11] Oakley R, Cidlowski J. The biology of the glucocorticoid receptor: New signaling mechanisms in health and disease. The Journal of Allergy and Clinical Immunology. 2013;**132**(5):1033-1044. DOI: 10.1016/j.jaci.2013.09.007

[12] Doe R, Goldman P, Severson S, Hruby H. Circadian variation of cytosol glucocorticoid receptors in human polymorphonuclear leukocytes (PMN) and mononuclear cells (MN) in a normal population. Journal of Steroid Biochemistry. 1986;**25**(4):483-487. DOI: 10.1016/0022-4731(86)90391-2

[13] Miyajima A, Kinoshita T. Cytokine signaling for proliferation, survival, and death in hematopoietic cells. lnternational Journal of Hematology. 1999;**69**(3):137-146 PMID: 10222650

[14] Iranmanesh A, Lizarralde C, Jonson M, et al. Dynamics of 24-hour endogenous cortisol secrtion and clearence in primary hypothyroidism assessed before and after partial thyroid hormon re-placement. The Journal of Clinical Endocrinology and Metabolism. 1990;**70**(1):155-161. DOI: 10.1210/jcem-70-1-155

[15] Persani L, Terzolo M, Asteria C. Circadian of thyrotropin bioactivity in normal subject and patients with primary hypothyroidism. The Journal of Clinical Endocrinology and Metabolism. 1995;**80**(99):2722-2728. DOI: 10.1210/jcem.80.9.7673415

[16] Ooka H, Fujita S, Yoshimoto E. Pituitary-thyroid activity and longevity in neonatally thyroxine-treated rats. Mechanisms of Ageing and Development. 1983;**22**:113-120. DOI: https://doi.org/10.1016/0047-6374(83)90104-5

[17] Ooka H, Shinkai T. Effects of chronic hyperthyroidism on the lifespan of the rat. Mechanisms of Ageing and Development. 1986;**33**:275-282 3713266

[18] Hauck S, Hunter W, Danilovich N, Kopchick J, Bartke A. Reduced levels of thyroid hormones, insulin, and glucose, and lower body core temperature in the growth hormone receptor/binding protein knockout mouse. Experimental Biology and Medicine (Maywood, N.J.). 2001;**226**:552-558 PMID: 11395925

[19] Rozing M, Westendorp R, de Craen A, et al. Leiden longevity study (LLS) group. Low serum free triiodothyronine levels mark familial longevity: The Leiden longevity study. Journal of Gerontology Series A: Biological Sciences and Medical Sciences. 2010;**65**:365-368. DOI: 10.1093/gerona/glp200

[20] Han C, He X, Xia X, Li Y, Shi X, Shan Z, Teng W. Subclinical hypothyroidism and type 2 diabetes: A systematic review and meta-analysis. PLoS One. 2015;**10**(8):e0135233. DOI: 10.1371/journal.pone.0135233

[21] Moller D, Flick T. Insulin resistance—Mechanisms, syndromes, and implication. New England Journal of Medicine. 1991;**325**:938-957. DOI: 10.1056/NEJM199109263251307

[22] Rincon M, Muzumdar R, Atzmon G, Barzilai N. The paradox of the insulin/IGF-1 signaling pathway in longevity. Mechanisms of Ageing and Development. 2004;**125**:397-403. DOI: 10.1096/fj.07-9261com

[23] Van Cauter E, Roland D, Desir D. Effect of gender and age on the levels and plasma cortisol. The Journal of Clinical Endocrinology and Metabolism. 1996;**81**(7):2468-2473. DOI: 10.1210/jcem.81.7.8675562

[24] Balligand T, Kelly R, Marsden P, et al. Control muscle function by endogenous nitric oxide signaling system. Proceedings of the National Academy of Sciences of United States of America. 1993;**90**:347-351 PMCID: PMC45657

[25] Oakley R, Cidlowski JJ. The biology of the glucocorticoid receptor: New signaling mechanisms in health and disease. Journal of Allergy and Clinical Immunology. 2013;**132**(5):1033-1044. DOI: 10.1016/j.jaci.2013.09.007

[26] Adcock I. Glucocorticoid-regulated transcription factors. Pulmonary Pharmacology & Therapeutics. 2001;**14**(3):211-219. DOI: 10.1006/pupt.2001.0283

[27] Mukaida N, Gussella G, Kasahara T, Ko Y, Zachariae C, Kawai T, Matsushima K. Molecular analysis of the inhibition of interleukin-8 production by dexamethasone in a human fibrosarcoma cell line. Immunology. 1992;**75**(4):674-679 PMCID: PMC1384849

[28] Folsom A, Kaye S, Sellers T, et al. Body fat distribution and 5-year risk of death in older women. JAMA. 1993;**269**:483-487. DOI: 10.1001/jama.1993.03500040049035

[29] Sepe A, Tchkonia T, Thomou T, Zamboni M, Kirkland J. Aging and regional differences in fat cell progenitors—A mini-review. Gerontology. 2011;**57**:66-75. DOI: 10.1159/000279755 Epub 2010 Jan 29

[30] Mayer J. Glucostatic mechanism of regulation of food intake. New England Journal of Medicine. 1953;**249**(1):13-16. DOI: 10.1056/NEJM195307022490104

[31] Kennedy G. The role of depot fat in the hypothalamic control of food intake in the rat. Proceedings of the Royal Society B. 1953;**140**(901):578-596 PMID: 13027283

[32] Nelson D, Cox M. Lehninger Principles of Biochemistry. 7th edition (1942) ed. New York/Houndmills, Basingstoke: W.H. Freeman/Macmillan Learning; 2017 NLM ID: 1017 03862

[33] Sivitz W, Fink B, Donohoue P. Fasting and leptin modulate adipose and muscle uncoupling protein: Divergent effects between messenger ribonucleic acid and protein expression. Endocrinology. 1999;**140**(4):1511-1519. DOI: 10.1210/endo.140.4.6668

[34] Paeger L, Karakasilioti I, Altmüller J, Frommolt P, Brüning J, Kloppenburg P. Antagonistic modulation of NPY/AgRP and POMC neurons in the arcuate nucleus by noradrenalin. eLife. 2000;**20**:6 pii: e25770. DOI:. DOI: 10.7554/eLife.25770

[35] Joly-Amado A, Cansell C, Denis R, Delbes A, Castel J, Martinez S, Luquet S. Best Practice & Research. Clinical Endocrinology & Metabolism. 2014;**28**(5):725-737. DOI: 10.1016/j.beem.2014.03.003

[36] Chen J, Tan B, Karteris E, Zervou S, Digby J, Hillhouse E, Vatish M, Randeva H. Secretion of adiponectin by human placenta: Differential modulation of adiponectin and its receptors by cytokines. Diabetologia. 2006;**49**(6):1292-1302. DOI: 10.1007/s00125-006-0194-7

[37] Michalik L, Auwerx J, Berger J, Chatterjee V, Glass C, Gonzalez F, et al. International Union of Pharmacology. LXI. Peroxisome proliferator-activated receptors. Pharmacological Reviews. 2006;**58**(4):726-741. DOI: 10.1124/pr.58.4.5

[38] Yin Y, Li Y, Zhang W. The growth hormone secretagogue receptor: Its intracellular signaling and regulation. International Journal of Molecular Sciences. 2014;**15**(3):4837-4855. DOI: 10.3390/ijms15034837

[39] Cummings D, Purnell J, Frayo R, Schmidova K, Wisse B, Weigle DA. Preprandial rise in plasma ghrelin levels suggests a role in meal initiation in humans. Diabetes. 2001;**50**(8):1714-1719. DOI: 10.2337/diabetes.50.8.1714

[40] Erikson G, Bodian D, Rueda M, Molparia B, Scott E, Scott-Van ZA, Topol S, et al. Whole-genome sequencing of a healthy aging cohort. Cell. 2016;**165**(4):1002-1011. DOI: 10.1016/j.cell.2016.03.022

[41] Barzilai N, Atzmon G, Schechter C, Schaefer E, Cupples A, Lipton R, Cheng S, Shuldiner A. Unique lipoprotein phenotype and genotype associated with exceptional longevity. Journal of the American Medical Association. 2003;**290**(15):2030-2040. DOI: 10.1001/jama.290.15.2030

[42] Suh Y, Atzmon G, Cho M-O, Hwang D, Liu B, Leahy D, Barzilai N, Cohen P. Functionally-significant insulin-like growth factor-I receptor mutations in centenarian. Proceedings of the National Academy of Sciences. 2008;**105**(9):3438-3442. DOI: 10.1073/pnas.0705467105

[43] Barzilai N, Gabriely I, Atzmon G, Suh Y, Rothenberg D, Bergman A. Genetic studies reveal the role of the endocrine and metabolic systems in aging. The Journal of Clinical Endocrinology and Metabolism. 2010;**95**:4493-4500. DOI: 10.1210/jc.2010-0859

[44] Bush W, Moore J. Chapter 11: Genome-wide association studies. Public Library of Science for Computational Biology. 2012;**8**(12):e1002822. DOI: 10.1371/journal.pcbi.1002822

[45] Harrison D, Strong R, Sharp Z, Nelson J, et al. Rapamycin fed late in life extends lifespan in genetically heterogeneous mice. Nature. 2009;**460**(7253):392-395. DOI: 10.1038/nature08221

[46] Cellini E, Nacmias B, Olivieri F, Ortenzi L, Tedde A, Bagnoli S, Petruzzi C, Franceschi C, Sorbi S. Cholesteryl ester transfer protein (CETP) I405V polymorphism and longevity in Italian centenarians. Mechanisms of Ageing and Development. 2005;**126**(6-7):826-828. DOI: 10.1016/j.mad.2005.01.009

[47] Koike N, Hida A, Numano R, Hirose M, Sakaki Y, Tei H. Identification of the mammalian homologues of the drosophila timeless gene, Timeless1. FEBS Letters. 1998;**441**(3):427-431. DOI: 10.1016/S0014-5793(98)01597-X

[48] Hao H, Allen D, Hardin P. A circadian enhancer mediates PER-dependent mRNA cycling in *Drosophila melanogaster*. Molecular and Cellular Biology. 1997;**17**(7):3687-3693 PMCID: PMC232220

[49] Gotter A, Manganaro T, Weaver D, Kolakowski L, Possidente B, Sriram S, MacLaughlin D, Reppert S. A time-less function for mouse timeless. Nature Neuroscience. 2000;**3**(8):755-756. DOI: 10.1038/77653

[50] Young M, Kay S. Time zones: A comparative genetics of circadian clocks. Nature Reviews. Genetics. 2001;**2**(9):702-715. DOI: 10.1038/35088576

[51] Gustafson C, Partch C. Emerging models for the molecular basis of mammalian circadian timing. Biochemistry. 2015;**54**(2):134-149. DOI: 10.1021/bi500731f

[52] Unsal-Kaçmaz K, Mullen T, Kaufmann W, Sancar A. Coupling of human circadian and cell cycles by the timeless protein. Molecular and Cellular Biology. 2005;**25**(8):3109-3116. DOI: 10.1128/MCB.25.8.3109-3116.2005

[53] Gadaleta M, González-Medina A, Noguchi E. Timeless protection of telomeres. Current Genetics. 2016;**62**(4):725-730. DOI: https://doi:10.1007/s00294-016-0599-x

[54] Pedrazzoli M, Ling L, Finn L, Kubin L, Young T, Katzenberg D, Mignot EA. Polymorphism in the human timeless gene is not associated with diurnal preferences in normal adults. Sleep Research Online. 2000;**3**:73-76 PMID: 11382904

[55] Mühlbauer E, Wolgast S, Finckh U, Peschke D, Peschke E. Indication of circadian oscillations in the rat pancreas. FEBS Letters. 2004;**564**(1-2):91-96. DOI: https://doi:10.1016/S0014-5793(04)00322-9

[56] Clymer B, Fisher K, Kelly D, White M, Lewis R. Abstract 1252: TIMELESS is a KSR1-like effector of Ras-driven colon tumorigenesis. Cancer Research. 2016;**76**(14 Supplement):1252. DOI: https://doi:10.1158/1538-7445.am2016-1252

[57] Li J, Miralles F, Simavorian T, Bartocci C, Tsai J, Karlseder J, Lazzerini D. TZAP: A telomere-associated protein involved in telomere length control. Science. 2017;**355**(6325):638-641. DOI: https://doi:10.1126/science.aah6752

[58] Zee R, Castonguay A, Barton N, Germer S, Martin M. Mean leukocyte telomere length shortening and type 2 diabetes mellitus: A case-control study. Translational Research. 2010;**155**:166-169. DOI: 10.1016/j.trsl.2009.09.012

[59] Salpea K, Talmud P, Cooper J, Maubaret C, Stephens J, Abelak K, Humphries S. Association of telomere length with type 2 diabetes, oxidative stress and UCP2 gene variation. Atherosclerosis. 2010;**209**:42-50. DOI: 10.1016/j.atherosclerosis.2009.09.070

[60] Fyhrquist F, Tiitu A, Saijonmaa O, Forsblom C, Groop P. Telomere length and progression of diabetic nephropathy in patients with type 1 diabetes. Journal of Internal Medicine. 2010;**267**:278-286. DOI: 10.1111/j.1365-2796.2009.02139.x

[61] Astrup A, Tarnow L, Jorsal A, Lajer M, Nzietchueng R, Benetos A, Rossing P, Parving H. Telomere length predicts all-cause mortality in patients with type 1 diabetes. Diabetologia. 2010;**53**:45-48. DOI: 10.1007/s00125-009-1542-1

[62] Adaikalakoteswari A, Balasubramanyam M, Ravikumar R, Deepa R, Mohan V. Association of telomere shortening with impaired glucose tolerance and diabetic macroangiopathy. Atherosclerosis. 2007;**195**:83-89. DOI: 10.1016/j.atherosclerosis.2006.12.003

[63] Al-Attas O, Al-Daghri N, Bamakhramah A, Sabico S, Huang T, McTernan P. Telomere length in relation to insulin resistance, inflammation and obesity among Arab youth. Acta Paediatrica. 2010;**99**:896-899. DOI: 10.1111/j.1651-2227.2010.01720.x

[64] Kuhlow D, Florian S, von Figura G, Weimer S, Schulz N, Petzke K, Zarse K, Pfeiffer A, Rudolph K, Ristow M. Telomerase deficiency impairs glucose metabolism and insulin secretion. Aging. 2010;**2**:650-658. DOI: 10.18632/aging.100200

[65] Klass M. Aging in the nematode *Caenorhabditis elegans*: Major biological and environmental factors influencing life span. Mechanisms of Ageing and Development. 1977;**6**:413-429 PMID: 926867

[66] Friedman D, Johnson T. A mutation in the age-1 gene in *Caenorhabditis elegans* lengthens life and reduces hermaphrodite fertility. Genetics. 1988;**118**:75-86 PMCID: PMC1203268

[67] Kenyon C, Chang J, Gensch E, Rudner A, Tabtiang R. A *C. elegans* mutant that lives twice as long as wild type. Nature. 1993;**366**(6454):461-464. DOI: 10.1038/366461a0

[68] Korc M. Diabetes mellitus in the era of proteomics. Molecular & Cellular Proteomics. 2002;**2**:399-404. DOI: 10.1074/mcp.R300005-MCP200

[69] Sarvilina I, Karkistchenko V, Gorshkova Y. Interdisciplinary Research in Medicine. Tekhnosfera Publisher; ISBN 978-5-94836-149-9; 2007, 368 pp

[70] Drawnel M, Boccardo S, Prummer M, Delobel F, et al. Disease modeling and phenotypic drug screening for diabetic cardiomyopathy using human induced pluripotent stem cells faye. Cell Reports. 2014;**9**(3):810-820. DOI: 10.1016/j.celrep.2014.09.055

[71] Ly D, Lockhart D, Lerner R, Schultz P. Mitotic misregulation and human aging. Science. 2000;**287**(5462):2486-2492. DOI: https://doi:10.1126/science.287.5462.2486

[72] Clark L, Lyons C. Electrode systems for continuous monitoring in cardiovascular surgery. Annals of the New York Academy of Sciences. 1962;**102**:29-45. DOI: https://doi:10.1111/j.1749-6632.1962.tb13623.x

[73] Wisniewski N, Reichert M. Methods for reducing biosensor membrane biofouling. Colloids and Surfaces B: Biointerfaces. 2000;**18**:197-219. DOI: https://doi.org/10.1016/S0927-7765(99)00148-4

[74] Cosnier S., Szunerits S., Marks R., Novoa A. et al. A comparative physical study of two different hydrophilic synthetic latex matrices for the construction of a glucose biosensor. Europe PMC. 2001;**55**(5):889-897. PMID: 18968439

[75] Revzin A, Sirkar K, Simonian A, Glucose PM. Lactate, and pyruvate biosensor arrays based on redox polymer/oxidoreductase nanocomposite thin-films deposited on photolithographically patterned gold microelectrodes. Analytica Chimica Acta. 2002;**466**(2):201-212. DOI: https://doi.10.1021/ac991041k

[76] Gough D, Armour J, Baker D. Advances and prospects in glucose assay technology. Diabetologia. 1997;**40**:S102-S107. DOI: 10.1007/s001250051418

[77] Thome-Duret V, Reach G, Gangnerau M, Klein J, Zhang Y, Hu Y, Wilson G. Use of a subcutaneous glucose sensor to detect decreases in glucose concentration prior to observation in blood. Analytical Chemistry. 1996;**68**:3822-3826. DOI: 10.1021/ac960069i

[78] Updike S, Shults M, Gilligan B, Rhodes RA. Subcutaneous glucose sensor with improved longevity, dynamic range, and stability of calibration. Diabetes Care. 2000;**23**:208-208. DOI: https://doi:org/10.2337/diacare.23.2.208

[79] Yin M., Huang B., Ping Zhang A., Tam H-Y, Ye X-S. Integrated microfluidic biochip with nanocoating self-assembled fiber-optic sensor. 2015 IEEE 15th International Conference on Nanotechnology (IEEE-NANO). 2015. p. 858-860. DOI: https://doi:10.1109/NANO.2015.7388748

[80] Krapfenbauer K. Identification of beta cell dysfunction at the pre-symptomatic stage of diabetes mellitus by novel analytical system: Liquid biopsy measurements in femtograms. The EPMA Journal. 2017;**8**:35-41. DOI: 10.1007/s13167-017-0079-5

[81] Snel B, Lehmann G, Bork P, Huyen M. STRING: A web-server to retrieve and display the repeatedly occuring neighborhood of a gene. Nucleic Acids Research. 2000;**28**:3442-3444. DOI: 10.1093/nar/28.18.3442

[82] Punta M, Coggill P, Eberhardt R, Mistry J, Tate J, Boursnell C, Pang N, Forslund K, Ceric G, Clements J, et al. The Pfam protein families database. Nucleic Acids Research. 2012;(40 (Database)):D290-D301. DOI: 10.1093/nar/gkr1065

[83] Amanchy R, Periaswamy B, Mathivanan S, Reddy R, Tattikota S, Pandey A. A curated compendium of phosphorylation motifs. Nature Biotechnology. 2007;**25**(3):285-286. DOI: https://doi:10.1038/nbt0307-285

[84] Zaytseva N, Shamkhalova M, Shestakova M, Matskeplishvili S, et al. Contrast-induced nephropathy in patients with type 2 diabetes during coronary angiography: Risk-factors and prognostic value. Diabetes Research and Clinical Practice. 2009;**86**(Suppl 1):S63-S69. DOI: 10.1016/S0168-8227(09)70012-9

[85] Ibragimov V, Sarvilina I, Batjushin M. The search of molecular prognostic markers of diabetic nephropathy in patients with type 2 diabetes mellitus. International Journal of Biomedicine. 2016;**6**(1):65-69. DOI: 10.21103/Article6(1)_OA14

[86] Haneda M, Utsunomiya K, Koya D, et al., Joint Committee on Diabetic Nephropathy. A new classification of Diabetic Nephropathy 2014: A report from Joint Committee on Diabetic Nephropathy. Journal of Diabetes Investigation. 2015;**6**(2):242-246. DOI: 10.1111/jdi.12319

9

Diabetes Mellitus in South Asia

Viduranga Y. Waisundara and Naofumi Shiomi

Abstract

The prevalence rates of diabetes mellitus and its complications in South Asia are much higher than in other developed and developing countries; therefore, diabetes mellitus has become a serious problem in this region. While the prevalence of diabetes mellitus in South Asia is remarkable, its characteristics and causes have not been well-elucidated. More than 85% of the diabetic population in South Asia suffer from type 2 diabetes, and the causes can be divided into two categories: internal/traditional causes and causes induced by rapid development. Factors such as age, gender, diet and lifestyle changes, including a lack of physical activity caused by modernization and urbanization, are major contributory factors. The majority of the healthcare costs associated with diabetes are due to its later complications and are not preventable. Therefore, inexpensive treatment at an early stage of diabetes is important. In this review, the following are recommended as preventive measures of the incidence of the disease: (1) induction of UCP1 through the diet, (2) increasing the intake of antidiabetic bioactive components and/or food and (3) evolution of the consensus through educational programs and government policy. National strategies and interventions should be implemented immediately for both the primary and secondary prevention of diabetes mellitus and its complications in order to advocate healthy living among the South Asian populations.

Keywords: diabetes mellitus, diabetic complications, India, South Asia, Sri Lanka

1. Introduction

Diabetes mellitus (hereafter referred to as "diabetes") develops under unusual conditions where the glucose level in the blood cannot be controlled. The disease is characterized by several symptoms such as thirst, polyuria and blurred vision [1]. Ketoacidosis or a nonketotic-hyperosmolar state caused by a chronic higher blood glucose level leads to stupor and coma in advanced cases and can even cause death in severe cases. There are four clinically defined categories of diabetes: type 1 diabetes (T1DM), type 2 diabetes (T2DM), gestational diabetes (GDM) and other specific types of the disease [2, 3]. In T1DM, also known as insulin-dependent diabetes (IDDM), the body is unable to produce insulin because of the autoimmune destruction of pancreatic islet beta cells (β cells), and as a result, the glucose levels in the blood cannot be maintained at normal concentrations. It ranks as the most common chronic childhood disease. T2DM or noninsulin-dependent diabetes (NIDDM) is characterized by both impaired insulin secretion and impaired insulin action. This type is associated with aging, obesity, a family history of diabetes, physical inactivity and certain ethnicities, although the causes of some of these factors are not well-explored. In GDM, the most widely accepted definition is diabetes that develops by varying insulin sensitivity during pregnancy or diabetes first recognized during pregnancy; in the former case, treatment with insulin can often be finished after pregnancy, as this type of diabetes is acute. Among these categories, T2DM accounts for about 85–95% of diabetes cases worldwide.

Diabetes research has mainly focused on people living in developed countries as a disease caused by obesity. However, the prevalence rate of diabetes has been increasing in many developing and newly-industrialized nations as well. In this review, we focused on South Asia as one such region. The prevalence rate of diabetes and its complications in South Asia is higher than in other areas, such as Europe [4], and diabetes has recently become a serious health issue leading to death [5]. Therefore, comprehensive knowledge about the prevalence rate and causes of diabetes in South Asian countries is desired. As part of this review, we investigated the present state, characteristics and causes of diabetes in South Asia and proposed strategies for its prevention. We hope that this appraisal will encourage recognition of the serious state of diabetes among South Asians and become an effective index for eventually solving this issue.

2. An overview of the prevalence of diabetes in South Asians

South Asia comprises the Indian subcontinent and is home to a diverse population of ethnic, linguistic and religious groups. The total population of South Asia is about 1.5 billion, representing more than 20% of the global population. The countries that fall under this regional demarcation include India, Pakistan, Sri Lanka, Nepal, Bhutan, Maldives, Afghanistan and Bangladesh. With deviating definitions based on often substantially different reasons (usually political), the British Indian Ocean Territory, Mauritius, Iran and the Tibet Autonomous Region are sometimes included as part of the South Asian subcontinent as well. Nevertheless, for the purpose of this review, we defined South Asia as India, Pakistan, Sri Lanka, Nepal, Bhutan, Maldives, Afghanistan and Bangladesh and focused on the diabetes status of the people living in these countries.

A recent study using a Diabetes Population Risk Tool in Canada showed that South Asians have the highest risk of developing diabetes [6], and another study estimated that the prevalence rate of diabetes in South Asians was around four times higher than in other ethnic groups [7]. The total number of people with diabetes in the world is estimated to increase from 171 million in 2000 to 366 million by 2030 [8]; this number among South Asians is predicted to reach 46 million in India, 14 million in Pakistan and 11.1 million in Bangladesh by 2030 [9].

A huge number of people (3.8 million) annually lose their lives due to diabetic complications, a value almost equivalent to the loss of life associated with AIDS [7]. **Table 1** shows the diabetic populations and its prevalence rates in South Asian countries based on the data of the International Diabetes Federation, which was estimated by a statistical investigation of the relevant populations primarily 20–79 years of age [10]. The results suggest that the diabetic populations and the prevalence rates of diabetes in most South Asian countries are thus expected to dramatically increase at a high rate until 2035. In India in particular, which has a large population and is rapidly advancing economically, 109 million people are predicted to develop diabetes by 2035 (**Table 1**). This will place India at the epicenter of this global epidemic [11]. In addition to this upward trend in the prevalence rate, the number of deaths and the economic burden due to diabetes in South Asians have been rapidly increasing. As shown in **Table 1**, around 43–870 USD per person is paid to cure diabetes and its complications. With the rising rate of incidence, people in South Asia will have to compensate for much higher diabetes-related expenditures in the near future, which will constitute a heavy burden upon the respective countries [12, 13].

Countries	A (in 1000s)	B (%)	C	D (USD)	E (in 1000s)	F (%)
Afghanistan	13086.9	6.15	18,514	102	27768.7	6.63
Bangladesh	94378.5	6.34	111,371	43	133493.5	8.18
Bhutan	474.0	4.94	124	150	656.9	6.90
India	774920.8	8.63	1,039,980	95	1042007.9	10.46
Maldives	214.0	7.97	109	870	332.9	5.94
Nepal	15307.4	4.58	14,778	60	23032.1	5.44
Pakistan	102124.6	6.80	87,548	56	158355.1	8.08
Sri Lanka	14155.4	8.32	16,384	123	16398.4	9.47

A, total adult population (20–79 years) in 2014; B, diabetes prevalence per total adult population in 2014; C, deaths number by the disease related to diabetes in 2014; D, mean diabetes-related expenditure per person in 2014; E, estimation of total adult population in 2035; F, diabetes prevalence per total adult population in 2035.

Table 1. Prevalence of diabetes in South Asia in 2014 and its estimated prevalence in 2035.

3. High prevalence rates of complications related to diabetes in South Asians

3.1. Prevalence rate of macrovascular complication

Diabetes is known to be strongly associated with many other disease and complications, and those ultimately lead to organ and tissue damage. The prevalence rates of macrovascular complications and atherosclerosis are especially high in diabetic patients, inducing adverse effects of ischemic heart disease [14], peripheral vascular disease and cerebrovascular disease. Diabetes is suspected to induce macrovascular complications and atherosclerosis. High blood glucose and insulin concentrations in diabetic patients induce structural and functional alterations and chronic inflammation at the arterial cell walls. Macrophages gather and invade the inflammation portion, forming plaque. This advanced plaque buildup is known as atherosclerosis. The main disease leading to death in diabetic patients is cardiovascular disease, with cerebrovascular disease and diabetic stroke being the second and third highest causes of death. The ratio of stroke in diabetic patients is two- to fourfold higher than in nondiabetic patients, and diabetics show a greater possibility of recurrence of stroke [15]. Furthermore, peripheral arterial disease (PAD), which is characterized by the occlusion of the arteries in the limb region and results in functional impairment and disability with intermittent claudication and pain, is also closely related to diabetes [15]. In most unfortunate cases, PAD causes foot ulceration, ultimately requiring amputation [16]. It is known that diabetic patients have a 25-times-greater risk of amputation than nondiabetes population.

It has been reported that Asian patients with diabetes are at a higher risk of developing macrovascular complications, such as cardiovascular disease, than other ethnicities [17]. For instance, a study conducted in Pakistan revealed that 30.5% of the young adult patients diagnosed with ischemic stroke were diabetic—a much higher percentage than in Western settings [18]. Another study performed in ischemic stroke patients of <45 years of age in Sri Lanka revealed that 5% of the study group with ischemic stroke had diabetes [19]. A prospective study was also conducted in 2403 patients with ischemic stroke and 783 patients with intracerebral hemorrhaging in India as a representative South Asian country [20]. That report mentioned that Asian diabetic patients had a high risk of early death due to ischemic stroke [20]. Furthermore, reports on the risks of cardiovascular disease and coronary in the Indian subcontinent have suggested that a leading cause of those diseases was diabetes [21, 22].

3.2. Prevalence rates of diabetic retinopathy, nephropathy and neuropathy

Another serious complication in diabetic patients is dysfunction of the eyes, kidneys and nerves. Diabetic retinopathy, a typical peripheral microvascular complication, induces acute damage to the retina of the eye [23]. Diabetic retinopathy is divided into two categories: background and proliferative retinopathy [22]. In background retinopathy, slight hemorrhaging develops in the middle layers of the retina, appearing as dots. In proliferative retinopathy, the formation of new blood vessels occurs on the surface of the retina, and white areas on the retina are a sign of this type of disease. Several studies have shown that the occurrence of diabetes retinopathy is influenced by chronic insulin resistance and a high blood glucose concentration, which occur in obese patients [24]. A poorly controlled blood-sugar level is the most significant factor associated with the development of retinopathy. The prevalence rate of retinopathy in diabetic patients in South Asia has been explored in several studies. One study investigated the rate in patients newly diagnosed with diabetes in India and found that the rate was lower (5–7%) than in both Western countries and neighboring countries such as Pakistan (15%), Nepal (19.3%) and Sri Lanka (15%) [25]. However, a similar study conducted in an urban population in Chennai, India, revealed that the prevalence of diabetic retinopathy per diabetic patient was 18%, although the prevalence of diabetic retinopathy in the general population was only 3.5%. Furthermore, men were shown to be at a higher risk than women in that investigation [26].

Diabetes nephropathy is also a serious complication. High blood pressure induced by both atherosclerosis and the function of adipose tissue causes the dysfunction of renal tissue. In the early stages, albumin in the urine is excreted at 30–299 mg per 24 h, which is called "microalbuminuria" and leads to renal failure at the final stage. A study found that one-quarter of patients with T1DM suffers from microalbuminuria or its advanced stage, diabetes nephropathy [15]. Some studies have reported on the prevalence rate of diabetic nephropathy in South Asians [27]. A study conducted in 10 countries in Asia, including Pakistan, found that the ratio of patients developing microalbuminuria per diabetic patient was alarmingly high (58.6%) [28]. A similar study conducted in an urban setting in South India revealed that the prevalence rate of microalbuminuria per diabetic patients was 26.3%, although the prevalence rate of overt nephropathy was only 2.2% in the study subjects [29]. These studies suggested that duration of the diabetes and hypertension is highly correlated with the development of nephropathy in South Asians.

Microalbuminuria caused by diabetes also induces peripheral nerve dysfunction, and half of diabetic patients consequently develop diabetic neuropathy [15]. The American Diabetic Association has stated that diabetic neuropathy is a sign of peripheral nerve dysfunction [30]. Among the symptoms of diabetic neuropathy, autonomic neuropathy is the most common. This symptom leads to an abnormal heart rate, loss of vascular control and cardiovascular autonomic dysfunction. Cardiac neuropathy caused by diabetes is the second-most common manifestation, depending on age, hypertension, smoking status and obesity. The prevalence rate of diabetic neuropathy in South Asia has been investigated. A study conducted in Sri Lanka reported that the prevalence rate of distal peripheral neuropathy (DPN) among T2DM patients was 24% (females and males: 26% and 20%, respectively). The prevalence rate of neuropathy among T2DM patients in South India was 19.1%, and this number is gradually increasing [31]. A similar study conducted in Indian states reported that the prevalence rate of diabetic neuropathy was 26.1% and was significantly associated with age, glycated hemoglobin and duration of diabetes [30]. Overall, **Figure 1** shows a schematic illustration of the

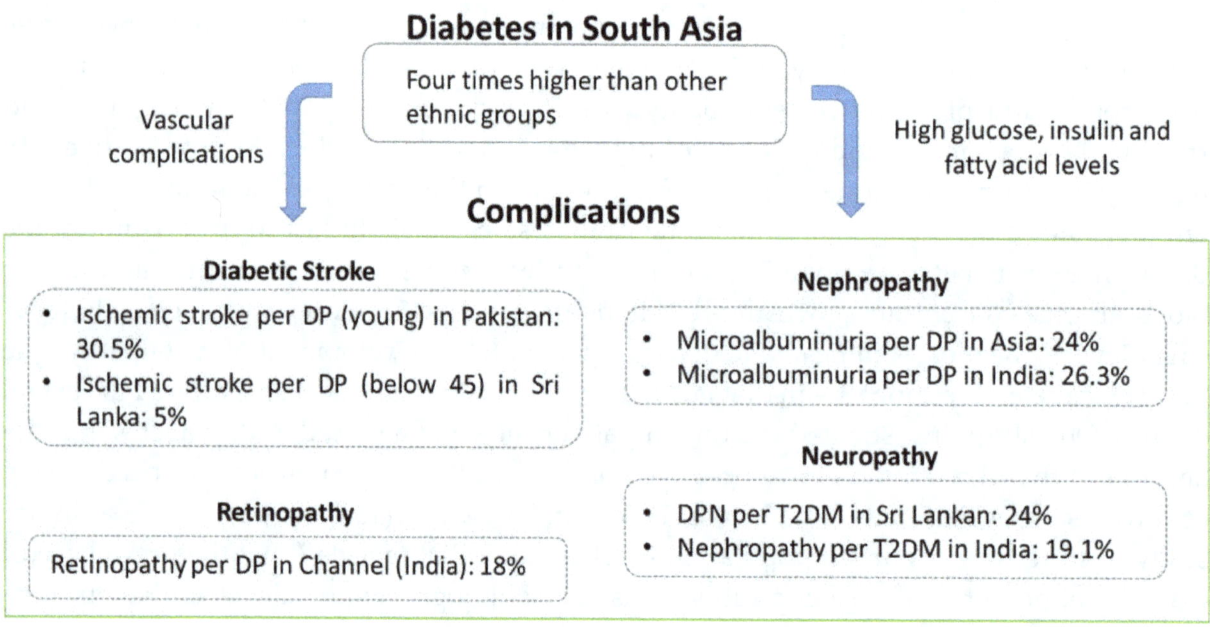

Figure 1. Prevalence rates of diabetes and its complications in South Asia (DP: diabetic patients).

typical course of diabetes and its complications in South Asia, as explained in this section. It is evident that the prevalence rates of diabetes and its complications in South Asians are much higher than in other countries. Therefore, recognition of this critical situation is duly warranted in order to mitigate the propagation of the disease condition.

4. Causes of the high prevalence rate of diabetes in South Asians

4.1. Physiological and traditional causes

4.1.1. Genetic factors

In this section, we explore why the prevalence rate of diabetes in South Asia is so much higher than in other developed or developing countries. Among the causes, genetic factors seem to be important, as a study suggested that 30–70% of the diabetes risk could be attributed to genetic variants (SNPs of diabetic genes) [32]. Genetic variants causing diabetes have been screened since the 1990s [33]. Around 50 genetic variants, known as "obese genes" or "thrifty genes" have been identified, and the relationship between diabetes and genetic variants of β3-adrenalin receptor—a thrifty gene—have been examined in particular detail. Individuals with a variant genotype of a thrifty gene proactively store fat in the body by reducing the energy metabolism; this is beneficial in times of nutrient scarcity [34, 35]. Asian populations are much more likely to possess thrifty genotypes than Europeans. The reason for this is believed to be because South Asian populations have not had sufficient time to adapt from this variant genotype to a normal genotype, as Europeans evolved in environments where they were relatively unaffected by famine cycles [32].

Several studies have reported that South Asians have several risk factors for disorder of glucose consumption and insulin resistance. For instance, features of insulin resistance, such as hypertriglyceridemia, and increased abdominal or visceral fat have been seen even in nonobese Asian populations [36–38], and South Asians have more adiposity than Europeans and residents of other parts of the world with the same body weight [39, 40]. Furthermore, South Asians are more insulin resistant than other races [36, 41]. Studies conducted in India as representative South Asians have reported that Indians were at a higher risk of glucose intolerance than Europeans, even in groups with a low waist circumference [42, 43]. Insulin resistance and compensatory hyperinsulinemia have been found even in children and adolescents of Asian-Indian origin [44]. These studies firmly suggest that South Asians have a special variant genotype of the thrifty gene strongly inducing insulin resistance and unusual glucose consumption. The Asian Indian phenotype—a thrifty gene seen among Pima Indians, is the most likely candidate for this special variant among the recognized thrifty genes based on the findings from several studies [36, 37]. Studies have shown that migrant Asian-Indians had a higher risk of developing diabetes and related metabolic abnormalities than other ethnic groups [37] and that the prevalence rate of diabetes and its adverse health effects has risen more rapidly among native and migrant populations in South Asia than in any other geographic region. However, another study that included 20,119 participants from

South Asia revealed a considerable degree of genetic contribution to the onset of T2DM [45]. The researchers identified novel six loci (GRB14, ST6GAL1, VPS26A, HMG20A, AP3S2 and HNF4A) showing correlations with T2DM [45]. Therefore, the diabetic constitution in South Asia is suspected to be related to other genes in addition to the Asian Indian phenotype.

4.1.2. Effects of family history, age and gender

Individuals' profiles are important to consider when examining the prevalence rate of diabetes [46]. The incidence of the disease in a patient's family is often involved in a given individual's risk, as the variant genotype of thrifty genes is passed down from parents to offspring. Studies comparing the effect of family with others estimated that the risk factors for diabetes in offspring with a single diabetic parent and two diabetic parents are, respectively, 3.5- and 6-fold higher than those without parental diabetes [47]. Among patterns of inheritance, diabetes and its related traits are both polygenic and heterogeneous, with multiple genes involved in different combinations [48]. However, the number of risk genes and their relative contributions are complicated and remain somewhat uncertain. A relationship is known to exist between diabetes and age, probably because the β-cells of older individuals have a reduced proliferative capacity and secreting activity, reduced expression of cell cycle activators, increased expression of cell cycle inhibitors, reduced pdx1 expression and increased amylin aggregation [49]. This decreased functional status is exacerbated in diabetic patients by increased rates of beta cell apoptosis [38]. In addition, in South Asia, elderly people tend to have a decreased muscle mass due to sedentary lifestyles [17].

In South Asians, diabetes does not always develop in the elderly, and the characteristics are remarkable. An investigation on the prevalence rate of diabetes in various age groups of South Asians showed that the diabetes population was highest among those ≥60 years of age for both males and females. However, the rate of diabetes among relatively young individuals was found to be higher in South Asians than Caucasians [37]. Furthermore, in India, the prevalence rate of diabetes peaks at 60–69 years of age [42], and Indian people develop the disease even in their youth [41]. Similar results to those in India were found in Pakistan and Sri Lanka [47]. The development of diabetes in younger generations is likely caused by changes in lifestyle brought about by urbanization [42]. The prevalence rate of diabetes (5.02%) was found to be associated with age-adjusted impaired glucose intolerance (5.27%) in a rural community in Sri Lanka [47]. Diabetes develops at any age, and the change in the prevalence over time is hypothesized to be associated with the rural to urban population shift [49].

The prevalence rate is also related to gender in South Asia. Diabetes is the second leading cause of death among South Asian women with diabetes, although it is only the ninth leading cause globally [9]. A relationship was reported between age and gender in Bangladesh diabetes patients [50]. The proportion of female diabetic patients (31.2%) was higher than that of male diabetic patients (28.5%) among subjects 31–50 years of age. Among subjects >50 years of age, the diabetic male population was 18.1% and that of the female population was 12.9%. However, below 31 years of age, only 3.3% of the male population had diabetes, whereas 6% of the female population was diabetic [51]. A study conducted in four provinces of Sri Lanka showed that the prevalence of severe obesity among males was 2.4%, whereas that among females was 8.8%. Further, the report found that, in all categories of overweight, the prevalence was greater in women than in men in all provinces [50]. Women with diabetes are also more likely to suffer a heart attack at a younger age than those without diabetes.

Gestational diabetes may be the main reason why there is a high prevalence rate of diabetes in women in South Asia, because the prevalence rate of GDM in South Asia is much higher than that in Europe [52, 53]. One cause of the high prevalence rate in South Asia is considered to be genetic factors. Several studies have suggested that South Asians basically have a constitution that is conducive to the development of GDM [53, 54]. Another cause is the influence of sociocultural and socioeconomic factors [55]. Weight and physical activity should be carefully controlled in order not to develop GDM before and during pregnancy. However, actions based on incorrect knowledge and bad traditional habits for pregnancy, which are taught from a person's mother, can lead to an increase in weight and a decrease in physical stress [55]. To make matters worse, GDM often causes miscarriages or birth defects, and the children born from mothers developing GDM also have a tendency to develop diabetes. Therefore, the prevention of GDM is very important to stop the passing of diabetes from mother to children and to decrease the development of diabetes among women in South Asia. It is hoped that future studies on diabetes in South Asia will focus on gestational and neonatal diabetes, and programs to prevent GDM should be established in the field at all governmental levels.

4.1.3. Chronic and heavy intakes of alcohol and smoking

Chronic drinking of large amounts of alcohol exacerbates a potential risk factor of diabetes [50]. The liver is an important organ for consuming and supplying glucose. As the chronic intake of high concentrations of ethanol induces alcoholic liver injury and inhibits the capacity to control the blood glucose level, the liver accumulates triglycerides. Such a liver condition is known as "alcoholic fatty liver." The serum levels of acetaldehyde, an intermediate metabolite of ethanol, are increased by the decrease in the detoxification capacity under conditions of alcoholic fatty liver, often severely adversely affecting the β-cells in the pancreas. Dysfunction of the liver and β-cells causes hyperglycemia, dyslipidemia and diabetes. In all South Asian countries, chronic and heavy drinking is traditionally common in poor rural regions; in addition, alcohol consumption is on the rise with rapid globalization and socioeconomic development. For instance, alcohol use among Indians has been increasing because the lifestyle patterns have been rapidly changing due to migration to urban regions and socioeconomic changes [56]. Public health policies regarding alcohol consumption are needed to stem this tide of change.

Cigarette smoking is an indirect but important risk factor for diabetes [57]. Studies have reported that a smoking habit increased the risk of developing diabetes by 44% [58], and smokers are 30–40% more likely to develop diabetes than nonsmokers [59]. Several studies have attempted to elucidate the relationship. Smoking reduces the insulin sensitivity because nicotine included in cigarettes has the ability to inhibit insulin secretion via neuronal nicotinic acetylcholine receptors. Furthermore, smoking damages cells by increasing the amount of reactive oxygen [60], and inflammation occurs at the damaged portion, causing swelling of cells. Smoking is also associated with an increased risk of abdominal obesity [39]. These harmful effects cause metabolic disorders of glucose and lipids and increase the risk of diabetes as a result. The percentage of regular smokers in adult males of South Asia is estimated to be very high (50–60%). India is the second-largest producer and consumer of tobacco products. Many persons in India use smokeless tobacco products such as betel quid, as these are non-taxable, and those products are commonly used in rural areas of the country [58]. Concurrent use of alcohol and tobacco, which is also extremely common among South Asian populations, has a synergistic effect on the enhancement of diabetes risk [56]. With the spread of chewing tobacco, smoking is being taken up by younger and younger individuals. An investigation in 7735 British men of 40–59 years of age suggested that the consumption of tobacco, either as a smoker or user of chewing tobacco, is occurring at lower ages, and 47% of men and 14% of women who admitted to consuming tobacco had started at age 15 [57]. Reducing heavy smoking rates and the concurrent intake of alcohol are important targets for preventing diabetes and its complications among South Asians [59]. Changes in the policy and effective education programs for tobacco use in addition to alcohol use must be implemented as soon as possible.

4.2. Causal factors of diabetes induced by rapid globalization and development

4.2.1. Urbanization

Unprecedented urbanization of rural areas of South Asia is a major environmental factor involved in the increasing rate of diabetes [61]. **Table 2** shows the ratio of urban/rural localization among diabetics based on data from the International Diabetes Federation. The urban prevalence of diabetes in Sri Lanka is lower than that in rural areas [5], and similar incidences can be seen in India, Pakistan, Nepal and Afghanistan. In contrast, in countries such as Bangladesh, Bhutan and the Maldives, where urbanization has not rapidly occurred, an opposite trend is shown [5]. This is a characteristic of importance, as the prevalence rate of diabetes is generally high in urban areas (12.4%) followed by the midland (8.1%), highland (5.8%) and coastal areas (2.5%) in developing countries. To further highlight this anomaly, in Japan—which is a developed country—the prevalence rate in urban areas is similar to that in rural areas.

	Effects of gender on diabetes*		Effects of area on diabetes**	
Countries	Female (in 1000s)	Female/male (–)	Urban (in 1000s)	Urban/rural (–)
Afghanistan	407.00	1.02	228.59	0.40
Bangladesh	3261.80	1.20	3053.02	1.50
Bhutan	9.60	0.69	12.11	1.17
India	31384.00	0.88	30571.31	0.89
Maldives	8.00	0.88	4.75	1.51
Nepal	196.40	0.38	244.02	0.57
Pakistan	3369.70	0.94	2934.76	0.78
Sri Lanka	569.60	0.94	330.11	0.41

* Data from Diabetes Atlas in 2014.

** Data from Diabetes Atlas in 2013.

Table 2. Ratio of diabetes by gender and area of South Asia.

Rapid urbanization gives important variation of rural area where agriculture had been the principle profession [9]. Urbanization has reduced the physical activity and altered dietary habits by changing the lifestyle among residents of rural areas through means such as increased mechanization of the agriculture industry, automation of daily activities, popularization of television and increased computer usage, which has accordingly increased the proportion of obese persons [9, 10]. Studies have shown that the prevalence rate of diabetic complications is associated with wealth/income, education and office-based occupations in South Asia [62]. Socially deprived urban South Asian communities have a lower prevalence of diabetes and obesity than developed countries [1], and a study performed in Sri Lanka reported that the majority of patients developing diabetic neuropathy resided in rural areas (75.3%) with a monthly income exceeding Sri Lankan Rs. 12,000 (87.6%) [31]. The inhabitants of South Asian countries who reside in rural areas and show a low prevalence of diabetes are involved in agriculture and engage in intense physical labor. These results suggest that the affluence accompanying urbanization leads to a luxurious—and by extension—more sedentary lifestyle, thereby increasing the rate of diabetes [63].

4.2.2. Increase in the rate of obesity due to changes in the diet

Obesity is a major determinant of T2DM. Many recent studies elucidated the mechanism underlying the development in T2DM. White adipocytes secrete adipokines, such as leptin, adiponectin and TNF-α. Leptin and adiponectin enhance the capacity of glucose consumption by increasing the noradrenalin secretion, but TNF-α inhibits it via the inhibition of insulin receptor and transport of GLUT4 [64]. As the secretion of leptin and adiponectin is decreased and the secretion of TNF-α is increased in white adipose tissues highly accumulating triglyceride, the glucose intake is inhibited [65]. Furthermore, the pressure on blood vessels induced by hypertrophic white adipose tissues causes an inflammatory response, and the enhanced concentration of free fatty acids in the blood by obesity causes the dysfunction of mitochondria in muscle cells and β-cells of the pancreas [66, 67]. These harmful effects induce disorder of glucose consumption and insulin resistance, thereby resulting in the development of T2DM.

Urbanization in South Asia is a major contributory factor to obesity [68, 69]. Investigations conducted among rural communities in Sri Lanka showed a strong relationship between diabetes and excess body weight, and the prevalence rate of obesity in diabetic patients (21%) was higher ($P < 0.05$) than in nondiabetic individuals (10.5%) [70]. Obesity is no longer a disease of affluent and therefore majority of the populations in South Asia in the wake of rapid changes in lifestyle among more rural populations [58]. As previously stated, migration toward rural areas of South Asia induced dramatic changes to the diet within a decade. Traditional dietary patterns are now being lost, and a significant transition to energy-rich diets is occurring in South Asia. The diet has shifted from relatively monotonous food products like indigenous staple grains or starchy roots, locally grown legumes, other vegetables and fruits, along with limited foods of animal origin (except for prosperous subpopulations), to more varied diets that include more preprocessed foods with higher fat and lower carbohydrate content, more foods of animal origin, edible oils and more added sugars, especially in the form of processed drinks and foods, and often more alcohol. These changes in diet have caused a rapid increase in the obese population of South Asia.

The amounts of fats and carbohydrates as well as the total calories strongly influence the rate of obesity, and the body mass index (BMI), glycemic index (GI) and glycemic load (GL) can be used as indices to estimate the amounts of fats and carbohydrate. Many nations in South Asia tend to have relatively high-GI and high-GL diets. For example, white rice, which is a daily staple of the South Asian diet, has a higher GI than whole-grain rice. A recent meta-analysis found that a single increment in white rice serving per day increased the risk of diabetes by 11% [71]. Furthermore, large portion sizes and predominantly starch-based diets in South Asians, which correspond to a high GL, are also associated with obesity. Reducing the carbohydrate portion sizes and increasing the portion of vegetables is necessary to reduce the diabetes risk, as high-GI and high-GL diets contribute to obesity [71, 72].

4.2.3. Increase in undesirable lifestyles and a shortage of education programs

Poor lifestyles, such as a short sleeping time, watching TV for a prolonged period and physical inactivity brought about by urbanization, may function as factors exacerbating and triggering the development of diabetes. The sleep duration among Asians is relatively short. In a meta-analysis of data from 23 countries, adolescents in Asia were sleeping 40–60 min less each night than Americans and 60–120 min less each night than Europeans [73]. Some studies have suggested that this short duration of sleep in Asians was associated with an increased risk of diabetes, childhood obesity and cardiometabolic abnormalities [73, 74]. As sleep-disordered breathing induces a twofold increase in the risk of diabetes [73], a short duration of sleep may induce a condition similar to that of sleep-disordered breathing.

Inactive behaviors (watching TV or playing on a PC for a prolonged period and sedentary careers) may also be associated with diabetes in South Asians. Prolonged stints of watching TV are independent of the metabolic activity for obesity, but wasting so much time with this behavior tends to be associated with an unhealthy diet, including increased consumption of snacks, sugary beverages and fast food [38]. Furthermore, this lifestyle is associated with physical inactivity due to a decrease in the metabolic capacity when performing such daily work. Therefore, watching TV for a prolonged period consequently increases the prevalence rate of obesity and diabetes. In addition, many studies in South Asians have revealed a rapid shift to careers in the service sector due to economic growth and the advent of new technologies. This has led to careers involving long durations of sitting, thereby resulting in a marked decline in physical activity [38]. People in a high socioeconomic class are more prone to developing diabetes than those in lower economic classes. Of special note, a study in adults in Sri Lanka revealed a strong association between physical inactivity and diabetes [75].

Education about diabetes is much more lacking among South Asians than in Europeans, and this low consciousness of diabetes has consequently contributed to an increase in the rate of diabetes in South Asians. A study conducted in Bangladesh found that individuals with more education had a 1.67-fold lower risk of developing diabetes than those with little or no education [75]. In that study, employees who had often been educated about diabetes had a lower probability of having diabetes themselves than unemployed individuals [75]. Another study in Sri Lankans showed that a higher educational level may be associated with better diabetes-related outcomes [70]. Therefore, education starting from elementary school may be an effective and practical way of reducing the rate of diabetes. The World Diabetes Foundation has already implemented prevention programs at the national level to educate students in urban and semi-urban areas in South Asian countries about the risk of diabetes, in view of these shortcomings [76].

Figure 2 shows a schematic illustration of the characteristics of diabetes in South Asia described in this chapter. The causes underlying the high prevalence of diabetes in South Asians can be distilled down to four main factors. First, South Asians have the thrifty gene derived from Asian Indian populations that induces insulin resistance and disorder of glucose consumption; they therefore develop a T2DM constitution. Second, obese populations are increasing due to dietary changes and a decrease in physical activity in the wake of remarkable economic progress, which causes T2DM. Third, traditional bad habits such as chronic heavy smoking and drinking, which cause T1DM and T2DM, are increasingly being adopted due to increased income caused by economic progress. Fourth, the recognition to diabetes is poor because of a lack of relevant policies and the education system.

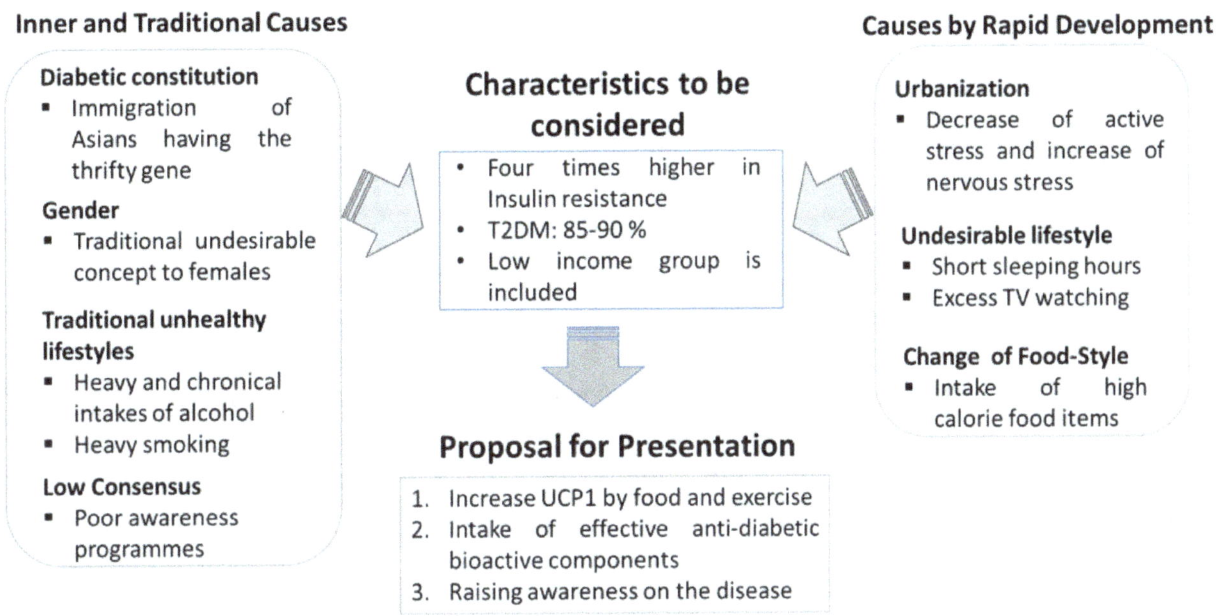

Figure 2. Causes of diabetes in South Asia and suggestions for their prevention.

5. Strategies for preventing diabetes in South Asia

As we suggested in the previous sections, the implementation of preventive strategies for diabetes is necessary as soon as possible. Preventive treatment should be performed as early as possible in subjects at risk of developing diabetes, as complete recovery is extremely difficult once diabetes develops. Second, the recovery of the glucose consumption capacity and insulin sensitivity are the most important targets for treatment because most diabetic patients in South Asia have T2DM, which is mainly caused by disorders in these activities. Furthermore, inexpensive treatments are necessary, as diabetic patients in South Asians tend not to be very wealthy. Given these aspects, we propose three strategies herein for reducing the prevalence rate of diabetes. The first strategy involves the induction of uncoupling protein 1 (UCP1) by changing the diet and lifestyle. UCP1, which is expressed only in brown adipocytes, plays a role in nonshivering heat generation using the proton potential of the inner membrane of mitochondria. Through the effects of UCP1, fatty acid is effectively metabolized to compensate for the loss of energy. Recently, the effects of UCP1 on glucose and insulin resistance were examined using fatty mouse and UCP1 transgenic mouse models [77–79]. The results of those studies suggest that increasing the concentration of UCP1 is the most effective way to rescue subjects with preliminary T2DM. The induction of UCP1 is relatively easy because muscle cells and white adipocytes can be differentiated to brown adipocyte by the stimulation of cool temperatures and exercise [80, 81] or by consuming herbal and/or complementary medicines [66]. We therefore think that the induction of brown adipocytes is the most inexpensive and effective way of preventing the development of diabetes at the early stage in South Asia.

The second strategy involves qualitative improvements in the diet by proactively consuming functional compounds or food products containing antidiabetic bioactives. Many effective compounds for protecting against obesity have been identified. For example, consuming fish instead of meat is good for protecting against obesity because DHA contained in fish can reduce fat and cholesterol. Proactively consuming food containing polyphenols, such as green tea, soybean products and berries, and carnitine, such as fish [82–84], is also effective for similar reasons. Superfoods that contain high levels of these effective compounds and functional foods with artificially enhanced levels have been enthusiastically studied, and many inexpensive functional foods and supplements are now available in developed countries [85, 86]. The proactive consumption of superfoods and functional foods through the daily diet without expensive drugs is extremely effective for protecting against obesity and diabetes.

The final and most important strategy involves changing the consensus. If most South Asians with obese constitutions continue their bad habits, such as chronic heavy smoking and drinking and consuming high-calorie and oily foods, the rapid increase in the prevalence rate of diabetes cannot be effectively curbed. In Japan, the consensus regarding obesity and metabolic syndrome has recently been enhanced by a trend toward anti-obesity and education via TV and books; in this way, the rising tide of obesity is being stemmed little by little. This is a strategy which could be easily implemented in South Asia as well. Therefore, revising the consensus can be effective, even in South Asians. In a case report from Ballabgarh, India, a five-step model (identify the problem, understand the problem, evaluate feasible and cost-effective intervention) is addressed to the issue [87], but statistics clearly display that such efforts are not sufficient, and further education toward diabetes and national strategies and interventions to protect against obesity and diabetes should be implemented immediately.

6. Conclusion

We focused on the issue of the recent increase in the diabetes prevalence in South Asia and described the results consequently obtained in associated studies. First, we investigated the prevalence of diabetes and its complications in South Asia. Existing studies and statistics suggest that the prevalence was much higher in this region than in other developed and developing countries and that this prevalence is rapidly increasing despite already being a serious problem in the subcontinent. This high prevalence rate will induce increased diabetes-related expenditures and incur a heavy financial and social burden in the near future for people in South Asia.

Second, we examined why South Asians show a higher prevalence rate of diabetes than other populations and explored the reasons for its rapid increase in prevalence. One potential internal cause is a constitution based on obesity, which is induced by the thrifty gene characteristic of Asians. Another potential internal cause is the adoption of traditional bad habits, such as chronic heavy smoking and drinking. These factors may cause T2DM even in nonobese subjects and T1DM even in older individuals. A potential environmental cause is urbanization. Rapid development gives rise to an undesirable diet and lifestyle, which can cause obesity in South Asians, especially those living in rural areas.

Finally, we proposed effective prevention strategies based on the above analyses. Primary prevention through the promotion of a healthy diet and lifestyle should be a priority, and the prevalence rate may be able to be drastically decreased by making changes to one's diet and lifestyle. However, if South Asians fail to recognize the impending diabetes crisis, this condition will unfortunately become much more serious in the near future. The implementation of public health strategies aimed at mitigating the obesogenic environment is critical.

Acknowledgements

The authors extend their gratitude to Mrs. Nilakshi Jayawardena, Ms. Mindani Watawana and Mrs. Chaminie B. Gunawardhana, who were former Research Assistants/Postgraduate Students at the National Institute of Fundamental Studies, Kandy, Sri Lanka. This work was partially supported by grants-in-aid from the School of Human Sciences at Kobe College, Japan.

Author details

Viduranga Y. Waisundara[1] and Naofumi Shiomi[2*]

*Address all correspondence to: n-shiomi@mail.kobe-c.ac.jp

1 Technology Degree Programme, Faculty of Applied Sciences, Rajarata University, Mihintale, Sri Lanka

2 School of Human Sciences, Department of Biosphere Sciences, Kobe College, Hyogo, Japan

References

[1] Mohan V, Sandeep S, Deepa R, Shah B, Varghese C. Epidemiology of type 2 diabetes: Indian scenario. Indian Journal of Medical Research. 2007;**125**:217-230

[2] Seidell JC. Obesity, insulin resistance and diabetes—A worldwide epidemic. British Journal of Nutrients. 2000;**83**:S5-S8. DOI: 10.1017/S000711450000088X

[3] Ahmed RG. Evolutional interactions between diabetes and development. Diabetes Research and Clinical Practice. 2011;**92**:153-167

[4] Jayawardena R, Ranasinghe P, Byrne NM, Soares MJ, Katulanda P, Hills AP. Prevalence and trends of the diabetes epidemic in South Asia: A systematic review and meta-analysis. BMC Public Health. 2012;**12**:380. DOI: 10.1186/1471-2458-12-380

[5] International Diabetes Federation. Diabetes Atlas. 6th ed. [Internet]. 2013. Available from: https://www.idf.org/e-library/epidemiology-research/diabetes-atlas/19-atlas-6th-edition.html [Accessed: 17 February 2016]

[6] Misra A, Vikram NK. High prevalence of obesity and associated risk factors in urban children in India and Pakistan highlights immediate need to initiate primary prevention program for diabetes and coronary heart disease in schools. Diabetes Research and Clinical Practice. 2006;**71**:101-102

[7] Rosella LC, Mustard CA, Stukel TA, Corey P, Hux J, Roos L, Manuel DG. The role of ethnicity in predicting diabetes risk at the population level. Ethnicity and Health. 2012;**17**(4):419-437. DOI: 10.1080/13557858.2012.654765

[8] Wild S, Roglic G, Green A, Sicree R, King H. Global prevalence of diabetes estimates for the year 2000 and projections for 2030. Diabetes Care. 2004;**27**(5):1047-1053. DOI: 10.2337/diacare.27.5.1047

[9] Kakar ZA, Siddiqui MA, Amin RA. Prevalence and risk factors of diabetes in adult population of South Asia. Clinical Medicine of Diagnosis. 2013;**3**:18-28. DOI: 10.5923/j.cmd.20130302.02

[10] International Diabetes Federation. Diabetes Atlas. 6th ed. [Internet]. 2014. Available from: http://www.idf.org/atlasmap/atlasmap [Accessed: 17-02-2016]

[11] Hu FB. Globalization of diabetes the role of diet, lifestyle, and genes. Diabetes Care. 2011;**34**:1249-1257. DOI: 10.2337/dc11-0442

[12] Hogan P, Dall T, Nikolov P. Economic costs of diabetes in the US in 2002. Diabetes Care. 2003;**26**:917-932. DOI: 10.2337/diacare.26.3.917

[13] Paterson AD, Rutledge BN, Cleary PA, Lachin JM, Crow RS. The effect of intensive diabetes treatment on resting heart rate in type 1 diabetes: The diabetes control and complications trial/epidemiology of diabetes interventions and complications study. Diabetes Care. 2007;**30**:2107-2112

[14] Fowler MJ. Microvascular and macrovascular complications of diabetes. Clinical Diabetes. 2008;**26**:77-82. DOI: 10.2337/diaclin.26.2.77

[15] Cade WT. Diabetes-related microvascular and macrovascular diseases in the physical therapy setting. Physical Therapy. 2008;**88**:1322-1335. DOI: 10.2522/ptj.20080008

[16] Calle-Pascual AL, Redondo MJ, Ballesteros M, Martinez-Salinas MA, Diaz JA, De Matias P, et al. Non-traumatic lower extremity amputations in diabetic and non-diabetic subjects in Madrid, Spain. Diabetes Metabolism. 1997;**23**:519-523

[17] Misra A, Khurana L, Vikram NK, Goel A, Wasir JS. Metabolic syndrome in children: Current issues and South Asian perspective. Nutrition. 2007;**23**:895-910. DOI: 10.1016/j.nut.2007.08.018

[18] Razzaq AA, Khan BA, Baig SM. Ischemic stroke in young adults of South Asia. JPMA. 2002;**52**(9):417-422

[19] De Silva R, Gamage R, Wewelwala C, Gunarathna D, Kittner S, Sirisena D, et al. Young strokes in Sri Lanka: An unsolved problem. Journal of Stroke Cerebrovascular Disease. 2009;**18**(4):304-308. DOI: 10.1016/j.jstrokecerebrovasdis.2008.11.004

[20] Wong KS. Risk factors for early death in acute ischemic stroke and intracerebral hemorrhage: A prospective hospital-based study in Asia. Asian acute stroke advisory panel. Stroke. 1999;**30**(11):2326-2330. DOI: 10.1161/01.STR.30.11.2326

[21] Goyal A, Yusuf S. The burden of cardiovascular disease in the Indian subcontinent. Indian Journal of Medical Research. 2006;**124**(3):235-244

[22] Ali MK, Narayan KMV, Tandon N. Diabetes and coronary heart disease: Current prospective. Indian Journal of Medical Research. 2010;**132**:584-597

[23] Shah CA. Diabetic retinopathy: A comprehensive review. Indian Journal of Medical Science. 2008;**62**(12):500-519

[24] Kaštelan S, Tomić M, Antunica AG, Ljubić S, Rabatić JS, Karabatić M. Body mass index: A risk factor for retinopathy in type 2 diabetic patients. Mediators Inflammation. 2013;**2013**:436329. DOI: 10.1155/2013/436329

[25] Sivaprasad S, Gupta B, Crosby-Nwaobi R, Evans J. Prevalence of diabetic retinopathy in various ethnic groups: A worldwide perspective. Survival Ophthalmology. 2012;**57**(4):347-70. DOI: 10.1016/j.survophthal.2012.01.004

[26] Raman R, Rani PK, Reddi Rachepalle S, Gnanamoorthy P, Uthra S, Kumaramanickavel G, et al. Prevalence of diabetic retinopathy in India, diabetic retinopathy epidemiology and molecular genetics study report 2. Ophthalmology. 2009;**116**(2):311-318. DOI: 10.1016/j.ophtha.2008.09.010

[27] Ashok S, Ramu M, Deepa R, Mohan V. Prevalence of neuropathy in type 2 diabetic patients attending a diabetes centre in South India. Journal of Association Physicians India. 2002;**50**:546-550

[28] Wu AYT, Kong NCT, De Leon FA, Pan CY, Tai TY, Yenug VT, et al. An alarmingly high prevalence of diabetic nephropathy in Asian type 2 diabetic patients: The microalbuminuria prevalence (MAP) study. Diabetologia. 2005;**48**(1):17-26. DOI: 10.1007/s00125-004-1599-9

[29] Unnikrishnan R, Rema M, Pradeepa R, Deepa M, Shanthirani CS, Deepa R, et al. Prevalence and risk factors of diabetic nephropathy in an urban South Indian population the Chennai Urban Rural Epidemiology Study (CURES 45). Diabetes Care. 2007;**30**(8):2019-2024. DOI: 10.2337/dc06-2554

[30] American Diabetes Association. Standards of medical care in diabetes. Diabetes Care. 2007;**30**:S4-S41

[31] Katulanda P, Ranasinghe P, Jayawardena R, Constantine GR, Sheriff MR, Matthews DR. The prevalence, patterns and predictors of diabetic peripheral neuropathy in a developing country. Diabetology & Metabolic Syndrome. 2012;**4**(1):21. DOI: 10.1186/1758-5996-4-21

[32] Mahendran Y. Identification of biomarkers for type 2 diabetes [dissertation]. University of Eastern Finland; 2014

[33] Singh S. The genetics of type 2 diabetes mellitus: A review. Journal of Science and Research. 2011;**55**:35-48

[34] Neel JV. Diabetes mellitus: A "thrifty" genotype rendered detrimental by "progress"? Bulletin World Health Organization. 1999;**77**:694-703

[35] Qi L, Cornelis MC, Zhang C, van Dam RM, Hu FB. Genetic predisposition, western dietary pattern, and the risk of type 2 diabetes in men. American Journal of Clinical Nutrients. 2009;**89**:1453-1458. DOI: 10.3945/ajcn.2008.27249

[36] Abate N, Chandalia M. Ethnicity, type 2 diabetes & migrant Asian Indians. Indian Journal of Medical Research. 2007;**125**:251-258

[37] Poulsen P, Kyvik KO, Vaag A, Beck-Nielsen H. Heritability of type II (non-insulin-dependent) diabetes mellitus and abnormal glucose tolerance—A population-based twin study. Diabetologia. 1999;**42**:139-145

[38] Hertel JK. Genetic risk factors for type 2 diabetes and related traits [dissertation]. University of Bergen; 2012

[39] Lowton J, Ahmed N, Hanna L. "I can't do any serious exercise": Barriers to physical activity amongst people of Pakistani origin with type 2 diabetes. Health Education Research. 2014;**21**:43-54. DOI: 10.1093/her/cyh042

[40] Basit A, Shera AS. Prevalence of metabolic syndrome in Pakistan. Pakistan Journal of Medical Science. 2008;**6**:171-174. DOI: 10.1089/met.2008.0005

[41] Raji A, Seely EW, Arky RA, Simonson DC. Body fat distribution and insulin resistance in healthy Asian Indians and Caucasians. Journal of Clinical Endocrinology Metabolism. 2001;**86**:5366-5371. DOI: 10.1210/jcem.86.11.7992

[42] King H, Aubert RE, Herman WH. Global burden of diabetes, 1995-2025: Prevalence, numerical estimates, and projections. Diabetes Care. 1998;**21**:1414-1431. DOI: 10.2337/diacare.21.9.1414

[43] Nikkila EA, Taskinen MR. Ethanol-induced alterations of glucose tolerance, post-glucose hypoglycemia, and insulin secretion in normal, obese, and diabetic subjects. Diabetes. 1975;**24**:933-943

[44] Ramachandran A, Snehalatha C, Yamuna A, Murugesan N, Narayan KM. Insulin resistance and clustering of cardiometabolic risk factors in urban teenagers in Southern India. Diabetes Care. 2007;**30**:1828-1833. DOI: 10.2337/diab.24.10.933

[45] Kooner JS, Saleheen D, Sim X, Sehmi J, Zhang W, Frossard P, et al. Genome-wide association study in people of South Asian ancestry identifies six novel susceptibility loci for type 2 diabetes. Nature Genetics. 2011;**43**(10):984-989. DOI: 10.1038/ng.921

[46] Global Health Estimates (GHE). 2014 Summary Tables: Deaths by Course, Age and Sex, by World Bank Region, 2000-2012 [Internet]. Geneva: World Health Organization; 2014. Available from http://www.who.int/healthinfo/global_burden_disease/en/ (Accessed 17 February 2016)

[47] Snehalatha C, Viswanathan V, Ramachandran A. Cut off values for normal anthropometric variables in Asian Indian adults. Diabetes Care. 2003;**26**:1380-1384. DOI: 10.2337/diacare.26.5.1380

[48] Doria A, Patti M-E, Kahn CR. The emerging genetic architecture of type 2 diabetes. Cell Metabolism. 2008;**8**(3):186-200. DOI: 10.1016/j.cmet.2008.08.006

[49] International Federation for Diabetes [Internet]. 2014. Available from: http://www.idf.org/sites/default/files/Atlas-poster-2014_EN.pdf [Accessed: 30-04-2015]

[50] Black SA. Diabetes, diversity, and disparity: What do we do with the evidence? American Journal of Public Health. 2002;**92**:543-548

[51] Al Sharmin A, Haque M. Susceptible factors of type two diabetes in a population of Bangladesh. HRPUB. 2016;**4**(1):38-45. DOI: 10.13189/ujph.2016.040106

[52] Petry CL. Gestational diabetes: Risk factors and recent advances in its genetics and treatment. British Journal of Nutrients. 2010;**104**:775-787. DOI: 10.1017/S0007114510001741

[53] Bellamy L, Casas JP, Hingorani AD, Williams D. Type 2 diabetes mellitus after gestational diabetes: A systematic review and meta-analysis. Lancet. 2009;**23**(373):1773-1779. DOI: 10.1016/S0140-6736(09)60731-5

[54] Dornhorst A, Paterson CM, Nicholls JS, Wadsworth J, Chiu DC, Elkeles RS, Johnston DG, Beard RW. High prevalence of gestational diabetes in women from ethnic minority groups. Diabetics Medicine. 1992;**9**:820-825. DOI: 10.1111/j.1464-5491.1992.tb01900.x

[55] Trisha G, Megan C, Nur A et al. Socio-cultural influences on the behaviour of South Asian women with diabetes in pregnancy: Qualitative study using a multi-level theoretical approach. BMC Medicine. 2015;**13**:120. DOI: 10.1186/s12916-015-0360-1

[56] Ronald CW, Ma RCW, Chan JCN. Type 2 diabetes in East Asians: Similarities and differences with populations in Europe and the United States. Annals of the New York Academy of Sciences. 2013;**1281**:64-91. DOI: 10.1111/nyas.12098

[57] Wannamethee SG, Shaper G, Perry IJ. Smoking as a modifiable risk factor for type 2 diabetes in middle-aged men. Diabetes Care. 2001;**24**(9):1590-1595. DOI: 10.2337/diacare.24.9.1590

[58] Kabir Z, Clancy L, Connolly GN. Tobacco control efforts: Where is India now? The Lancet. 2007;**370**(9582):134

[59] Caballero AE. Competence in diabetes mellitus care: an urgent need. Insulin. 2007;**2**:80-91. DOI: 10.1016/S1557-0843(07)80019-4

[60] Diano S, Horvath TL. A sympathetic view on free radicals in diabetes. Neuron. 2010;**66**(6):809-811

[61] Wijewardene K, Mohideen MR, Mendis S, Fernando DS, Kulathilaka T. Prevalence of hypertension, diabetes and obesity: baseline findings of a population-based survey in four provinces in Sri Lanka. Ceylon Medical Journal. 2005;**50**:62-70. DOI: 10.4038/cmj.v50i2.1571

[62] Ghaffar A, Reddy KS, Singhi M. Burden of non-communicable diseases in South Asia. British Medicine of Journal. 2004;**328**:807-810. DOI: 10.1136/bmj.328.7443.807

[63] Popkin BM, Horton SU, Kim S. The nutrition transition and prevention of diet-related diseases in Asia and the Pacific. Food and Nutrient Bulletin. 2011;**22**:3-10

[64] Ouchi N, Ohashi K, Shibata R, Murohara T. Adipocytokines and obesity-linked disorders. Nagoya Journal of Medical Science. 2012;**74**:19-30

[65] Shiomi N, Itoh M, Watanabe K. Characteristics of beige adipocytes induced from white adipocytes by Kikyo extract. Journal of Biomedical Science and Engineering. 2016;**9**(7):342-353. DOI: 10.4236/jbise.2016.97029

[66] Lowell BB, Shulman GI. Mitochondrial dysfunction and type 2 diabetes. Science. 2005;**307**(5708):384-387. DOI: 10.1126/science.1104343

[67] Shiomi N, Watanabe K. Effects of oleic acid on murine macrophage dysfunction. Journal of Biomedical Science and Engineering. 2013;**6**:654-660. DOI: 10.4236/jbise.2013.66080

[68] Gupta M, Prabhu K, Parijatham BO, Šlaiselvi VS, Rajendran SM, Rose J. Prevalence of diabetes mellitus in South India: A retrospective analysis. JIMSA. 2012;**25**:239-240

[69] Venkatachalam J, Muthu RE, Singh Z, Sathya GR. Alcohol consumption and diabetes: A case control study in a rural area of Kanchipuram district of Tamil Nadu. IOSR-JDMS. 2013;**4**(6):83-86

[70] Fernando DJS, Siribaddana S, De Silva D. Impaired glucose tolerance and diabetes mellitus in a suburban Sri Lankan community. Postgraduate Medical Journal of Sri Lanka. 1994;**70**:347-349

[71] Bhopal R, Hayes L, White M, White M, Unwin N, Harland J, Ayis S, et al. Ethnic and socio-economic inequalities in coronary heart disease, diabetes and risk factors in Europeans and South Asians. Journal of Public Health Medicine. 2002;**24**:95-105

[72] Forouhi NG, Sattar N, Tillin T, Mckeigue PM, Chaturvedi N. Do known risk factors explain the higher coronary heart disease mortality in south Asian compared with European men? Prospective follow-up of the Southall and Brent studies, UK. Diabetologia. 2006;**49**:2580-2588. DOI: 10.1007/s00125-006-0393-2

[73] Chowdhury MAB, Uddin MJ, Khan HMR, Haque MR. Type 2 diabetes and its correlates among adults in Bangladesh: A population based study. BMC Public Health. 2015;**15**:1070. DOI: 10.1186/s12889-015-2413-y

[74] Lopez AD, Mathers CD, Ezzati M, Jamison DT, Murray CJL. Global and regional burden of disease and risk factors, 2001: Systematic analysis of population health data. The Lancet. 2006;**367**:1747-1757. DOI: 10.1016/S0140-6736(06)68770-9

[75] Katulanda P, Jayawardana R, Ranasinghe P, Rezvi Sheriff MH, Matthews DR. Physical activity patterns and correlates among adults from a developing country: The Sri Lanka Diabetes and Cardiovascular Study. Public Health Nutrients. 2013;**16**(9):1684-1692. DOI: 10.1017/S1368980012003990

[76] Newsletter Q2_07_Primary Prevention in Indian Schools [Internet]. World Diabetes Foundation. Available at http://www.worlddiabetesfoundation.org/composite-1279.htm [Accessed: 13-02-2016]

[77] Arechaga I, Ledesma A, Rial E. The mitochondrial uncoupling protein UCP1: A gated pore. IUBMB Life. 2001;**52**:165-173. DOI: 10.1080/15216540152845966

[78] Kontani Y, Wang Y, Kimura K, Inokuma KI, Saito M, Suzuki-Miura T, Wang Z, Sato Y, Mori N, Yamashita H. UCP1 deficiency increases susceptibility to diet-induced obesity with age. Aging Cell. 2005;**4**:147-155. DOI: 10.1111/j.1474-9726.2005.00157.x

[79] Zhou Y, Yang J, Huang J, Li T, Xu D, Zuo B, Hou L, et al. The formation of brown adipose tissue induced by transgenic over-expression of PPARγ2. Biochemical and Biophysics Research and Communication. 2014;**446**(4):959-964. DOI: 10.1016/j.bbrc.2014.03.033

[80] Vegiopoulos A, Müller-Decker K, Strzoda D, Schmitt I, et al. Cyclooxygenase-2 controls energy homeostasis in mice by de novo recruitment of brown adipocytes. Science. 2010;**328**:1158-1161

[81] Cypess AM, Chen YC, Sze C, Wang K, English J, Chan O, Holman AR, Tal I, Palmer MR, Kolodny GM, Kahn CR. Cold but not sympathomimetics activates human brown adipose tissue in vivo. Proceedings of the National Academic Science USA. 2012;**109**:10001-10005. DOI: 10.1073/pnas.1207911109

[82] Wang S, Moustaid-Moussa N, Chen L, Mo H, Shastri A, et al. Nov-el insights of dietary polyphenols and obesity. Journal of Nutritional Biochemistry. 2014;**25**:1-18. DOI: 10.1016/j.jnutbio.2013.09.001

[83] Derosa G, Maffioli P, Ferrari I, D'Angelo A, Fogari E, Palumbo I, Randazzo S, Cicero AF. Orlistat and L-carnitine compared to orlistat alone on insulin resistance in obese diabetic patients. Endocrine Journal. 2011;**57**:777-786. DOI:10.1507/endocrj.K10E-049

[84] Shiomi N, Maeda M, Mimura M. Compounds that inhibit triglyceride accumulation and TNF-α secretion in adipocytes. Journal of Biomedical Science and Engineering 2011;**4**(11):684-691. DOI: 10.4236/jbise.2011.411085

[85] Waisundara V, Shiomi N, editors. Superfood and Functional Food—An Overview of Their Processing and Utilization. InTech, Rijeka, Croatia; 2017. DOI: 10.5772/63180

[86] Shiomi N, Waisundara V, editors. Superfood and Functional Food—The Development of Superfoods and Their Roles as Medicine. InTech, Rijeka, Croatia; 2017. DOI: 10.5772/65088

[87] Krishnan A, Nongkynrih B, Kapoor SK, Pandav C. A role for INDEPTH Asian sites in translating research to action for non-communicable disease prevention and control: A case study from Ballabgarh, India. Global Health Action. 2009;**2**:76-83

Author	Country	Type of study	Universe	Prevalence %
Adeleye et al. [13]	Southwest of Nigeria	Based on the clinic	160	11.9
Ipadeola et al. [14]	Southwest of Nigeria	Based on the clinic	235	14.0
Agyei-Frempong et al. [15]	Ghana	Based on the clinic	120	11.7
Otieno et al. [16]	Kenya	Based on the clinic	124	5.7
Hwangbo et al. [17]	Korea	Based on the clinic	462	4.3
Tuomi et al. [18]	Finland	Based on population density	1122	9.3
Bosil et al. [19]	Italy	Based on population density	2076	2.8
Zinman et al. [20]	North America and Europe	Based on population density	4134	4.2
Arikan et al. [21]	Turkey	Based on the clinic	54	31.0
Brahmkshatriya et al. [22]	India	Based on the clinic	500	5.0
Lerman et al. [23]	Mexico	Based on the clinic	83	3.6

Table 1. Prevalence of positive glutamic acid decarboxylase antibodies (late autoimmune diabetes in adults) in subjects with type 2 diabetes among different population groups.

3. Genetics

Pathological studies have proposed that LADA and type 1 DM share physiopathological and genetic aspects; such as genes (HLA, INS VNTR and PTPN22) and with respect to DM type 2 (TCF7L2) [26], which suggest that it may represent a genetic admixture of the two types of diabetes, especially when non-insulin requiring.

It is known that LADA has a higher frequency of human histocompatibility antigens (HLA) characteristic of DM type 1: HLA-DR3 (28% of patients), DR4 (27%) and DR 3/4 (22%), in comparison with the general population [26, 27].

The dilemma persists in the fact whether this genetic mixture represents a totally different disease syndrome or is part of a continuum of an autoimmune process.

It is important to mention that in all the genome-wide association studies directed to the exome sequencing carried out until now or the sequencing of the whole genome exome, they have not yet been carried out in large cohorts of adult autoimmune patients.

As mentioned, both diseases have specific antibodies. Concomitantly, a decrease in the frequency and activation of "natural killer" cells in peripheral blood compared with healthy individuals has been demonstrated, which translates into a defect in the immune response [28].

4. Why are LADA and non-diabetic type 1?

Taking into account its subsequent and less aggressive presentation, different arguments have been formulated that explain the appearance of LADA. See **Table 2**.

4.1. When to think about LADA?

Some characteristics have been related, which in order of frequency associated with the disease in comparison with type 2 diabetics are: age of onset <50 years, symptoms of acute onset, BMI <25 kg/m^2 and personal or family history of autoimmune disease.

It is described that the presence of 2 or more of these criteria presents a 90% sensitivity and 71% specificity for the identification of LADA patients [25, 30].

In case of suspicion, specific antibodies should be requested to confirm the diagnosis.

1. Less marked exposure to environmental factors.
2. Lower specific antibody titers.
3. Intermittent crisis of autoimmune aggression.
4. Greater capacity to regenerate beta cells and protection against the apoptotic process.
5. Acquired immunotolerance.

The last three points would be the result of a better protection/risk gene balance compared to type 1 diabetics [3, 29].

Table 2. Postulates of Pozzilli and Di Mario [3], which differentiates LADA from DM type 1.

1. Appearance in adulthood, usually after 30 years
2. Presence of specific auto antibodies, anti-GAD the most prevalent
3. There is no need for insulin therapy at the onset of the disease, which should last at least 6 months

Table 3. LADA diagnostic criteria, proposed by Immunology of Diabetes Society (IDS).

Characteristics	DM type 1	LADA	DM type 2
Age of onset of the disease	Childhood or adulthood	Adulthood	Adulthood
Metabolic syndrome	Similar general population	Similar general population	80 and 90%
Ketoacidosis	Frequent	Infrequent	Absent
Autoimmunity	Present (ICA predominates)	Present (predominates anti GAD)	Absent
Insulin therapy	Since the diagnosis	Approximately 6 months without therapy requirement	Late

Source: Pollak et al. [31].

Table 4. Characteristics of DM type 1, LADA and DM type 2.

However, in order to clarify and have a more unified concept at the time of diagnosis, The Immunology of Diabetes Society (IDS) [4] has proposed 3 criteria for diagnosis, including: diagnosis of diabetes according to criteria established at a higher age at 30 years, independence of insulin for at least 6 months after diagnosis and positivity of antibodies against GADA (**Tables 3** and **4**).

5. Clinical presentation and relationship with chronic diseases

Andersen et al. mentions that patients with LADA have a higher body mass index (BMI) than type 1 diabetics, but less than type 2. The condition of normal weight is the most frequent nutritional status [32].

However, it is not a Sine Qua Non standard in its diagnosis.

5.1. Metabolic characteristics

Patients with adult onset autoimmune diabetes generally have a better metabolic profile than those with type 2 diabetes, with lower levels of triglycerides, higher HDL cholesterol and lower BMI, waist/hip ratio, and blood pressure [18, 33–37].

5.1.1. Body mass index and LADA

A clinical point of view that persists is that patients with LADA are usually thin at the time of diagnosis [5] similar to children with diabetes type 1. However, documentation of BMI in LADA populations of European extraction does not support this point of view. Most of the larger LADA cohort studies report an average BMI in categories of overweight or obesity (BMI > 25.0 kg/m^2) [20, 38–40] and most report a BMI similar to the diabetes type 2 cohorts [20, 38, 40]. Therefore, a normal BMI (<25.0 kg/m^2) should not be a diagnostic criterion for LADA.

5.1.2. Metabolic syndrome and LADA

The increase in the prevalence of metabolic syndrome (MetS) worldwide is alarming, even more so if we take into account that it is considered a risk factor for the development of diabetes, or a pre-diabetic state. The impact of MetS has been demonstrated by the increase in subclinical atherosclerotic disease in patients with the syndrome, even without the diagnosis of diabetes [41]. In countries such as the United States and Mexico, the prevalence of MetS is around 25% of its adult population [42].

Through a cross-sectional population-based study conducted by Wong-McClure et al. they claim that the general prevalence of MetS in Central America is high, being higher in Honduras (21.1%, CI: 16.4–25.9) than in the other countries of the isthmus [43].

Given the presented and due to the absence of data in primary care in Honduras [44], a descriptive study is carried out; in which the prevalence of MetS was determined using the criteria of the third report of the Group of Experts in Adult Treatment (Adult Treatment Panel III) of the National Program of Education on Cholesterol or by its acronym in English «National Cholesterol Education Program-Adult Treatment Panel III (NCEP-ATPIII) [45] being 65.8%.

Multiple studies on MetS and its relationship with DM type LADA estimate that at least 30% of patients diagnosed with type LADA have metabolic disorders [36].

Given the age of onset and the frequency of this syndrome in the adult population, the coexistence of both pathologies is not infrequent. It is estimated that approximately 42% of patients may present with metabolic syndrome, a figure lower than in type 2 DM, in which the association reaches 84% [36].

It is probable that some patients present insulin resistance (IR) although the importance of this phenomenon in the onset of the disease is not clear. It has been shown that adiponectin levels are similar to individuals without DM, suggesting that IR is not part of the etiopathogenesis of the disease [46].

In turn, the presence of dyslipidemia and hypertension is higher than in type 1 diabetics [47], but less frequent than in type 2 diabetics, which could result in an intermediate cardiovascular risk between both types.

5.1.3. DM type 2 and LADA

Multiple studies have found that patients with LADA require treatment with insulin more frequently and earlier after diagnosis than those with type 2 diabetes who are negative for antibodies. GADA positivity in adult patients with diabetes who do not require insulin is associated with decreased fasting C-peptide and a decrease in peptide-C response to oral glucose [12, 18, 48, 49].

It is mentioned that, the magnitude of this insulin response is inversely related to the GADA title [18]. Curiously, insulin secretion was similar in patients recently diagnosed with LADA and DM type 2, as mentioned in two large studies conducted by Zinman et al. and Lundgren et al. [20, 50]

A metabolic study of insulin secretion and insulin sensitivity, conducted by Juhl et al. in 2014; confirmed the lack of weight difference in the groups with LADA and DM type 2 [51].

However, despite these early characteristics, over time, the increased propensity to reduce the function of b cells in LADA becomes evident [12, 18, 48].

Among GADA-positive patients, these altered metabolic parameters tend to be significantly better in those with high GADA titer compared to low GADA titer, but without a clear distinction between groups [18, 33–35].

These wide differences in metabolic parameters translate into negative GADA patients with more signs of metabolic syndrome than positive GADA patients, regardless of whether the latter have LADA or adults with diabetes onset Type 1 [34, 35, 51].

The formal examination of insulin resistance indicates that patients with LADA are more insensitive to insulin than healthy controls, but their insensitivity to insulin is comparable to or lower than that of patients with DM type 2 and is dependent on BMI [20, 40, 50, 52].

6. Clinical features

At the time of diagnosis, the clinical phenotype of patients with apparent autoimmune diabetes can be remarkably broad, ranging from diabetic ketoacidosis to the characteristics of diabetes that can be controlled only with diet.

The classification of these patients also covers a range that may seem arbitrary; for example, in the European Action LADA study, patients with GADA who started taking insulin in the first month of diagnosis were designed as classic type 1 diabetes, those who started with insulin in 6 months were not published and those who started with insulin 6 months or later were designed LADA. Compared with patients with type 2 diabetes, patients with adult onset autoimmune diabetes, even when they do not require insulin (LADA), have a lower age at the time of diabetes, lower BMI and waist/hip ratio, but a higher Pronounced loss of C-peptide and an increased likelihood of treatment with insulin [18, 35, 48].

Phenotypically, patients with high GADA titres tend to have these same characteristics, but they are more marked and more similar to classic type 1 diabetes, with younger patients at the time of diagnosis being thinner with a high risk of progression to treatment with insulin.

Patients with a low GADA titer are phenotypically more similar to those with DM type 2 diabetes. These differences are also observed in the metabolic syndrome, which is more frequent in type 2 diabetes than type 1 and LADA diabetes, and more prevalent in low-grade patients than patients with GADA high titer [18, 33, 35, 48].

Because the high GADA titer tends to be associated with multiple diabetes-associated autoantibodies (DAA), it is not surprising that the NIRAD study found that among patients with adult diabetes, more DAA were detected plus these patients needed insulin treatment and had an earlier age [53].

However, there is sufficient overlap for these clinical parameters between patient groups to make it impossible to accurately distinguish autoimmune diabetes from adult type 2 diabetes in clinical characteristics only when considering individual patients [4, 54].

7. Complications

The frequency of ketoacidosis has not been documented in LADA, but it is assumed to be very low. Chronic vascular complications associated with type 1 diabetes and type 2 diabetes are also present in LADA [55].

7.1. Chronic complications

Few studies have addressed this issue. Cabrera-Rode et al. describe a lower incidence of retinopathy, nephropathy and peripheral vascular disease, in comparison with type 2 diabetics, although without significant differences given the small number of patients. Recently, a study in Korea, with more than 300 patients (5.3% classified as LADA, 70% in insulin therapy), reveals that the risk of developing microvascular complications is similar to diabetic patients type 1 and 2 [55, 56].

7.2. Diabetes microvascular and macrovascular complications

It has been observed that the prevalence of microvascular complications in LADA is broadly similar to that observed in patients with type 2 diabetes, however in a small study conducted by Myhill et al., reported a lower risk of nephropathy [51, 55–57].

It is important to mention that patients with LADA generally have a more favorable cardiovascular risk profile than those with type 2 diabetes. However, to date, different studies have found no evidence of a lower risk of macrovascular disease in patients with DM type LADA [51, 55, 57].

The independent associations of hypertension, hyperlipidemia, obesity and hyperglycemia with macrovascular disease in diabetic patients are well established. Interestingly, hypertension, hyperlipidemia and obesity were less frequent in LADA than in type 2 diabetes [55], but the rates of macrovascular complications were similar. Possible explanations include differences in pathogenesis or treatment.

Given the autoimmune pathology, patients with LADA may have greater systemic inflammation, involved in vascular pathology [58].

It is a fact that patients with LADA can be treated suboptimally because they often start treatment with insulin later than clinically indicated, due to unrecognized insulin deficiency, detection of specific antibodies and a reluctance to change oral therapies to injections.

They are also likely to have a shorter duration of treatment with metformin, an oral agent associated with a lower rate of ischemic heart disease in the UKPDS [59].

Although these studies were small, there is no evidence to support a less aggressive treatment policy for cardiovascular risk factors in patients with LADA.

8. Therapeutic update for DM type LADA

Currently there is no established intervention for patients with LADA-type DM, despite the fact that they represent a considerable number of patients with diabetes. Considering that these patients present hyperglycemia, there is no doubt that they require specific therapy to control blood glucose levels.

Therefore, there is no doubt that the best therapeutic option in patients with LADA (while trials are expected to prevent the depletion of B cells) is to achieve good metabolic control and prevent chronic complications.

As a cornerstone in the treatment it is important to keep in mind that glycemic control is a strong risk factor for the development of cardiovascular disease in patients with LADA at a higher level than in patients with type 2 diabetes and could be related to the lower prevalence of the metabolic syndrome in the first ones [60].

Different studies show that insulin therapy is the ideal treatment to achieve a better metabolic control in subjects with type LADA DM.

This procedure is useful to reduce the destruction of β-cells when there is a break in their activity, which determines a decrease in the expression of pancreatic antigens in β-cells [3, 61–68].

The application of an early insulin treatment in subjects with LADA who present a discrete insulin secretion is beneficial, and influences the preservation of pancreatic β-cell function. The early and correct identification of the LADA is necessary to define the adequate therapeutic behavior and improve the prognosis of these individuals.

In patients initially diagnosed as type 2 diabetic, a number of therapeutic options are possible that coincide with present available treatments of hyperglycemia.

It is at this moment where conjecturing or establishing a therapeutic goal is a challenge; because alternatives have been sought for the management of our patients, among which are mentioned.

8.1. Sulfonylureas

Beside diet, sulfonylureas are largely used in patients with type 2 diabetes. Sulfonylureas stimulate insulin secretion by promoting closure of the ATP-dependent potassium channels on pancreatic b-cells.

They are effective as blood glucose reducers, however, there is experimental evidence that they can increase the immune response, so they are considered imprudent, as they could accelerate the progression towards insulin dependence [3, 22].

In 1996, Kobayashi and 114 others observed that the administration of small doses of insulin was an effective treatment in individuals with recently diagnosed LADA, which is expressed by a high rate of negative conversion of the AHF and an increase in the levels of C-peptide. In serum, on the other hand, when a sulfonylurea (glibenclamide) is used alone in these diabetics, the persistence of the ICA is maintained and there is a progressive decrease in the levels of C-peptide in the serum.

8.2. Biguanides

Treatment with metformin has no direct action on the β cell, and it could be indicated in patients with LADA with clinical characteristics of metabolic syndrome or with obesity. This treatment allowed a good control of HbA1c and caused a drastic decrease in insulinemia [69]. In these cases, a combination therapy of metformin with insulin could also be considered.

Nevertheless, one potential problem associated with the use of metformin is the development of lactic acidosis in a patient at high risk of becoming insulin-dependent.

8.3. Glitazones

Theoretically they could have their value in the treatment, not only to improve the sensitivity of the insulin but also to exert an anti-inflammatory effect that would favor the preservation of the β cell mass [2, 70].

There is interesting evidence that glitazones increase insulin synthesis and the insulin content of islet cells as well as improve the secretory response of islets [71].

Zhou and others have demonstrated the efficacy of treatment with rosiglitazone in combination with insulin, which helps preserve the function of the cell compared to insulin alone in LADA [2, 70, 71].

Sitagliptin is a potent DPP-4 inhibitor which results in the delay of degradation of incretin hormones (glucagon-like peptide-1 (GLP-1) and gastric inhibitory peptide (GIP)), thereby improving beta-cell function and resulting in better glycemic control in patients with T2D.

Recent studies demonstrate that the use of sitagliptin in individuals with T1D improved overall the glycemic control and reduced insulin requirements without altering the amount of endogenous insulin production [72].

A prospective study of 1-year duration demonstrated maintenance of beta-cell function through the administration of sitagliptin in patients with recent-onset LADA [73]. A similar study proved that c-peptide secretion and glycemic control was improved by the use of another DPP-4 inhibitor, saxagliptin, versus placebo in LADA patients [74, 75]. All these accumulating evidences support the hypothesis that this may be a class effect; however, further studies are required.

8.4. Potential strategies for preventing b-cell destruction in LADA

A clinical trial showed that insulin therapy was the best treatment in this type of diabetic, and that the use of glibenclamide produced a persistence of the ICA (the ICA persisted in 100% of the subjects with LADA treated with glibenclamide + insulin), and that its exclusion decreased the presence of these antibodies (the ICA disappeared in 75% of the individuals with LADA treated only with insulin) [76, 77].

The use of glibenclamide or another sulphonylurea is not recommended in the treatment of these patients or their combination with insulin [65, 66], since it could contribute to the persistence of the autoimmune process and the probable progressive destruction of pancreatic cells.

Finally, a meta-analysis on pharmacological treatment [71], with a total of 8 publications (735 patients), concludes that:

- There are no benefits in the metabolic control when associating hypoglycemics with insulin therapy.
- Better metabolic control with insulin compared to sulfonylureas.
- Insulin dependence earlier in patients treated with sulfonylureas.
- Preservation of initial C peptide with early insulin therapy or rosiglitazone, which would position these therapies as the choice.

9. Conclusions

9.1. Summary: knowledge and uncertainty

Patients with DM type LADA are more likely to have lower C-peptide, associated with fewer signs of metabolic syndrome; higher levels of HbA1c, faster progress to insulin therapy. It is not yet clear how DM type LADA is associated with the loss of insulin secretion capacity.

9.2. Summary: knowledge and uncertainty

There are no clear clinical features that distinguish autoimmune diabetes from type 2 diabetes. However, there is a tendency for adult patients with GADA, even when they do not require insulin, being younger at the time of diagnosis and thinner with a greater tendency to progress to treatment with insulin. Within a cohort of positive GADA adult patients, the GADA title and the number of LADA patients impact the clinical and biochemical differences of type 2 diabetes. The clinical phenotype should drive the management strategy.

Author details

Javier Eduardo Escober Torres

Address all correspondence to: jetorres.9307@gmail.com

Universidad Nacional Autónoma de Honduras, Tegucigalpa, Honduras

References

[1] American Diabetes Association. Classification and diagnosis of diabetes. Diabetes Care. 2016;**39**(Suppl 1):S13-S22

[2] Stenstrom G, Gottsa A, Bakhtadze E, Berger B, Sundkvist G. Latent autoimmune diabetes in adults: Definition, prevalence, cell function, and treatment. Diabetes. 2005;**54**(2):68-72

[3] Pozzilli P, Di Mario U. Autoimmune diabetes not requiring insulin at diagnosis (latent autoimmune diabetes of the adult): Definition, characterization, and potential prevention. Diabetes Care. 2001;**24**:1460-1467

[4] Fourlanos S, Dotta F, Greenbaum C, Palmer J, Rolandsson O, Colman P, et al. Latent autoimmune diabetes in adults (LADA) should be less latent. Diabetologia. 2005;**48**:2206-2212

[5] Van Deutekom A, Heine R, Siemsek S. The islet autoantibody titres: Their clinical relevance in latent autoimmune diabetes in adults (LADA) and the classification of diabetes mellitus. Diabetic Medicine. 2008;**25**:117-125

[6] Palmer J, Hampe C, Chiu H, Goel A, Brooks-Worrell B. Is latent autoimmune diabetes in adults distinct from type 1 diabetes or just type 1 diabetes at an older age? Diabetes. 2005;**54**(2):62-67

[7] Irvine WJ, Gray RS, McCallum CJ, Duncan LJP. Clinical and pathogenic significance of pancreatic-islet-cell antibodies in diabetics treated with oral hypoglycaemic agents. Lancet. 1977;**14**:1025-1027

[8] Naik RG, Brooks-Worrell BM, Palmer JP. Latent autoimmune diabetes in adults. The Journal of Clinical Endocrinology and Metabolism. 2009;**94**:4635-4644

[9] Groop LC, Bottazzo GF, Doniach D. Islet cell antibodies identify latent type I diabetes in patients aged 35-75 years at diagnosis. Diabetes. 1986;**35**:237-41.5

[10] Schiel A, Müller UA. GAD autoantibodies in a selection-free population of insulin-treated diabetic patients: Indicator of a high prevalence of LADA? Diabetes Research and Clinical Practice. 2000;**49**:33-40

[11] Xiuying Q, Jing S, Jing W, Peizhong P, Zhongliang X, Madonna M, et al. Prevalence and correlates of latent autoimmune diabetes in adults in Tianjin, China: A population-based cross-sectional study. Diabetes Care. 2011;**34**:66-70

[12] Turner R, Stratton I, Horton V, Manley S, Zimmet P, Mackay IR, et al. UKPDS 25: Autoantibodies to islet-cell cytoplasm and glutamic acid decarboxylase for prediction of insulin requirement in type 2 diabetes. UK Prospective Diabetes Study Group. Lancet. 1997;**350**:1288-1293

[13] Adeleye OO, Ogbera AO, Fasanmade O, Ogunleye OO, Dada AO, Ale AO, et al. Latent autoimmune diabetes mellitus in adults (LADA) and it's characteristics in a subset of Nigerians initially managed for type 2 diabetes. International Archives of Medicine. 2012;**5**:23

[14] Ipadeola A, Adeleye JO, Akinlade KS. Latent autoimmune diabetes amongst adults with type 2 diabetes in a Nigerian tertiary hospital. Primary Care Diabetes. 2015;**9**:231-236

[15] Agyei-Frempong MT, Titty FV, Owiredu WK, Eghan BA. The prevalence of autoimmune diabetes among diabetes mellitus patients in Kumasi, Ghana. Pakistan Journal of Biological Sciences. 2008;**11**:2320-2325

[16] Otieno CF, Huho AN, Omonge EO, Amayo AA, Njagi E. Type 2 diabetes mellitus: Clinical and aetiologic types, therapy and quality of glycaemic control of ambulatory patients. East African Medical Journal. 2008;**85**:24-29

[17] Hwangbo Y, Kim JT, Kim EK, Khang AR, Oh TJ, Jang HC, et al. Prevalence and clinical characteristics of recently diagnosed type 2 diabetes patients with positive anti-glutamic acid decarboxylase antibody. Diabetes and Metabolism Journal. 2012;**36**:136-143

[18] Tuomi T, Carlsson A, Li H, Isomaa B, Miettinen A, Nilsson A, et al. Clinical and genetic characteristics of type 2 diabetes with and without GAD antibodies. Diabetes. 1999;**48**:150-157

[19] Bosil EP, Garancini MP, Poggiali F, Bonifacio E, Gallus G. Low prevalence of islet autoimmunity in adult diabetes and low predictive value of islet autoantibodies in the general adult population of Northern Italy. Diabetologia. 1999;**42**:840-844

[20] Zinman B, Kahn SE, Haffner SM, O'Neill MC, Heise MA, Freed MI; ADOPT Study Group. Phenotypic characteristics of GAD antibody-positive recently diagnosed patients with type 2 diabetes in North America and Europe. Diabetes. 2004;**53**:3193-3200

[21] Arikan E, Sabuncu T, Ozer EM, Hatemi H. The clinical characteristics of latent autoimmune diabetes in adults and its relation with chronic complications in metabolically poor controlled Turkish patients with type 2 diabetes mellitus. Journal of Diabetes and its Complications. 2005;**19**:254-258

[22] Brahmkshatriya PP, Mehta AA, Saboo BD, Goyal RK. Characteristics and prevalence of latent autoimmune diabetes in adults (LADA). ISRN Pharmacology. 2012;**2012**:580202

[23] Lerman I et al. Baja prevalencia de autoinmunidad (anticuerpos anti GAD +) en pacientes adultos con diabetes mellitus tipo 2 de inicio temprano. Revista de Endocrinología y Nutrición. 2010;**18**(4):170-175

[24] The Expert Committee on the Diagnosis and Classification of Diabetes Mellitus. Report of the expert committee on the diagnosis and classification of diabetes mellitus. Diabetes Care. 1998;**21**(Suppl 1):S3-519

[25] Naik RG, Palmer JP. Latent autoimmune diabetes in adults (LADA). Reviews in Endocrine & Metabolic Disorders. 2003;**4**:233-241

[26] Cervin C, Lyssenko V, Bakhtadze E, Lindholm E, Nilsson P, Tuomi T, et al. Genetic similarities between latent autoimmune diabetes in adults, type 1 diabetes, and type 2 diabetes. Diabetes. 2008;**57**:1433-1437

[27] Leslie R, Williams R, Pozzilli P. Clinical review: Type 1 diabetes and latent autoimmune diabetes in adults: One end of the rainbow. The Journal of Clinical Endocrinology and Metabolism. 2006;**91**(5):1654-1659

[28] Hosszufalusi N, Vatay A, Rajczy K, Prohaszka Z, Pozsonyi E, Horvath L. Similar genetic features and different islet cell autoantibody pattern of latent autoimmune diabetes in adults (LADA) compared with adult-onset type 1 diabetes with rapid progression. Diabetes Care. 2003;**26**:452-457

[29] Grant SF, Thorleifsson G, Reynisdottir I, Benediktsson R, Manolescu A, Sainz J, et al. Variant of transcription factor 7–like 2 (TCF7L2) gene confers risk of type 2 diabetes. Nature Genetics. 2006;**38**:320-323

[30] Fourlanos S, Perry C, Stein M, Stankovich J, Harrison L, Colman P. A clinical screening tool identifies autoimmune diabetes in adults. Diabetes Care. 2006;**29**:970-975

[31] Pollak F et al. Diabetes autoinmune (latente) del adulto. Revista Médica de Chile. 2012;**140**:1476-1481

[32] Lutgens M, Meijer M, Peeters B, Poulsen M, Rutten M, Bots M, et al. Easily obtainable clinical features increase the diagnostic accuracy for latent autoimmune diabetes in adults: An evidence-based report. Primary Care Diabetes. 2008;**2**(4):207-211

[33] Andersen M, Lundgren V, Turunem J, Forsblom C, Isomaa B, Groop P, et al. Latent autoimmune diabetes in adults differs genetically from classical type 1 diabetes diagnosed after the age of 35 years. Diabetes Care. 2010;**33**(9):2064-2010

[34] Buzzetti R, Di PS, Giaccari A, Petrone A, Locatelli M, Suraci C, et al. High titer of autoantibodies to GAD identifies a specific phenotype of adult-onset autoimmune diabetes. Diabetes Care. 2007;**30**:932-938

[35] Zhou Z, Xiang Y, Ji L, Jia W, Ning G, Huang G, et al. Frequency, immunogenetics, and clinical characteristics of latent autoimmune diabetes in China (LADA China study): A nationwide, multicenter, clinic-based cross-sectional study. Diabetes. 2013;**62**:543-550

[36] Hawa MI, Kolb H, Schloot N, Beyan H, Paschou SA, Buzzetti R, et al. Adult-onset autoimmune diabetes in Europe is prevalent with a broad clinical phenotype: Action LADA 7. Diabetes Care. 2013;**36**:908-913

[37] Hawa MI, Thivolet C, Mauricio D, Alemanno I, Cipponeri E, Collier D, et al. Metabolic syndrome and autoimmune diabetes: Action LADA 3. Diabetes Care. 2009;**32**:160-164

[38] Leslie RD, Pozzilli P. Type I diabetes masquerading as type II diabetes. Possible implications for prevention and treatment. Diabetes Care. 1994;**17**:1214-1219

[39] Lohmann T, Nietzschmann U, Kiess W. 'Lady-like': Is there a latent autoimmune diabetes in the young? Diabetes Care. 2000;**23**:1707-1708

[40] Davis TM, Zimmet P, Davis WA, Bruce DG, Fida S, Mackay IR. Autoantibodies to glutamic acid decarboxylase in diabetic patients from a multi-ethnic Australian community: The Fremantle Diabetes Study. Diabetic Medicine. 2000;**17**:667-674

[41] Carlsson A, Sundkvist G, Groop L, Tuomi T. Insulin and glucagon secretion in patients with slowly progressing autoimmune diabetes (LADA). The Journal of Clinical Endocrinology and Metabolism. 2000;**85**:76-80

[42] Garber AJ, Handelsman Y, Einhorn D, Bergman DA, Bloomgarden ZT, Fonseca V, et al. Diagnosis and management of prediabetes in the continuum of hyperglycemia: When do the risks of diabetes begin? A consensus statement from the American College of Endocrinology and the American Association of Clinical Endocrinologists. Endocrine Practice. 2008;**14**(7):933-946

[43] Won KB, Chang HJ, Kim HC, Jeon K, Lee H, Shin S, et al. Differential impact of metabolic syndrome on subclinical atherosclerosis according to the presence of diabetes. Cardiovascular Diabetology. 2013;**12**:41

[44] Wong-McClure RA, Gregg EW, Barceló A, Lee K, Abarca-Gómez L, Sanabria-López L, et al. Prevalence of metabolic syndrome in Central America: A cross-sectional population-based study. Revista Panamericana de Salud Pública. 2015;**38**(3):202-208

[45] Escober Torres J et al. Síndrome metabólico: primer estudio de prevalencia en atención primaria, Honduras. Endocrinología, Diabetes y Nutrición. 2017;**64**:273-276. http://dx.doi.org/10.1016/j.endinu.2017.02.003

[46] Executive summary of the Third Report of The National Cholesterol Education Program (NCEP) Expert panel on detection, evaluation, and treatment of high blood cholesterol in adults (Adult treatment panel III). JAMA. 2001;**285**:2486-2492

[47] Brophy S, Davies H, Stephens J, Prior S, Atkinson M, Bain S, et al. Adiponectin levels in people with Latent Autoimmune Diabetes—A case control study. BMC Research Notes. 2010;**3**:317

[48] Weslley P, Sepulveda J, Amim R, Alvarenga T, Calsolari M, Cavalcanti S. Comparison of clinical and laboratory characteristics between adult-onset type 1 diabetes and latent autoimmune diabetes in adults. Diabetes Care. 2005;**28**(7):1803-1804

[49] Radtke MA, Midthjell K, Nilsen TI, Grill V. Heterogeneity of patients with latent autoimmune diabetes in adults: Linkage to autoimmunity is apparent only in those with perceived need for insulin treatment: Results from the Nord-Trondelag Health (HUNT) study. Diabetes Care. 2009;**32**:245-250

[50] Lundgren VM, Isomaa B, Lyssenko V, Laurila E, Korhonen P, Groop LC, et al. GAD antibody positivity predicts type 2 diabetes in an adult population. Diabetes. 2010;**59**:416-422

[51] Juhl CB, Bradley U, Holst JJ, Leslie RD, Yderstraede KB, Hunter S. Similar weight-adjusted insulin secretion and insulin sensitivity in short-duration late autoimmune diabetes of adulthood (LADA) and Type 2 diabetes: Action LADA 8. Diabetic Medicine. 2014;**31**:941-945

[52] Hawa MI, Buchan AP, Ola T, Wun CC, DeMicco DA, Bao W, et al. LADA and CARDS: A prospective study of clinical outcome in established adult-onset autoimmune diabetes. Diabetes Care. 2014;**37**:1643-1649

[53] Tripathy D, Carlsson AL, Lehto M, Isomaa B, Tuomi T, Groop L. Insulin secretion and insulin sensitivity in diabetic subgroups: Studies in the prediabetic and diabetic state. Diabetologia. 2000;**43**:1476-1483

[54] Lampasona V, Petrone A, Tiberti C, Capizzi M, Spoletini M, Di PS, et al. Zinc transporter 8 antibodies complement GAD and IA–2 antibodies in the identification and characterization of adult-onset autoimmune diabetes: Non Insulin Requiring Autoimmune Diabetes (NIRAD) 4. Diabetes Care. 2010;**33**:104-108

[55] Juneja R, Hirsch IB, Naik RG, Brooks-Worrell BM, Greenbaum CJ, Palmer JP. Islet cell antibodies and glutamic acid decarboxylase antibodies, but not the clinical phenotype, help to identify type 1(1/2) diabetes in patients presenting with type 2 diabetes. Metabolism. 2001;**50**:1008-1013

[56] Roh M-O, Jung C-H, Kim B-Y, Mok J-O, Kim C-H. The prevalence and characteristics of latent autoimmune diabetes in adults (LADA) and its relation with chronic complications in a clinical department of a university hospital in Korea. Acta Diabetologica. 2013 Apr;**50**(2):129-134. 2010 Oct 16 (online)

[57] Myhill P, Davis WA, Bruce DG, Mackay IR, Zimmet P, Davis TM. Chronic complications and mortality in community-based patients with latent autoimmune diabetes in adults: The Fremantle Diabetes Study. Diabetic Medicine. 2008;**25**:1245-1250

[58] Ridker PM. High-sensitivity C-reactive protein and cardiovascular risk: Rationale for screening and primary prevention. The American Journal of Cardiology. 2003;**92**:17K-22K

[59] UK Prospective Diabetes Study (UKPDS) Group. Effect of intensive blood-glucose control with metformin on complications in overweight patients with type 2 diabetes (UKPDS 34). Lancet. 1998;**352**:854-865

[60] Isomaa B, Almgren P, Henricsson M, et al. Chronic complications in patients with slowly progressing autoimmune type 1 diabetes (LADA). Diabetes Care. 1999;**22**:1347-1353

[61] Leslie RDG. Intervention in patients with type 1 diabetes masquerading as type II diabetes. Diabetes, Nutrition & Metabolism. 1996;**9**:319-324

[62] Bjork E, Kampe E, Karlsson A, Pipeleers DG, Anderson A, Hellerstrom C, et al. Glucose regulation of the autoantigen GAD65 in human pancreatic islet. The Journal of Clinical Endocrinology and Metabolism. 1992;**75**:1574-1576

[63] Keller RJ, Eisenbarth GS, Jackson RA. Insulin prophylaxis in individuals at high risk of type 1 diabetes. Lancet. 1993;**341**:927-928

[64] Malone JI. The role of exogenous insulin in the pathogenesis of autoimmune diabetes mellitus. In: Rifkin H, Colwell JA, Taylor SI, editors. Diabetes. Amsterdam, The Netherlands: Elsevier Science Publisher; 1991. pp. 1022-1025

[65] Kobayashi T, Nakanishi K, Murase T, Kosaka K. Small doses of subcutaneous insulin as a strategy for preventing slowly progressive β-cell failure in islet cell antibody-positive patients with clinical features of NIDDM. Diabetes. 1996;**45**:622-626

[66] Cabrera-Rode E, Perich P, Díaz-Horta O, Tiberti C, Molina G, Arranz C, et al. Slowly progressing type 1 diabetes: Persistence of islet cell autoantibodies is related to glibenclamide treatment. Autoimmunity. 2002;**35**:469-474

[67] Cabrera-Rode E, Perich P, Licea M. Latent autoimmune diabetes in adults (LADA) or slowly progressing type 1 diabetes: Type 1 or type 1.5 diabetes? Revista de la Asociación Latinoamericana de Diabetes. 2002;**X**:76-84

[68] Maruyama T, Tanaka S, Shimada A, Funae O, Kasuga A, Kanatzuka A, et al. Insulin intervention in slowly insulin-dependent (type 1) diabetes mellitus. The Journal of Clinical Endocrinology and Metabolism. 2008 Jun;**93**(6):2115-2121. Disponible en: http://jcem.endojournals.org/cgi/rapidpdf/jc.2007-2267v1 Consultado, 28 de noviembre de 2008

[69] Loriz Peralta O, Campos Bonilla B, Granada Ybern ML, Sanmarti Sala A, Arroyo J e investigadores asociados del Catalonian Overweight and Diabetes Pilot Study Group (CODIPS). Detección de diabetes tipo LADA en pacientes diabéticos con exceso ponderal ¿Es adecuado el tratamiento con metformina? Atencion Primaria. 2007;**39**:133-137

[70] Masuda K, Okamoto Y, Tsuura Y, Kato S, Misura T, Tsuda K, Horikoshi H, Ishida H, Seino Y. Effects of troglitazone (CS-045) on insulin secretion in isolated rat pancreatic cells and HIT cells: An insulinotropic mechanism distinct from glibenclamide. Diabetologia. 1995;**38**:24-30

[71] Beales PE, Pozzilli P. Thiazolidinediones for the prevention of diabetes in the non-obese diabetic (NOD) mouse: Implications for human type 1 diabetes. Diabetes/Metabolism Research and Reviews. 2002;**18**:114-117

[72] Kumar K, Shaikh A, Prusty P. Addition of exenatide or sitagliptin to insulin in new onset type 1 diabetes: A randomized, open label study. Diabetes Research and Clinical Practice. 2013;**100**:55-58. DOI: 10.1016/j.diabres.2013.01.020

[73] Zhao Y, Yang L, Xiang Y, Liu L, Huang G, Long Z, Li X, Leslie RD, Wang X, Zhou Z. Dipeptidyl peptidase 4 inhibitor sitagliptin maintains β-cell function in patients with recent-onset latent autoimmune diabetes in adults: One year prospective study. The Journal of Clinical Endocrinology and Metabolism. 2014;**99**:E876-E880. DOI: 10.1210/jc.2013-3633

[74] Buzzetti R, Pozzilli P, Frederich R, Iqbal N, Hirshberg B. Saxagliptin improves glycaemic control and C-peptide secretion in latent autoimmune diabetes in adults (LADA). Diabetes/Metabolism Research and Reviews. 2016;**32**:289-296. DOI: 10.1002/dmrr.v32.3

[75] Zhou Z, Li X, Huang G, Peng J, Yang L, Yan X, Wang J. Rosiglitazone combined with insulin preserves islet beta cell function in adult-onset latent autoimmune diabetes (LADA). Diabetes/Metabolism Research and Reviews. 2005;**21**:203-208

[76] Törn C, Gupta M, Nikitina Zake L, Sanjeevi CB, Landin-Olsson M. Heterozygosity for MICA5.0/MICA5.1 and HLA-DR3-DQ2/DR4-DQ8 are independent genetic risk factors for latent autoimmune diabetes in adults. Human Immunology. 2003;**64**:902-909

[77] Borg H, Gottsater A, Fernlund P, Sundkvist G. A 12 years prospective of the relationship between islet antibodies and β-cell function at and after the diagnosis in patients with adult onset diabetes. Diabetes. 2002;**51**:1754-1762

11

Body Temperature Regulation during Exercise and Hyperthermia in Diabetics

Ryosuke Takeda and Kazunobu Okazaki

Abstract

Thermoregulatory function, that is, heat dissipative responses such as skin blood flow (SkBF) and sweating to an increased body temperature, is critical during physical work or exercise in warm and hot conditions and during hyperthermia. Thermoregulatory function is associated with individual somatotype, fitness level, normal aging, and physiological status and diseases. Individuals with type 2 diabetes have decreased thermoregulatory responses compared with healthy counterparts, characterized by decreased SkBF and sweating. The decreased SkBF and sweating would be associated with the reduction in nitric oxide bioavailability and endothelial functions in skin vasculatures, also with central mechanisms, and so on. Aerobic exercise training and/or acclimation to the heat improve heat dissipative responses in healthy subjects. The effects of exercise training in type 2 diabetics on glycemic control are well established while it remains unclear that high levels of aerobic fitness or exercise training in diabetics improve thermoregulatory function during heat stress.

Keywords: thermoregulation, sweat rate, skin blood flow, plasma volume, aging, diabetes

1. Introduction

Individuals are more likely to become exhausted and to develop heat-related illnesses when physical work or sporting activities are performed for a prolonged time in warm and hot conditions or direct sunlight compared to in cooler conditions. Thermoregulation is one of the most important physiological functions for when individuals are exposed to extreme hot environments. The incidence of heat-related illnesses is particularly great if physical work or exercise is performed at higher intensities and in higher ambient temperatures (T_a) and relative humidity (RH) [1]. In addition, the incidence is greater in persons who are dehydrated, who are not acclimated to hot environments, or who have low levels of physical fitness and daily activity even if they are healthy [1]. More importantly, the incidence is greater in individuals with obesity, diabetes mellitus, and cardiovascular diseases, due to impaired thermoregulatory responses [1, 2]. It is also greater in individuals with attenuated thermoregulatory responses, such as those with skin grafts, spinal cord injuries, and multiple sclerosis [3–5]. Moreover, an extreme hot environment can be dangerous for the elderly (even those who are healthy) because of the normal aging process [1, 2]. Over the last two decades, the morbidity and mortality of heat-related illnesses has rapidly increased in Japan because of the rapidly aging population and global warming [6]. This chapter first discusses thermoregulation during work and exercise in warm and hot conditions and the possible physiological effects of humoral and other important factors on thermoregulation. Second, the effects of diseases such as diabetes on thermoregulatory responses are discussed.

2. Thermoregulation in warm and hot conditions

Core body temperature is determined by the heat equilibrium between heat gain and loss [1]. Typically, core body temperature is elevated when we face continuous whole-body work and exercise. This is because only approximately 20% of the energy produced in contracting muscles is used for muscle contraction; the remaining 80% is converted to heat energy, and therefore exercise causes an increase in muscle temperature. The heat is distributed to the body by the circulation and increases body temperatures. Therefore, greater exercise intensities are associated with greater heat production during exercise. However, although core body temperature elevates rapidly within several minutes of starting exercise, heat dissipation mechanisms are activated sufficiently to balance heat production and eventually the increase in core body temperature reaches a steady state. The cutaneous vasculature and sweat glands are thermoregulatory effectors of the skin and promote heat loss by increasing skin blood flow (SkBF) via cutaneous vasodilation and by sweating, respectively [1]. The heat generated in contracting muscles is transferred, because of circulation of blood, to the skin surface; thus, skin surface temperature is elevated by the increased SkBF. The heat transferred to the skin surface is released to the surrounding air according to the thermal gradient between the skin and the air (non-evaporative heat dissipation). Therefore, in a cool environment, non-evaporative heat dissipation is effective; however, in warm environments, when T_a is higher than skin temperatures (~30°C), it becomes ineffective or even negative and acts as a source of heat gain. Conversely, sweating enhances heat loss via sweat evaporation from the skin surface to the air (evaporative heat dissipation). Evaporative heat dissipation is determined according to the gradient of water vapor between the skin surface and the surrounding air. Therefore, it is available regardless of T_a and is the main and critical heat loss mechanism when T_a exceeds ~30°C; however, it is attenuated in a humid environment. Consequently, when heat gain exceeds heat loss during high-intensity work and/or exercise in a hot and humid environment, core body temperature increases rapidly. Therefore, these conditions increase susceptibility to heat-related illnesses.

Physiologically, SkBF and sweating are regulated by body core and skin temperatures (thermal factors) and also other (non-thermal) factors [1]. Body core temperature is monitored continuously by central thermoreceptors. On the other hand, skin temperatures are monitored continuously by the peripheral thermoreceptors. These receptors send received thermal information through an afferent pathway to the thermoregulatory center in the preoptic/anterior hypothalamus [1]. When the hypothalamic thermoregulatory center determines that core and skin temperatures are elevated compared to the set point, SkBF and sweating are increased through the reflex efferent pathways of sympathetic nerve systems [1]. In humans, SkBF and sweating are neutrally controlled via two distinct skin sympathetic nerves. A sympathetic adrenergic vasoconstrictor system is one of the neural control mechanisms for SkBF and the other is a separate sympathetic cholinergic vasodilator system [1]. Sweating is controlled by sympathetic cholinergic nerves [1]. In addition, non-thermal factors modify the thermal reflex, including central commands, mechano- and metabo-reflexes, arterial and cardiopulmonary baroreflexes, blood volume and osmolality, and mental stimuli [1]. During exercise, they exert different effects on SkBF and sweating responses [1]. Typically, SkBF at the same levels of core and skin temperatures is lower during exercise than resting conditions, and this restriction is greater at higher exercise intensities. Conversely, sweating at the same levels of core and skin temperatures is likely to be higher during exercise than resting conditions.

When levels of dehydration worsen, the risk of heat-related illnesses is much higher during work or exercise in a hot environment [7]. Rothstein and Towbin [8] described for the first time the effects of dehydration on thermoregulation in humans. They reported that an ~0.3°C increase in rectal temperature is caused by every 1% body weight loss by sweating in breaks between exercises when soldiers march in the desert. This is because, as non-thermal factors, dehydration-induced hypovolemia and hyperosmolality limit the response to enhance SkBF and sweating to increased body temperature. Decreased body fluid volume and increased osmolality change dramatically during exercise even in a cool environment. Indeed, plasma volume (PV) is decreased with an increased intensity of exercise. In maximal exercise, the decrease in PV is reached by approximately 300–500 mL (8–15%). Increased capillary fluid filtration from the intravascular to the extravascular spaces due to an increase in blood pressure and peripheral vasodilation during exercise causes the PV change. Additionally, metabolites accumulated in the intracellular fluid of contracting muscles such as lactic acid increases free-water shift from the plasma to the intracellular fluid through the interstitium based on the osmotic gradient [9]. It is estimated to be ~1 L of the volume shifted to the contracting muscles at maximal exercise. About half of this water is from PV [10]. In addition, plasma osmolality (P_{osm}) is increased from ~285 mosmol/kgH_2O at rest to over 300 mosmol/kgH_2O at maximal exercise due to accumulated metabolites. These humoral changes are not caused by dehydration due to sweating; rather, they are associated with the exercise itself. Because they are observed within several minutes after the start of exercise, in addition, when exercise is performed in warm and hot conditions, hypohydration due to the decrease in PV and hyperosmolality due to the increase in P_{osm} during exercise is exacerbated because of increased SkBF and sweating for thermoregulation. Enhanced SkBF induces a reduction in venous return to the heart due to pooling of excessive blood in dilated peripheral vasculature of the skin [11]. Additionally, ~10% of the sweat volume is lost from plasma fluids, and P_{osm} is increased according to sweat rate because sweat is hypotonic compared to body fluids. These humoral changes enhance the load on the circulation and act as limiting factors for thermoregulation.

Nadel et al. [12] first showed that isotonic hypovolemia (change in PV, −700 mL; body weight, −2.7%) achieved by diuretic administration before exercise induced upward shift of the esophageal temperature (T_{es}) threshold for the onset of cutaneous vasodilation by 0.4°C during exercise at 55% of maximal oxygen consumption rate (VO_{2max}) in a hot environment (T_a 35°C). It also reduced the SkBF at peak value by about 50% compared to control condition. Besides, Mack et al. [13] reported that an acute reduction in venous return to the heart induced by application of −40 mmHg lower body negative pressure (LBNP) decreased SkBF and elevated T_{es} during exercise at an intensity corresponding to a heart rate of 125 beats/min in a warm environment (T_a, 28°C). In contrast, all techniques to acutely increase venous return during exercise, including isotonic hypervolemia with saline infusion [11], postural change from upright to supine position [14, 15], head-out water immersion [16], or continuous negative pressure breathing [17], enhanced the response to increase SkBF to an increased core body temperature during exercise. From these observations, the response to increase SkBF to an increased core body temperature during exercise is attenuated by dehydration-induced hypovolemia via the cardiopulmonary baroreflex. Recently, Ogawa et al. [18] reported that the efferent sympathetic signals to skin vasculature, that is, the skin sympathetic nerve activity (SSNA), component synchronized with the cardiac cycle was decreased by postural change from supine to 30° head-up tilt during hyperthermia (T_{es} increased ~0.7°C) with passive heating and that the responses were correlated with the decrease in cutaneous vasodilation. With these data, they suggested that the SSNA component synchronized with the cardiac cycle was likely to contribute to the suppression of cutaneous vasodilatation.

Previous studies have suggested that the response to increase sweat rate during exercise is also attenuated by hypovolemia. Fortney et al. [19] presented that the ability to enhance sweating of the chest and forearm to an increase in T_{es}, but not the T_{es} threshold at the start of sweating during cycle ergometer exercise (65–70% VO_{2max}) in a warm environment (T_a, 30°C; RH, 40%), was attenuated by isotonic hypovolemia (9% reduction in plasma volume induced by diuretics) prior to exercise. Additionally, Mack et al. [13] showed that LBNP at the level of −40 mmHg during exercise dampened the sweat rate and SkBF to increased T_{es}. Dodt et al. [20] also observed decreased skin sympathetic nerve activity following LBNP in passively heated subjects. In contrast, Kamijo et al. [21] reported that isotonic hypovolemia induced by diuretic (−10%) before exercise dampened increases in SkBF, similar to the results of Nadel et al. [12]. However, it did not dampen the increase in sweat rate during exercise at 60% VO_{2max} in a warm environment (T_a, 30°C; RH, 45%). Thus, the effects of hypovolemia on sweat rate are still debatable.

Plasma hyperosmolality suppresses the response to increase SkBF and sweating during exercise. Fortney et al. [22] showed that 10 mosmol/kgH_2O increases in P_{osm} achieved by hypertonic saline infusion before exercise caused an increased T_{es} thresholds for cutaneous vasodilation and sweating by 0.2°C. In addition, the sensitivity to increase SkBF in response to increased T_{es} decreased during exercise at 70% VO_{2max} in a warm environment (T_a, 30°C; RH, 40%). Additionally, onset of SkBF and sweat rate responses to increased core body temperature is delayed by plasma hyperosmolality. Takamata et al. [23] showed a linear upward shift of the T_{es} thresholds with several levels of increase in P_{osm} by hypertonic saline infusion. They suggested with these data that T_{es} thresholds for cutaneous vasodilation and sweating during passive heat stress (lower-leg water immersion, 42°C) at rest shifted upward by 0.044°C and 0.034°C per 1 mosmol/kgH_2O increase, respectively. More intriguingly, they also suggested that the upward shift in T_{es} thresholds during exercise were caused by an increased P_{osm} induced by exercise. The increased T_{es} thresholds at a given increase in P_{osm} during exercise were identical to those during resting passive heat stress [23]. Mitono et al. [24] supported this evidence by indicating that when the increase in P_{osm} during exercise was attenuated by hypotonic saline infusion prior to exercise, the delayed onset of cutaneous vasodilation in response to increased T_{es} during exercise was normalized. It has been suggested that the response of the thermoregulatory center was attenuated by plasma hyperosmolality via osmoreceptors.

As described above, dehydration is a limiting factor for heat loss mechanisms during exercise in the heat. These mechanisms prevent cardiovascular failure caused by reduction in venous return to the heart due to blood pooling in dilated peripheral skin vasculature and reductions in PV due to sweating. Indeed, it has been reported that, when drinking such a small amount of water so as not to change PV and P_{osm} in dehydrated individuals, thirst sensation and plasma vasopressin secretion induced by increased P_{osm} are released rapidly by a stimulation of oropharyngeal reflexes [25, 26]. It also simultaneously releases the dehydration-induced attenuated responses of SkBF [21] and SR [26].

3. Effects of exercise training on thermoregulation in warm and hot conditions

Thermoregulatory responses are improved by aerobic and endurance exercise training, resulting in reduced physiological strain and therefore enhanced cardiovascular and exercise capacities during exercise in warm and hot conditions. These adaptations are remarkable when exercise training is performed in the heat [1]. After a 10-day training period in a cool condition (T_a, 20°C), SkBF and sweat rate responses to increased T_{es} during exercise (T_a, 25°C) are enhanced. After a subsequent 10-day training period in a hot condition (T_a, 35°C), these responses improved further [27]. The increased SkBF and sweating responses are characterized by the early start of cutaneous vasodilation and sweating responses to increased T_{es} [28, 29] and the increased sensitivity to increase SkBF and sweat rate in response to an increased T_{es} compared with before exercise training [28, 29]. It is suggested that the mechanisms of the increase in thermoregulatory responses with exercise training are similar to those following acclimations to repeated heat exposures, including adaptations of the thermoregulatory center and thermoregulatory effectors [1, 12] as well as an increase in VO_{2max} [30] and PV [28, 31, 32].

It is suggested that the exercise-induced PV expansion is primarily associated with an increase in total volume of extracellular fluid [33]. An increase in plasma protein (mainly albumin content) also contributes by drawing fluids into the intravascular space from the interstitium [33–35]. Facilitated Na^+ and water reabsorption [33, 36] and an enhancement of voluntary fluid intake with increased thirst sensation [37] (associated with an activated renin-angiotensin-aldosterone system and vasopressin release) during and after exercise or dehydration are suggested as mechanisms of training-induced increases in extracellular fluid volume [38].

Increases in plasma protein may be due to activated hepatic plasma protein synthesis [39, 40] and enhanced translocation of protein to the intravascular space from the interstitium [41] coincide with a restricted transcapillary escape ratio of protein [42].

PV expansion by exercise training results in a reduction in lactic acid concentration in the blood at the same absolute intensity of exercise (an enhanced lactate threshold), which contributes to a suppression of increase in P_{osm} during exercise. This mechanism contributes to the downward shift of the body core temperature threshold for cutaneous vasodilation and sweating after training. Moreover, expanded PV increases venous return to the heart and cardiac filling pressure and therefore enhances cardiac stroke volume. It also improves the responses of SkBF and sweat rate to increased core body temperature during exercise [11, 16, 17]. Indeed, an increase in cardiac stroke volume and also the sensitivity of increase in SkBF to increased T_{es} during exercise in a warm condition (T_a, 30°C) was closely correlated to a PV expansion by a 10-day endurance training (60% VO_{2max} for 1 h/day at 30°C) [28]. Additionally, Goto et al. [43] reported the influences of protein and carbohydrate (CHO) supplementation just after exercise (Pro-CHO; 0.36 g protein/kg and 3.6 kcal) during the 5-day training period (70% VO_{2max} for 30 min/day) in a warm environment (T_a, 30°C) on PV and thermoregulatory responses. They suggested that, in the Pro-CHO group, plasma albumin content (Alb_{cont}) and therefore PV increased by ~10% and ~8%, respectively. These were significantly higher than the increase of ~4% in the placebo intake control group (CNT; 0.9 kcal and 0 g protein/kg body weight). They attributed the increase in Alb_{cont} to activated hepatic albumin synthesis following exercise due to the increased substance bioavailability [39, 40] and also the effects of insulin on protein synthesis in hepatocytes [44]. Most notably, the sensitivity of an increase in SkBF and sweat rate to increased T_{es} enhanced after training more in the Pro-CHO group compared with the CNT group. Additionally, both groups showed a significant decrease in heart rate and T_{es} during exercise after training period. However, these adaptations were more prominent in the Pro-CHO group than in the CNT group, indicating decreased cardiovascular and thermal strains after the training period with PV expansion.

In addition, Ikegawa et al. [31] supported the observations by Goto et al. [43] by presenting an increased PV with an early shift of the onset of the cutaneous vasodilation and sweating responses to an increased T_{es} after the same training protocol. Further, the early shift of the onset of the cutaneous vasodilation and sweating responses was wholly or partly diminished after the expanded PV by training was reduced to the pre-training level by using the diuretics. Furthermore, Ichinose et al. [28] showed that 10 days of exercise training (60% VO_{2max} for 60 min/day at 30°C) attenuated the sensitivity of the upward shift of T_{es} threshold for cutaneous vasodilation with the increased P_{osm} by hypertonic saline infusion, though the threshold for sweating was not changed. Furthermore, they suggested that increased PV after training correlated with the attenuated sensitivity to hyperosmolality in each individual, suggesting that the attenuation is associated with the stretch of cardiopulmonary baroreceptors induced by PV expansion. Thus, the enhanced thermoregulation and cardiovascular capacities after exercise training are closely associated with PV expansion in addition to the neural adaptation of the thermoregulatory center and thermoregulatory effectors [1, 12].

The Na^+ concentration of sweat is important to maintain PV during exercise. It decreases after exercise training or heat acclimation due to an enhanced Na^+ reabsorption at the sweat gland duct induced by an enhanced sensitivity to aldosterone [45]. To maintain PV during exercise, hypotonic sweat is advantageous because hypotonic sweat loss causes a greater increase in osmolality of extracellular fluid. It promotes the shift of water from intracellular to extracellular fluid space according to the osmotic gradient between the spaces [45]. This therefore attenuates the decreased PV and venous return to the heart. As a result, the decreased thermoregulatory responses with a sweating loss at a given volume are attenuated with low Na^+ concentration in sweat [46]. Moreover, the delayed onset of cutaneous vasodilation and sweating responses to increased T_{es} at a given increase in P_{osm} was attenuated in heat-acclimated individuals in whom an increased P_{osm} by sweating loss at a given volume was enhanced due to low Na^+ concentration in sweat [46].

4. Effects of biological aging on thermoregulation in warm and hot conditions

The susceptibility to heat related-illnesses in the elderly [6] is caused by a deterioration in thermoregulatory responses with aging [47, 48]. Previous studies have indicated that even healthy elderly individuals have an impaired thermal perception [49] and impaired autonomic [50, 51] and behavioral [52, 53] thermoregulatory responses. A recent study indicated that skin warmth detection thresholds in the extremities and the whole-body thermal sensation deteriorated with normal aging under both normothermic conditions and under passive heat-induced mild hyperthermic conditions [54]. Decreased VO_{2max} and cardiovascular capacity associate with the deteriorated thermoregulation with aging [51]. Nevertheless, elderly individuals with a similar level of VO_{2max} to young individuals are known to show an attenuated response of SkBF both during passive heat stress in whole-body or local-body parts and during exercise under a hot environment compared to young individuals [55, 56]. Specifically, Kenney et al. [56] used bretylium tosylate to block the local release of norepinephrine on the forearm skin. They suggested that the attenuated SkBF response to hyperthermia during exercise in a hot condition was caused not by an enhanced vasoconstrictor system but mainly by a decreased sensitivity of the active vasodilator system to increased T_{es}. In addition, the whole-body and local sweat rate in response to passive heat stress or exercise are attenuated in the elderly compared to young adults [57].

Several physiological changes with advancing age, for example, such as decreased PV and increased P_{osm} at baseline [58], diminished thirst sensation [58], and responses in antidiuretic hormone and aldosterone after thermal dehydration [38], are suggested to be associated with the decreased thermoregulatory responses in the elderly. Decreased renal concentrating ability [59] and lower reabsorptive ability of sweat gland ducts [59] with advancing age are also suggested to be associated with the deteriorated thermoregulatory responses with aging. Vasoconstriction of splanchnic organs during exercise, which enhances the redistribution of cardiac output to the skin vasculature, is associated with increased cutaneous vasodilation in youth, which is also attenuated with aging [60]. Furthermore, elderly individuals commonly take a variety of prescription drugs that may affect thermoregulatory responses and body fluid regulation [1]. Exercise training and heat acclimation can improve the blunted body fluid regulation and thermoregulation with aging, although generally the improvement of these is lower or limited relative to their younger counterparts.

5. Effects of type 2 diabetes on thermoregulation in warm and hot conditions

Type 2 diabetes typically presents later in life with a mean onset age of 54 years [61]. Type 2 diabetes is associated with multiple comorbidities, including obesity, dyslipidemia, metabolic syndrome, hypertension, and other markers of cardiovascular diseases in addition to the changes associated with aging. Most of the research examining ability of thermoregulation in type 2 diabetic patients has considered not only to estimate itself but also the responses to evaluate the severity of neuropathy along with other diabetes-related complications. Many studies have only measured the local heat dissipative responses of the hands and feet. It is generally reported that type 2 diabetic patients have attenuated SkBF responses evoked by pharmacological stimuli [62, 63], local skin heating [64, 65], and whole-body heating [64, 66]. Importantly, these effects appear to depend on physical fitness level. Type 2 diabetic engaging in physical activity has reduced impairments in skin vasodilation compared with type 2 diabetics who are not physically active [67]. Conversely, studies of local sweating in type 2 diabetics have generally found that these individuals have impaired sweating responses compared to their healthy counterparts [64, 68, 69], despite one study reporting otherwise [70]. The changes in regional sweating with type 2 diabetes are comparable to those observed with type 1 diabetes, such that there is relatively lower body anhidrosis along with euhydrosis or hyperhidrosis compared to the upper body [68]. While these studies have implications for whole-body temperature regulation during heat stress, the evidence regarding the impact of heat stress (as induced by warm and hot environments, physical activity, or both) on type 2 diabetics remains limited.

Kenny et al. [71] recently reported that relatively active type 2 diabetics who were otherwise generally healthy (good glycemic control and no diabetes-related complications) have significantly decreased whole-body heat loss during exercise for 60 min (~370 W of metabolic heat production or ~60% of the predetermined VO_{2max}) as assessed by whole-body direct calorimetry. During the exercise bout, due to the lower evaporative heat loss in type 2 diabetes, they stored ~1.5-fold more heat than their healthy counterparts. Regardless of the greater amount of heat accumulation during exercise, the diabetes-related impairment in the capacity to dissipate heat persisted into the 60-minute recovery. Healthy groups lost ~twofold more heat relative to the group with type 2 diabetes, which was associated with slightly and no statistically significant, but sustained difference in the rate of non-evaporative heat loss [71].

6. The mechanisms underlying type 2 diabetes-related impairments in heat dissipation

To date, few studies have examined the mechanisms underlying type 2 diabetes-related impairments in heat dissipation; however, some information may be gleaned from those studies aimed primarily at assessing the presence of neuropathies. The reduction in nitric oxide bioavailability in individuals with type 2 diabetes is well established [62, 63, 72, 73] and may be further exacerbated by the presence of atherosclerotic plaques which are known to adversely alter endothelial function through interfering with nitric oxide signaling [74]. In fact, one study reported that the relative nitric oxide-dependent vasodilation during whole-body passive heating was similar between healthy controls and type 2 diabetics; however, absolute SkBF was lower in the latter group [72]. Moreover, there is evidence to support an endothelium-independent component to the impairment in vasodilation as observed during exogenous administration of a nitric oxide donor (e.g., sodium nitroprusside) [63]. Importantly, these diabetes-related changes in SkBF appear to be closely associated with the duration of diabetes and/or the presence of related complications [62, 63]. There is little report on the central versus peripheral mechanisms that form the basis of diabetes-related SkBF responses; one study indicated that onset of vasodilation responses to increased core body temperature was delayed and it was the primary factor, explaining lower SkBF in patients with type 2 diabetes mellitus. This indicates that central mechanisms contribute to the modulation of SkBF [66].

The mechanisms responsible for diabetes-related impairments in sweating during heat stress remain incompletely understood and most of the information is provided from studies which have not examined thermoregulatory control. Petrofsky et al. [64] indicated that, during isometric handgrip exercise to exhaustion, sweating on the arms and legs was significantly lower, but only forehead sweat rate was actually higher in type 2 diabetics than the controls. The primary factors associated with this modulation in sweating include long-term diabetes, poorly controlled glycemia, and the presence of neuropathy. Diabetic neuropathy seems to have an important role in altering the sweat gland innervations [68, 75]. Luo et al. [75, 76] showed that the sweat glands in type 2 diabetics with poor glycemic control exhibit exacerbated reductions in periglandular nerve terminals and in the innervation index. Impairments in sweating during heat stress may also be related to the reduction in nitric oxide bioavailability since the role of nitric oxide-induced sweating during exercise has recently been proven [77, 78].

7. Effects of hyperglycemia on thermoregulation during thermal stress

Hyperglycemia can have an important negative impact on body core temperature regulation. Specifically, hyperglycemia can lead to increases in P_{osm} which have been independently associated with impairments in sweating and SkBF as described in the earlier section [79]. Furthermore, hyperglycemia can induce dehydration through osmotic diuresis [80] which can lead to hypovolemia without adequate fluid replacement. Recently, studies have demonstrated that the combination of hyper osmolality and hypovolemia augments any effects to further exacerbate impairments in heat dissipation in healthy individuals [81, 82]. In contrast, acute hyperglycemia (induced by hyperinsulinemic-hyperglycemic clamp) did not result in the impairment of NO-mediated skin microvascular function [83].

8. Effects of exercise training on thermoregulation in the elderly individuals

Several longitudinal studies have reported that heat dissipative responses during exercise in a hot environment are enhanced when aerobic training is performed under hot or even cool to thermoneutral conditions by initially sedentary elderly individuals [30, 60, 84] and young individuals [27–29]. Thomas et al. [30] reported that a 16-week aerobic training program increased

VO_{2max} by ≥5% and advanced onset of cutaneous vasodilation in response to an increased mean body temperature during exercise in a hot environment (T_a, 36°C) both in young and in elderly individuals. They also suggested that an enhanced sensitivity of the active vasodilator system contributes to the enhanced cutaneous vasodilation [30]. Additionally, Okazaki et al. [84] supported and extended these results by showing that onset of cutaneous vasodilation and sweating responses to an increased T_{es} during exercise in a warm environment (T_a, 30°C) were advanced after an 18-week aerobic and resistance training under cool to thermoneutral conditions in initially sedentary elderly individuals. The improvements in VO_{2max} were 20 and 10%, respectively, in each study. However, both studies indicated that the sensitivity of increase in SkBF and sweat rate to an increased mean body temperature or T_{es} did not increase after training. Further, Okazaki et al. [84] indicated that a diminished increase in PV following training period in elderly individuals was associated with the unchanged sensitivity, by showing a linear correlation between changes in the sensitivities and those in PV following the training period. Similarly, in young individuals, the increase in PV is considered to be the major mechanism which contributed to the improvement of thermoregulatory responses by exercise training as described in the earlier section. This results from increased venous return to the heart by increasing cardiac stroke volume and/or by suppressing baroreflex-induced reduction of skin vasodilation [11]. Additionally, Ho et al. [60] showed that splanchnic and renal vasoconstriction during exercise were increased in young individuals but not in elderly individuals following aerobic training period. Thus, in elderly people, exercise training improved VO_{2max} but generally diminished the enhancement of thermoregulation compared with younger counterparts [60, 84].

The primary limiting factor for the blunted increase in PV with aerobic training in elderly people is an attenuated increase in Alb_{cont} with exercise [35, 84, 85]. Other factors are likely to be a reduced fluid intake after thermal dehydration [38, 58] or water deprivation [86] with aging. Accordingly, enhanced albumin synthesis in the liver in response to exercise is one mechanism of the increased Alb_{cont} after aerobic training in the young individuals [39, 40]. In regard to this point, the response to increase Alb_{cont} after aerobic training is smaller in the elderly individuals. It may be affected, in part, by the attenuated hepatic albumin synthesis response to exercise [87, 88] due to decreased gene expression with normal aging. However, it is also reasonable that this is caused by insufficient protein intake for albumin synthesis in elderly people. Decreased daily activity with aging may be accustomed to low energy and protein diets in elderly people. Therefore, improvements would occur if substrates for plasma albumin synthesis are given immediately after exercise when albumin synthesis is reportedly enhanced [40, 88]. In this regard, one study showed that when young and elderly individuals ingested placebo (i.e., non-energy ingestion) just after acute high-intensity interval exercise, the ability of recovery of Alb_{cont} and PV after exercise was generally blunted in elderly individuals compered to young individuals. In contrast, Alb_{cont} and PV recovered more when they consumed a protein and CHO mixture compared to consumed placebo in both individuals [35].

Okazaki et al. [89] further determined the effects of protein and CHO intake just after exercise on PV and thermoregulatory responses during 8 weeks of aerobic training under cool to thermoneutral conditions in elderly individuals. In individuals consuming protein and CHO, Alb_{cont} and PV increased by 6%, and these increases were accompanied by enhanced sensitivities of SkBF and sweat rate (18 and 80%, respectively) to increased T_{es}. In contrast, they remained unchanged in individuals taking the placebo immediately after exercise [89].

Additionally, this enhanced sensitivity associated with a 10% increase in stroke volume during exercise [89]. Consequently, the improved PV expansion response induced by exercise along with post-exercise protein and CHO intake enhances the attenuated increase in cardiovascular and thermoregulatory capacity in elderly individuals compared with young counterparts. Recently, Kataoka et al. [90] reported the similar results in hypertensive elderly individuals (~160 mmHg for systolic and ~90 mmHg for diastolic blood pressure at rest) that PV and SkBF response to increased T_{es} both increased after aerobic training (60–75% of VO_{2peak} for 60 min/day, 3 days/week, for 8 weeks) with protein (10 g) and CHO (15 g) supplementation. Furthermore, they showed that despite the increased PV, arterial blood pressures rather decreased after training with an increased carotid arterial compliance and baroreflex sensitivity.

Recent studies have presented that aerobic training improves cutaneous vasodilation by local mechanisms in aged skin [91]. Black et al. [92] used L-NAME (an NO synthase inhibitor) during acetylcholine infusions to block NO production and demonstrated that, in initially sedentary elderly individuals, increase in vascular responsiveness following 12 and 24 weeks of aerobic training was induced by the increase in action of NO in the skin. There are similar results in a longitudinal study [93] although a cross-sectional study reported no effects [94].

The enhancement of the sweating function in summer occurred later and its reduction in winter occurred earlier, in an elderly group compared with a younger group despite a smaller seasonal variation range [95]. To prevent heat disorders in elderly individuals, it is strongly recommended that they engage in exercise training prior to the summer season. Regular exercise generally improves thermoregulatory capacity alongside VO_{2max}. Protein and CHO intake after exercise will also enable adequate training adaptations to be achieved.

9. Effects of exercise training on thermoregulation in diabetic patients

The effects of aerobic fitness along with short- and long-term exercise training have been widely studied in the context of glucoregulation in type 2 and type 1 diabetics. The effects of exercise training on glycemic control in type 2 diabetics are well established. A recent meta-analysis by Umpierre et al. [96] reported that structured exercise training (over 12 weeks) consisting of aerobic exercise, resistance training, or a combination is associated with enhanced glycemic control (~0.7% HbA1c reduction) in type 2 diabetics. They also reported that structured exercise training of more than 150 min per week is associated with greater HbA1c reduction (~0.9%) compared to 150 min or less per week [96]. Structured exercise training also has beneficial effects on diabetes-related complications [97]. Greater benefits are apparent in type 2 diabetics with higher HbA1c before the exercise intervention [97].

In healthy individuals, it has been suggested that higher levels of aerobic fitness and/or physically activity improve the capacity to dissipate heat during exercise [98, 99]. A recent study indicated that the age-related decline in aerobic fitness was associated with the decreased whole-body evaporative heat loss during exercise in the heat [100]. Moreover, a group of trained middle-aged males (~48 years) exhibited greater whole-body heat loss than an untrained group during exercise [100]. Other studies have also indicated that VO_{2max} decreased ~7% per decade in sedentary, active, and even endurance-trained populations [101]. Despite reports of the relationship between aerobic fitness and thermoregulatory capacity in healthy people, there are no reports in with either type 1 [102–104] or type 2 [71] diabetics because aerobic fitness has not been considered as a potential factor influencing thermoregulatory capacities. Therefore, the increased aerobic fitness with exercise training in diabetics would improve thermoregulatory control, autonomic nervous system function, and cardiovascular responses, especially during exercise-induced heat stress, as reported in healthy counterparts, however, the situation remains unclear.

10. Oral rehydration during exercise

Based on the physiological responses to warm and hot conditions described previously, it is suggested that dehydration prior to and during exercise should be prevented or countered. This would reduce extra thermal and cardiovascular strains during exercise in the heat and the risk of developing heat-related illnesses. In general, oral rehydration with solutions containing 0.1–0.2% of NaCl and 4–8% of CHO based on thirst sensation is recommended, but, during exercise, we need to prevent the addition of 2% of body weight reduction [7]. Elderly persons or persons who work or undertake high-intensity exercise in warm and hot conditions should start fluid ingestion prior to and during the early period of work before thirst is perceived [7]. Special care should be taken by diabetics so that hyper and hypoglycemia are not induced with oral rehydration during exercise and hyperthermic conditions.

11. Conclusions

The morbidity and mortality of heat-related illnesses would expand in the years to come worldwide because of the rapidly aging population and global warming. The decreased thermoregulatory capacity in type 2 diabetes is associated with the presence of neuropathies, reduced nitric oxide bioavailability, central mechanisms, and so on, while it would be improved with aerobic fitness with exercise training as in healthy counterparts. Thermoregulatory adaptations after exercise training are enhanced with PV expansion with a dietary supplementation conjunction with exercise in healthy individuals. Further researches are necessary to elucidate the effective strategy to improve thermoregulatory capacity as well as glycemic control in type 2 diabetes with or without complications with exercise training.

Author details

Ryosuke Takeda and Kazunobu Okazaki*

*Address all correspondence to: okazaki@sports.osaka-cu.ac.jp

Department of Environmental Physiology for Exercise, Osaka City University Graduate School of Medicine, Research Center for Urban Health and Sports, Osaka City University, Sumiyoshi, Osaka, Japan

References

[1] Taylor NAS, Kondo N, Kenney WL. The physiology of acute heat exposure, with implications for human performance in the heat. In: Taylor NAS, Groeller H, editors. Physiological Bases of Human Performance during Work and Exercise. Philadelphia: Elsevier; 2008. pp. 341-358

[2] Kenny GP, Yardley J, Brown C, Sigal RJ, Jay O. Heat stress in older individuals and patients with common chronic diseases. CMAJ. 2010;**182**:1053-1060

[3] Crandall CG, Davis SL. Cutaneous vascular and sudomotor responses in human skin grafts. Journal of Applied Physiology (Bethesda, Md.: 1985). 2010;**109**:1524-1530

[4] Davis SL, Wilson TE, White AT, Frohman EM. Thermoregulation in multiple sclerosis. Journal of Applied Physiology (Bethesda, Md.: 1985). 2010;**109**:1531-1537

[5] Price MJ, Campbell IG. Thermoregulatory responses of spinal cord injured and able-bodied athletes to prolonged upper body exercise and recovery. Spinal Cord. 1999;**37**: 772-779

[6] Nakai S, Shin-ya H, Yoshida T, Yorimoto A, Inoue Y, et al. Proposal of new guidelines for prevention of heat disorders during sports and daily actibities vased on age, clothing and heat acclimatization. Japanese Journal of Physical Fitness and Sports Medicine. 2007;**56**:437-444

[7] American College of Sports Medicine, Sawka MN, Burke LM, Eichner ER, Maughan RJ, et al. American College of Sports Medicine position stand. Exercise and fluid replacement. Medicine and Science in Sports and Exercise. 2007;**39**:377-390

[8] Rothstein A, Towbin EJ. Blood circulation and temperature of men dehydrating in the heat. In: Adolph EF, editor. Physiology of Man in the Desert. New York: Interscience; 1947. pp. 172-196

[9] Nose H, Takamata A, Mack GW, Oda Y, Okuno T, et al. Water and electrolyte balance in the vascular space during graded exercise in humans. Journal of Applied Physiology. 1991;**70**:2757-2762

[10] Lundvall J, Mellander S, Westling H, White T. Fluid transfer between blood and tissues during exercise. Acta Physiologica Scandinavica. 1972;**85**:258-269

[11] Nose H, Mack GW, Shi XR, Morimoto K, Nadel ER. Effect of saline infusion during exercise on thermal and circulatory regulations. Journal of Applied Physiology. 1990; **69**:609-616

[12] Nadel ER, Fortney SM, Wenger CB. Effect of hydration state of circulatory and thermal regulations. Journal of Applied Physiology. 1980;**49**:715-721

[13] Mack G, Nishiyasu T, Shi X. Baroreceptor modulation of cutaneous vasodilator and sudomotor responses to thermal stress in humans. The Journal of Physiology. 1995;**483**(Pt 2): 537-547

[14] Johnson JM, Rowell LB, Brengelmann GL. Modification of the skin blood flow-body temperature relationship by upright exercise. Journal of Applied Physiology. 1974;**37**:880-886

[15] Gonzalez-Alonso J, Mora-Rodriguez R, Coyle EF. Supine exercise restores arterial blood pressure and skin blood flow despite dehydration and hyperthermia. The American Journal of Physiology. 1999;**277**:H576-H583

[16] Nielsen B, Rowell LB, Bonde-Petersen F. Cardiovascular responses to heat stress and blood volume displacements during exercise in man. European Journal of Applied Physiology and Occupational Physiology. 1984;**52**:370-374

[17] Nagashima K, Nose H, Takamata A, Morimoto T. Effect of continuous negative-pressure breathing on skin blood flow during exercise in a hot environment. Journal of Applied Physiology (Bethesda, Md.: 1985). 1985;**84**:1845-1851

[18] Ogawa Y, Kamijo Y, Ikegawa S, Masuki S, Nose H. Effects of postural change from supine to head-up tilt on the skin sympathetic nerve activity component synchronised with the cardiac cycle in warmed men. Journal of Physiology-London. 2017;**595**:1185-1200

[19] Fortney SM, Nadel ER, Wenger CB, Bove JR. Effect of blood volume on sweating rate and body fluids in exercising humans. Journal of Applied Physiology. 1981;**51**:1594-1600

[20] Dodt C, Gunnarsson T, Elam M, Karlsson T, Wallin BG. Central blood volume influences sympathetic sudomotor nerve traffic in warm humans. Acta Physiologica Scandinavica. 1995;**155**:41-51

[21] Kamijo Y, Okumoto T, Takeno Y, Okazaki K, Inaki M, et al. Transient cutaneous vasodilatation and hypotension after drinking in dehydrated and exercising men. The Journal of Physiology. 2005;**568**:689-698

[22] Fortney SM, Wenger CB, Bove JR, Nadel ER. Effect of hyperosmolality on control of blood flow and sweating. Journal of Applied Physiology. 1984;**57**:1688-1695

[23] Takamata A, Nagashima K, Nose H, Morimoto T. Role of plasma osmolality in the delayed onset of thermal cutaneous vasodilation during exercise in humans. The American Journal of Physiology. 1998;**275**:R286-R290

[24] Mitono H, Endoh H, Okazaki K, Ichinose T, Masuki S, et al. Acute hypoosmolality attenuates the suppression of cutaneous vasodilation with increased exercise intensity. Journal of Applied Physiology. 2005;**99**:902-908

[25] Geelen G, Keil LC, Kravik SE, Wade CE, Thrasher TN, et al. Inhibition of plasma vasopressin after drinking in dehydrated humans. The American Journal of Physiology. 1984; **247**:R968-R971

[26] Takamata A, Mack GW, Gillen CM, Jozsi AC, Nadel ER. Osmoregulatory modulation of thermal sweating in humans: Reflex effects of drinking. The American Journal of Physiology. 1995;**268**:R414-R422

[27] Roberts MF, Wenger CB, Stolwijk JA, Nadel ER. Skin blood flow and sweating changes following exercise training and heat acclimation. Journal of Applied Physiology. 1977; **43**:133-137

[28] Ichinose T, Okazaki K, Masuki S, Mitono H, Chen M, et al. Ten-day endurance training attenuates the hyperosmotic suppression of cutaneous vasodilation during exercise but not sweating. Journal of Applied Physiology. 2005;**99**:237-243

[29] Takeno Y, Kamijo YI, Nose H. Thermoregulatory and aerobic changes after endurance training in a hypobaric hypoxic and warm environment. Journal of Applied Physiology (Bethesda, Md.: 1985). 2001;**91**:1520-1528

[30] Thomas CM, Pierzga JM, Kenney WL. Aerobic training and cutaneous vasodilation in young and older men. Journal of Applied Physiology. 1999;**86**:1676-1686

[31] Ikegawa S, Kamijo Y, Okazaki K, Masuki S, Okada Y, et al. Effects of hypohydration on thermoregulation during exercise before and after 5-day aerobic training in a warm environment in young men. Journal of Applied Physiology. 2011;**110**:972-980

[32] Okazaki K, Goto M, Nose H. Protein and carbohydrate supplementation increases aerobic and thermoregulatory capacities. The Journal of Physiology. 2009;**587**:5585-5590

[33] Convertino VA, Brock PJ, Keil LC, Bernauer EM, Greenleaf JE. Exercise training-induced hypervolemia: Role of plasma albumin, renin, and vasopressin. Journal of Applied Physiology. 1980;**48**:665-669

[34] Gillen CM, Lee R, Mack GW, Tomaselli CM, Nishiyasu T, et al. Plasma volume expansion in humans after a single intense exercise protocol. Journal of Applied Physiology. 1991;**71**:1914-1920

[35] Okazaki K, Hayase H, Ichinose T, Mitono H, Doi T, et al. Protein and carbohydrate supplementation after exercise increases plasma volume and albumin content in older and young men. Journal of Applied Physiology. 2009;**107**:770-779

[36] Nagashima K, Wu J, Kavouras SA, Mack GW. Increased renal tubular sodium reabsorption during exercise-induced hypervolemia in humans. Journal of Applied Physiology (Bethesda, Md.: 1985). 1985;**91**:1229-1236

[37] Greenleaf JE, Brock PJ, Keil LC, Morse JT. Drinking and water balance during exercise and heat acclimation. Journal of Applied Physiology: Respiratory, Environmental and Exercise Physiology. 1983;**54**:414-419

[38] Takamata A, Ito T, Yaegashi K, Takamiya H, Maegawa Y, et al. Effect of an exercise-heat acclimation program on body fluid regulatory responses to dehydration in older men. The American Journal of Physiology. 1999;**277**:R1041-R1050

[39] Nagashima K, Cline GW, Mack GW, Shulman GI, Nadel ER. Intense exercise stimulates albumin synthesis in the upright posture. Journal of Applied Physiology. 2000;**88**:41-46

[40] Yang RC, Mack GW, Wolfe RR, Nadel ER. Albumin synthesis after intense intermittent exercise in human subjects. Journal of Applied Physiology. 1998;**84**:584-592

[41] Mack GW, Yang R, Hargens AR, Nagashima K, Haskell A. Influence of hydrostatic pressure gradients on regulation of plasma volume after exercise. Journal of Applied Physiology (Bethesda, Md.: 1985). 1998;**85**:667-675

[42] Haskell A, Gillen CM, Mack GW, Nadel ER. Albumin infusion in humans does not model exercise induced hypervolaemia after 24 hours. Acta Physiologica Scandinavica. 1998;**164**:277-284

[43] Goto M, Okazaki K, Kamijo Y, Ikegawa S, Masuki S, et al. Protein and carbohydrate supplementation during 5-day aerobic training enhanced plasma volume expansion and thermoregulatory adaptation in young men. Journal of Applied Physiology. 2010; **109**:1247-1255

[44] Ahlman B, Charlton M, Fu A, Berg C, O'Brien P, et al. Insulin's effect on synthesis rates of liver proteins. A swine model comparing various precursors of protein synthesis. Diabetes. 2001;**50**:947-954

[45] Nose H, Mack GW, Shi XR, Nadel ER. Shift in body fluid compartments after dehydration in humans. Journal of Applied Physiology (Bethesda, Md.: 1985). 1988;**65**:318-324

[46] Takamata A, Yoshida T, Nishida N, Morimoto T. Relationship of osmotic inhibition in thermoregulatory responses and sweat sodium concentration in humans. American Journal of Physiology. Regulatory, Integrative and Comparative Physiology. 2001; **280**:R623-R629

[47] Blatteis CM. Age-dependent changes in temperature regulation—A mini review. Gerontology. 2012;**58**:289-295

[48] Kenny GP, Poirier MP, Metsios GS, Boulay P, Dervis S, et al. Hyperthermia and cardiovascular strain during an extreme heat exposure in young versus older adults. Temperature (Austin). 2017;**4**:79-88

[49] Guergova S, Dufour A. Thermal sensitivity in the elderly: A review. Ageing Research Reviews. 2011;**10**:80-92

[50] Holowatz LA, Kenney WL. Peripheral mechanisms of thermoregulatory control of skin blood flow in aged humans. Journal of Applied Physiology (Bethesda, Md.: 1985). 2010;**109**:1538-1544

[51] Kenney WL. Thermoregulation at rest and during exercise in healthy older adults. Exercise and Sport Sciences Reviews. 1997;**25**:41-76

[52] Kenney WL, Chiu P. Influence of age on thirst and fluid intake. Medicine and Science in Sports and Exercise. 2001;**33**:1524-1532

[53] Van Someren EJ, Raymann RJ, Scherder EJ, Daanen HA, Swaab DF. Circadian and age-related modulation of thermoreception and temperature regulation: Mechanisms and functional implications. Ageing Research Reviews. 2002;**1**:721-778

[54] Takeda R, Imai D, Suzuki A, Ota A, Naghavi N, et al. Lower thermal sensation in normothermic and mildly hyperthermic older adults. European Journal of Applied Physiology. 2016;**116**:975-984

[55] Kenney WL, Tankersley CG, Newswanger DL, Hyde DE, Puhl SM, et al. Age and hypohydration independently influence the peripheral vascular response to heat stress. Journal of Applied Physiology. 1985;**68**:1902-1908

[56] Kenney WL, Morgan AL, Farquhar WB, Brooks EM, Pierzga JM, et al. Decreased active vasodilator sensitivity in aged skin. The American Journal of Physiology. 1997; **272**:H1609-H1614

[57] Inoue Y, Shibasaki M, Ueda H, Ishizashi H. Mechanisms underlying the age-related decrement in the human sweating response. European Journal of Applied Physiology and Occupational Physiology. 1999;**79**:121-126

[58] Mack GW, Weseman CA, Langhans GW, Scherzer H, Gillen CM, et al. Body fluid balance in dehydrated healthy older men: Thirst and renal osmoregulation. Journal of Applied Physiology. 1994;**76**:1615-1623

[59] Geelen G, Corman B. Relationship between vasopressin and renal concentrating ability in aging rats. The American Journal of Physiology. 1992;**262**:R826-R833

[60] Ho CW, Beard JL, Farrell PA, Minson CT, Kenney WL. Age, fitness, and regional blood flow during exercise in the heat. Journal of Applied Physiology. 1997;**82**:1126-1135

[61] Surveillance CfDCaPN. Diabetes Publich Health Resource. GA: Atlanta; 2014

[62] Beer S, Feihl F, Ruiz J, Juhan-Vague I, Aillaud MF, et al. Comparison of skin microvascular reactivity with hemostatic markers of endothelial dysfunction and damage in type 2 diabetes. Vascular Health and Risk Management. 2008;**4**:1449-1458

[63] Williams SB, Cusco JA, Roddy MA, Johnstone MT, Creager MA. Impaired nitric oxide-mediated vasodilation in patients with non-insulin-dependent diabetes mellitus. Journal of the American College of Cardiology. 1996;**27**:567-574

[64] Petrofsky JS, Lee S, Patterson C, Cole M, Stewart B. Sweat production during global heating and during isometric exercise in people with diabetes. Medical Science Monitor. 2005;**11**:CR515-CR521

[65] Strom NA, Sawyer JR, Roberts SK, Kingsley-Berg SM, Charkoudian N. Local sensory nerve control of skin blood flow during local warming in type 2 diabetes mellitus. Journal of Applied Physiology (Bethesda, Md.: 1985). 2010;**108**:293-297

[66] Wick DE, Roberts SK, Basu A, Sandroni P, Fealey RD, et al. Delayed threshold for active cutaneous vasodilation in patients with type 2 diabetes mellitus. Journal of Applied Physiology (Bethesda, Md.: 1985). 2006;**100**:637-641

[67] Colberg SR, Stansberry KB, McNitt PM, Vinik AI. Chronic exercise is associated with enhanced cutaneous blood flow in type 2 diabetes. Journal of Diabetes and its Complications. 2002;**16**:139-145

[68] Fealey RD, Low PA, Thomas JE. Thermoregulatory sweating abnormalities in diabetes mellitus. Mayo Clinic Proceedings. 1989;**64**:617-628

[69] Rand SPJ, Zimmermann G. Diabetes: Sweat response and heart rate variability during electrical stimulation in controls and people with diabetes. Journal of Applied Research. 2008;**8**:48-54

[70] Berghoff M, Kilo S, Hilz MJ, Freeman R. Differential impairment of the sudomotor and nociceptor axon-reflex in diabetic peripheral neuropathy. Muscle & Nerve. 2006; **33**:494-499

[71] Kenny GP, Stapleton JM, Yardley JE, Boulay P, Sigal RJ. Older adults with type 2 diabetes store more heat during exercise. Medicine and Science in Sports and Exercise. 2013;**45**:1906-1914

[72] Sokolnicki LA, Roberts SK, Wilkins BW, Basu A, Charkoudian N. Contribution of nitric oxide to cutaneous microvascular dilation in individuals with type 2 diabetes mellitus. American Journal of Physiology. Endocrinology and Metabolism. 2007;**292**:E314-E318

[73] Fujii N, Meade RD, Akbari P, Louie JC, Alexander LM, et al. No effect of ascorbate on cutaneous vasodilation and sweating in older men and those with type 2 diabetes exercising in the heat. Physiological Reports. 2017;**5**:e13238

[74] Kawashima S, Yokoyama M. Dysfunction of endothelial nitric oxide synthase and atherosclerosis. Arteriosclerosis, Thrombosis, and Vascular Biology. 2004;**24**:998-1005

[75] Luo KR, Chao CC, Hsieh PC, Lue JH, Hsieh ST. Effect of glycemic control on sudomotor denervation in type 2 diabetes. Diabetes Care. 2012;**35**:612-616

[76] Luo KR, Chao CC, Chen YT, Huang CM, Yang NC, et al. Quantitation of sudomotor innervation in skin biopsies of patients with diabetic neuropathy. Journal of Neuropathology and Experimental Neurology. 2011;**70**:930-938

[77] McGinn R, Paull G, Meade RD, Fujii N, Kenny GP. Mechanisms underlying the postexercise baroreceptor-mediated suppression of heat loss. Physiological Reports. 2014; **2**:e12168

[78] Welch G, Foote KM, Hansen C, Mack GW. Nonselective NOS inhibition blunts the sweat response to exercise in a warm environment. Journal of Applied Physiology (Bethesda, Md.: 1985). 2009;**106**:796-803

[79] Suzuki A, Okazaki K, Imai D, Takeda R, Naghavi N, et al. Thermoregulatory responses are attenuated after fructose but not glucose intake. Medicine and Science in Sports and Exercise. 2014;**46**:1452-1461

[80] Dhatariya K. People with type 1 diabetes using short acting analogue insulins are less dehydrated than those with using human soluble insulin prior to onset of diabetic ketoacidosis. Medical Hypotheses. 2008;**71**:706-708

[81] Kenny GP, Jay O. Thermometry, calorimetry, and mean body temperature during heat stress. Comprehensive Physiology. 2013;**3**:1689-1719

[82] Lynn AG, Gagnon D, Binder K, Boushel RC, Kenny GP. Divergent roles of plasma osmolality and the baroreflex on sweating and skin blood flow. American Journal of Physiology. Regulatory, Integrative and Comparative Physiology. 2012;**302**:R634-R642

[83] Naylor LH, Yusof NM, Paramalingam N, Jones TW, Davis EA, et al. Acute hyperglycaemia does not alter nitric oxide-mediated microvascular function in the skin of adolescents with type 1 diabetes. European Journal of Applied Physiology. 2014;**114**:435-441

[84] Okazaki K, Kamijo Y, Takeno Y, Okumoto T, Masuki S, et al. Effects of exercise training on thermoregulatory responses and blood volume in older men. Journal of Applied Physiology. 2002;**93**:1630-1637

[85] Zappe DH, Bell GW, Swartzentruber H, Wideman RF, Kenney WL. Age and regulation of fluid and electrolyte balance during repeated exercise sessions. The American Journal of Physiology. 1996;**270**:R71-R79

[86] Phillips PA, Rolls BJ, Ledingham JG, Forsling ML, Morton JJ, et al. Reduced thirst after water deprivation in healthy elderly men. The New England Journal of Medicine. 1984; **311**:753-759

[87] Gersovitz M, Munro HN, Udall J, Young VR. Albumin synthesis in young and elderly subjects using a new stable isotope methodology: Response to level of protein intake. Metabolism. 1980;**29**:1075-1086

[88] Sheffield-Moore M, Yeckel CW, Volpi E, Wolf SE, Morio B, et al. Postexercise protein metabolism in older and younger men following moderate-intensity aerobic exercise. American Journal of Physiology. Endocrinology and Metabolism. 2004;**287**:E513-E522

[89] Okazaki K, Ichinose T, Mitono H, Chen M, Masuki S, et al. Impact of protein and carbohydrate supplementation on plasma volume expansion and thermoregulatory adaptation by aerobic training in older men. Journal of Applied Physiology. 2009;**107**:725-733

[90] Kataoka Y, Kamijo YI, Ogawa Y, Sumiyoshi E, Nakae M, et al. Effects of hypervolemia by protein and glucose supplementation during aerobic training on thermal and arterial pressure regulations in hypertensive older men. Journal of Applied Physiology (Bethesda, Md.: 1985). 2016;**121**:1021-1031

[91] Simmons GH, Wong BJ, Holowatz LA, Kenney WL. Changes in the control of skin blood flow with exercise training: Where do cutaneous vascular adaptations fit in? Experimental Physiology. 2011;**96**:822-828

[92] Black MA, Green DJ, Cable NT. Exercise prevents age-related decline in nitric-oxide-mediated vasodilator function in cutaneous microvessels. The Journal of Physiology. 2008;**586**:3511-3524

[93] Hodges GJ, Sharp L, Stephenson C, Patwala AY, George KP, et al. The effect of 48 weeks of aerobic exercise training on cutaneous vasodilator function in post-menopausal females. European Journal of Applied Physiology. 2010;**108**:1259-1267

[94] Tew GA, Saxton JM, Klonizakis M, Moss J, Ruddock AD, et al. Aging and aerobic fitness affect the contribution of noradrenergic sympathetic nerves to the rapid cutaneous vasodilator response to local heating. Journal of Applied Physiology. 2011;**110**:1264-1270

[95] Inoue Y, Nakao M, Okudaira S, Ueda H, Araki T. Seasonal variation in sweating responses of older and younger men. European Journal of Applied Physiology and Occupational Physiology. 1995;**70**:6-12

[96] Umpierre D, Ribeiro PA, Kramer CK, Leitao CB, Zucatti AT, et al. Physical activity advice only or structured exercise training and association with HbA1c levels in type 2 diabetes: A systematic review and meta-analysis. JAMA. 2011;**305**:1790-1799

[97] Snowling NJ, Hopkins WG. Effects of different modes of exercise training on glucose control and risk factors for complications in type 2 diabetic patients: A meta-analysis. Diabetes Care. 2006;**29**:2518-2527

[98] Buono MJ, Sjoholm NT. Effect of physical training on peripheral sweat production. Journal of Applied Physiology (Bethesda, Md.: 1985). 1988;**65**:811-814

[99] Havenith G, van Middendorp H. The relative influence of physical fitness, acclimatization state, anthropometric measures and gender on individual reactions to heat stress. European Journal of Applied Physiology and Occupational Physiology. 1990;**61**:419-427

[100] Stapleton JM, Poirier MP, Flouris AD, Boulay P, Sigal RJ, et al. Aging impairs heat loss, but when does it matter? Journal of Applied Physiology (Bethesda, Md.: 1985). 2015;**118**:299-309

[101] Wilson TM, Tanaka H. Meta-analysis of the age-associated decline in maximal aerobic capacity in men: Relation to training status. American Journal of Physiology. Heart and Circulatory Physiology. 2000;**278**:H829-H834

[102] Stapleton JM, Yardley JE, Boulay P, Sigal RJ, Kenny GP. Whole-body heat loss during exercise in the heat is not impaired in type 1 diabetes. Medicine and Science in Sports and Exercise. 2013;**45**:1656-1664

[103] Carter MR, McGinn R, Barrera-Ramirez J, Sigal RJ, Kenny GP. Impairments in local heat loss in type 1 diabetes during exercise in the heat. Medicine and Science in Sports and Exercise. 2014;**46**:2224-2233

[104] McGinn R, Carter MR, Barrera-Ramirez J, Sigal RJ, Flouris AD, et al. Does type 1 diabetes alter post-exercise thermoregulatory and cardiovascular function in young adults? Scandinavian Journal of Medicine & Science in Sports. 2015;**25**:e504-e514

12

Nutritional Management of Type 1 Diabetes

Shereen Abdelghaffar

Abstract

This chapter focuses on medical nutrition therapy (MNT) in type 1 diabetes mellitus (T1DM), which is vital to achieve metabolic control in patients suffering from this disease. The nutritional goals for people with T1DM are reviewed, which aim at maintaining near-normal blood glucose levels by coordinating insulin therapy, diet, and physical activity patterns. A nutrition prescription is given, and recommendations for appropriate MNT in type 1 diabetes are deduced. Glycemic targets in people with T1DM are highlighted; moreover, the principle of carbohydrate consistency and insulin adjustments with food intake are stressed upon. Meal planning approaches to achieve carbohydrate consistency, including carbohydrate counting, exchange system, and sample meal plans, are explained. Weight management, energy requirements, macronutrients and micronutrients needs, as well as nutritional management during exercise and supports take special attention in this chapter.

Information in this chapter is retrieved from evidence-based resources and evidence-based guidelines. If the latter are not available, information retrieved from high-quality research studies, consensus statements, and well-based experts opinions are included.

Keywords: Medical nutrition therapy, type 1 diabetes mellitus, carbohydrate consistency, meal plans

1. Introduction

Management of type 1 diabetes mellitus (T1DM) is a complex task, integrating multiple factors, but it is ultimately centered on the approach to nutrition. Proper attention to diet is a major factor in minimizing hypoglycemia and weight gain while achieving glycemic control; the latter has been shown to markedly diminish the likelihood of chronic diabetic complications, namely, neuropathy, nephropathy, retinopathy, and coronary artery disease (CAD), in patients with type 1 diabetes [1].

2. General principles of Medical Nutrition Therapy (MNT) in type 1 diabetes

MNT is an integral component of diabetes management and diabetes self-management education. Nutrition advice should be tailored for people with T1DM based on age, medical, lifestyle, and personal factors, taking into account associated diabetes complications and other concomitant conditions for every individual. Consideration should also be given to an individual's culture and beliefs, eating patterns, and food availability [2].

The following aspects should be highly considered:

i. **The nutrition prescription: ABC**

Optimally manage the "ABCs" of diabetes control:

- Glycated hemoglobin (**A**1C)
- **B**lood pressure
- Low-density lipoprotein (LDL)-**c**holesterol

ii. **The nutritional goals for people with type 1 diabetes [3]**

- Maintain blood glucose (BG) concentrations in as physiologically a normal range as possible, by coordinating diet and physical activity patterns and insulin therapy.
- Minimize episodes of hypoglycemia.
- Maintain optimal blood pressure and lipid levels.
- Manage weight appropriately by providing adequate calories, thus also ensuring normal growth and development for children and adolescents with T1DM both physically and emotionally.
- Manage risk factors and prevent complications of diabetes.
- Improve overall health through healthful food choices.
- Address individual nutrition needs, incorporating personal and cultural preferences [3].

iii. **General recommendations for MNT in type 1 diabetes**

Current nutrition recommendations for children and adolescents with diabetes mellitus are rooted in the same principles as those established for all healthy children and adolescents without diabetes. Individualized meal plans should emphasize a wide variety of healthy food choices to meet the recommended nutrient intakes for essential vitamins and minerals, energy, and fiber and to provide for normal growth and development [4].

The patient should be advised of the following:

- Adhering to the negotiated meal plan
- Adjusting food and/or insulin in response to hyperglycemia
- Adjusting insulin dose for meal size and content
- Appropriately treating hypoglycemia [5]

Glycemic targets in people with diabetes are as follows:

- Fasting BG: 90–130 mg%
- Two-hour postprandial (2 h pp); BG: less than 180 mg%
- Glucose excursion: 2 h pp more than BG before meal by 30–50 mg%
- HBA1c: less than 7 mg% [1]

MNT for type 1diabetes should consider five key aspects:

1. Establishing carbohydrate consistency at meals and snacks
2. Adjusting insulin for variations in blood glucose, food, or physical activity
3. Balancing caloric intake and expenditure for optimum weight management
4. Balancing the nutritional content of selected protein, carbohydrates, and fats
5. Adjusting meal-insulin timing [6]

2.1. Carbohydrate consistency

- Variations in food intake, particularly carbohydrate, should be minimized to avoid fluctuations in blood glucose. Reductions in medication or insulin doses are necessary when there is decrease in carbohydrate intake.
- When using a long-acting basal insulin and a rapid-acting insulin as bolus doses, this allows flexibility in adjustments of insulin dose according to carbohydrate intake. On the other hand, using fixed doses of short- and intermediate-acting insulin require more carbohydrate consistency in timing and amounts.
- Patients who use short-acting insulin analogs or who use insulin pumps may need to take additional bolus insulin injections with snacks that contain more than 10–15 g of carbohydrate [7].

2.2. Meal planning

There are several meal planning approaches to achieve carbohydrate consistency, including [8]

1. carbohydrate counting
2. the exchange system
3. sample meal plans

2.3. Carbohydrate counting

The methods for counting carbohydrate are as follows:

1. **Reading food labels:** looking at the grams of carbohydrates on the label.
2. **Using the exchange system:** estimation of carbohydrate content can be broken down into three food groups that are standardized for carbohydrate content according to particular portions, which are carbohydrate, meat and meat substitutes, and fat. Table1 shows calories and macronutrient content of exchange lists. The exchange lists also identify foods that are good sources of fiber and foods that have high sodium content [9].

Group	Carbohydrate (g)	Protein (g)	Fat (g)	Calories (Cals)
Carbohydrate group				
Starch	15	3	0–1	80
Fruit	15	0	0	60
Milk	15	8	Varies	90–150
Other carbohydrates	15	Varies	Varies	Varies
Nonstarchy vegetables	5	2	0	25
Meat and meat substitutes				
Very lean	0	7	0–1	35
Lean	0	7	3	55
Medium fat	0	7	5	75
High fat	0	7	8	100
Fat group	0	0	5	45

Table 1. Calories and macronutrient content of exchange lists

3. **Use sample meal plans:** These are defined meal menus that specify the time and amounts of food to be eaten at each meal and snack. Dietitians typically tailor the menus to incorporate food preferences and medical nutrition therapy (MNT) goals. Sample menus are created after review of a person's typical food intake; they are best suited for patients who have fairly routine eating habits and who do not eat a wide variety of foods. They also are appropriate for patients who need structured guidance on what to eat [10].

3. Insulin adjustments with food intake

3.1. Advanced carbohydrate counting

At a more advanced level, carbohydrate counting focuses on adjustment of food, insulin, and activity based on patterns from detailed logs. The patient needs to record the time of meals and snacks, the amount and type of food eaten, the amount of carbohydrate consumed, insulin dose, physical activity, and blood glucose results. Patients should first practice eating consistent amounts of carbohydrate at meals and snacks so that baseline insulin requirements can be matched to usual carbohydrate intake using pre- and postprandial blood glucose testing results. When pre- and postprandial blood glucose levels are in the target range, then insulin-to-carbohydrate ratios can be determined as follows [11]:

Insulin-to-carbohydrate ratios

- Divide the number of grams of carbohydrate eaten at the meal by the number of units of premeal insulin (e.g., 45 g carbohydrate divided by 3 units of insulin is a 1:15 ratio). Insulin-to-carbohydrate ratios can vary with time of day and are affected by stress, illness, and variations in physical activity.

- Insulin-to-carbohydrate ratios can also be calculated using the 450–500 rule:

450–500 rule—calculate the insulin-to-carbohydrate ratio as follows:

Regular insulin-to-carbohydrate ratio = 450 divided by total daily dose (TDD) of insulin.

Rapid acting insulin-to-carbohydrate ratio = 500 divided by TDD of insulin.

- Treatment of hypoglycemia: if the patient is hypoglycemic (blood glucose <70 mg/dL), 10–30 g of fast-acting carbohydrate should be taken. Retesting and retreating is mandatory, without overtreatment, till blood glucose rises >70 mg/dL, then the patient resumes the appropriately calculated insulin doses and carbohydrate requirements [12].

3.2. Weight management in T1DM

The relative importance of caloric intake for an individual patient is dependent on several factors, including the following:

- Current weight in relationship to desirable and healthy body weight (BW)
- Fat distribution and waist circumference
- Glycated hemoglobin (A1C)

Lowering caloric intake and inducing weight loss are of major importance for overweight (body mass index [BMI] ≥25–29.9 kg/m^2) and obese (BMI ≥30 kg/m^2) patients with diabetes because the risk of comorbidities associated with excess adipose tissue increases with BMI in these ranges [13].

In children and adolescents, energy needs can be evaluated by tracking weight gain, BMI, and growth patterns on pediatric growth charts from the Centers for Disease Control and Prevention (CDC) or national growth curves [14].

3.3. Weight gain with intensive insulin therapy

Weight gain is a potential adverse effect of intensive insulin therapy and occurs when insulin dosing matches nutritional intake and glycosuria is eliminated.

If A1C is high enough to promote glycosuria, then lowering calorie intake by an additional 250–300 calories per day is necessary to prevent weight gain with intensification of diabetes therapy. Other strategies to minimize weight gain with intensive therapy are to reduce insulin doses preferentially for patterns of hypoglycemia rather than increasing meal size or adding an undesired snack. To reduce calories further, it is helpful to reduce fat intake and try to keep carbohydrate intake consistent to minimize risk of hypoglycemia [15].

3.4. Total energy expenditure

Easiest way to calculate: 20–35 Cal/kg current weight/day

If the patient's current weight is more than 30% of his ideal BW, it is better to use adjusted BW (ABW)

- ABW = (current BW – ideal BW) × 0.25 + ideal BW

4. Estimating caloric needs to promote weight loss

If 500–1000 calories are subtracted from weight maintenance calories every day, this would lead to loss of 1–2 pounds per week. Low-calorie diets (less than 1200 kcal/day) should be avoided to be sure that nutritional needs are met [16]

4.1. Nutritional content in T1DM

- The optimal macronutrient composition of the diet for patients with diabetes is controversial.
- The mix of dietary carbohydrate, protein, and fat may be adjusted to meet the metabolic goals and individual preferences of the person with T1DM, but in general, daily energy intake should be targeted to include 50–55% carbohydrate, 10–15% protein, and 30–35% fat [3].
- Low-fat, low-carbohydrate, Mediterranean, and vegetarian diet are all acceptable.
- Individualized meal planning should include optimization of food choices to meet the recommended daily allowance (RDA)/dietary reference intake (DRI) for all micronutrients [3]

4.2. Carbohydrates (CHO)

- The RDA/DRI is 60 g for infants 0–6 months, 95 g for infants 7–12 months, and 130 g for children and adolescents. Diets containing less than 130 g of CHO for children older than 1 year may not provide adequate glucose as fuel for the central nervous system without relying on gluconeogenesis from ingested protein and fat. Low-carbohydrate diets also restrict intake of essential nutrients, energy, and fiber from carbohydrates found in whole grains, fruits, vegetables, dried peas and beans, legumes, nuts and seeds, and low-fat milk and yogurt.

- Monitoring carbohydrate, whether by carbohydrate counting, a choice, or experience-based estimation, remains a key strategy in achieving glycemic control. Monitoring carbohydrate intake is important as it directly determines postprandial blood sugar, and consequent insulin adjustment can improve glycemic control [16].
- For individuals with diabetes, the use of glycemic index and glycemic load may provide a modest additional benefit for glycemic control over that observed when total carbohydrate is considered alone. Meals with low glycemic index and glycemic load leads to better glycemic control.
- Carbohydrates from fruits, vegetables, whole grains, legumes, and low-fat milk are preferable.
- Nonnutritive sweeteners are safe when consumed within daily levels established by the US Food and Drug Administration (FDA). Consumption of nonnutritive sweeteners does not increase blood glucose concentrations or affect insulin response in adults, although no similar data are available in children. When calculating carbohydrate content of foods, one-half of the sugar alcohol content should be counted in the total carbohydrate content of the food. Careful reading of food labels is always recommended for foods containing nonnutritive sweeteners as they still contain carbohydrates [17].

4.3. Sucrose

- Intake of sucrose does not need to be restricted, although care should be taken to avoid excess calories; sucrose can be substituted for other carbohydrate sources in the meal plan or, if added, covered with insulin. Sucrose-containing foods typically provide additional calories from fats and are frequently devoid of essential nutrients. Nutrition therapy strategies should focus on consuming these foods in moderation in the context of a healthy well balanced diet. Use of added fructose as a sweetener is not recommended, as it may adversely affect lipids, but there is no need to avoid fructose occurring naturally in fruits and vegetables [18].

4.4. Fats

- Because of the increased risk of cardiovascular disease in people with T1 DM, nutrition therapy also emphasizes a diet low in *saturated fat*, as outlined by the National Cholesterol Education Program and the American Heart association, for all children and adolescents. Saturated fat intake should be less than 7% of total calories. Saturated fats (eg, in fatty and processed meats, butter, lard, hydrogenated fats, coconut and palm oils, cheese, ice cream, and other high-fat dairy products) can be replaced with monounsaturated (about 20%) and polyunsaturated fatty acids (eg, in fish, olive oil, nuts) (about 10%) due to their relatively cardioprotective profile. Sources include olive, canola and peanut oils; olives; nuts; seeds; and avocados.

- Reducing intakes of trans-fatty acids lowers low-density lipoprotein and increases high-density lipoprotein; therefore, intake of trans-fatty acids should be minimized. Added trans-fatty acids are found in margarine and processed and commercially prepared foods. Total cholesterol should be less than 200 mg daily. Dietary cholesterol is only found in foods of animal origin.
- Omega 3 fatty acids, specifically eicosapentaenoic acid (EPA) and docosahexaenoic acid (DHA), have emerged as important dietary adjuncts for individuals at risk of cardiovascular disease and in adults who have already experienced a cardiovascular event. The American Heart Association currently recommends marine-derived omega-3 fatty acids as a dietary adjunct to aid in reduction of serum triglycerides, which can safely be used in children with diabetes and hypertriglyceridemia. Eating two or more servings of fish per week is recommended to provide an excellent source of omega-3 fatty acids. Other potent sources are salmon, tuna, herring, sardines, mackerel, flax seeds and oil, various nuts, and canola and soybean oil [19].

4.5. Proteins

- In individuals with normal renal function, protein intake is based on the RDA for all children and adolescents. The usual daily intake of protein should be approximately 10–25% of total caloric intake (1.1 gm/kg/d).
- Patients should be encouraged to substitute lean meats, fish, eggs, beans, peas, soy products, low-fat dairy products, legumes and nuts, and seeds for red meat.
- Protein intake should not be used to treat hypoglycemia or prevent hypoglycemia overnight.
- In patients with microalbuminuria, a reduction of protein to 0.8–1 g/kg/d of body weight may slow the progression of nephropathy. Overt nephropathy necessitates reduction of protein to 0.8 g/kg/d [20].

4.6. Fiber

- Fiber intake should be at least 14 g per 1000 calories daily, or approximately 19–38 g of fiber/day. High-fiber diets have been demonstrated to decrease postprandial glucose concentrations among adolescents with T1DM. Dietary fiber is found in whole grains, fruits, vegetables, dried peas, beans, legumes, nuts, and seeds. Soluble fiber sources should be emphasized because studies in people without diabetes show that diets high in total and soluble fiber (7–13 g) can reduce total cholesterol by 2–3% and LDL cholesterol up to 7%. Potent sources of soluble fiber include oatmeal, oat cereal, lentils, apples, oranges, pears, oat bran, strawberries, nuts, flaxseeds, beans, dried peas, blueberries, cucumbers, celery, and carrots [21].

4.7. Sodium

- A reduced sodium intake of 2300 mg per day is advised, which is the same for healthy children and adolescents. However, for individuals with hypertension, further reduction to 1500 mg/day is recommended.

- Avoidance of processed foods, restaurant and fast foods, and soda beverages and preparations containing preservatives is advisable due to high content of sodium [19].

4.8. Micronutrients

- Routine supplementation with antioxidants, such as vitamins E and C and beta-carotene, is not advised because of lack of evidence of efficacy and concerns related to long term safety.
- Low serum 25-hydroxyvitamin D concentrations are globally associated with children and adolescents with T1DM. Vitamin D screening and supplementation should therefore be considered and should be meeting the RDA of 600 IU vitamin D per day.
- Supplementation with vitamins and micronutrients in general is not necessary if a well-balanced, healthy diet is consumed unless there are underlying deficiencies [21].

5. Glycemic index

A food's GI is a numeric value that reflects its glycemic response in comparison to that of a reference food, such as pure glucose. The GI of the reference food is set at 100. When glucose is used as a reference food, foods with GI>70 are considered high-glycemic index, while Foods with GI<55 are considered low-glycemic index. Some examples of low-glycemic index foods include nonstarchy vegetables, nuts, legumes, and certain grains such as barley and converted rice. High glycemic index foods include potatoes, candies, white bread, and other refined products made from grains [22].

6. Glycemic load

Glycemic load is the product of the glycemic index value of a food and its total carbohydrate content. The concept of the glycemic load was developed because the blood glucose response is influenced not only by the quality of the carbohydrate consumed (i.e., the glycemic index) but also by the quantity of carbohydrate consumed.

The glycemic index and glycemic load may have far greater health implications than glycemic control alone. Several prospective studies have associated diets high in glycemic index and glycemic load with an increased risk of developing type 2 diabetes, coronary heart disease, and some cancers. Data also suggest that low-glycemic load diets are particularly effective among the most susceptible individuals, those who are already overweight and insulin resistant [22].

7. Eating disorders

Eating disorders are relatively common in patients with diabetes, especially in female adolescents and young adults with diabetes. Dieting or omission of insulin for weight loss and binge eating are the most common. Eating disorders have a deleterious impact on glycemic control and on long-term outcome in these patients. It is important to evaluate patients with diabetes, especially young women, for an eating disorder (or misreporting of insulin administration) and arrange appropriate psychological and nutritional counseling and support when indicated [23,24].

8. Promoting dietary compliance

- Gradual behavioral and dietary changes should be advised to move the patient toward a more ideal diet and eating pattern.
- The patient's own food records and motivation to learn can be helpful in guiding decisions for meal planning approaches
- Motivating a patient to make a long-term commitment to dietary alterations is a challenge. Achieving and maintaining weight reduction is difficult in any obese patient. Compliance can occasionally be enhanced by the rapid and often dramatic improvements in glycemic control.
- Diabetes Education Workshops for small groups of patients is highly effective.
- Exercise can increase the degree of weight loss, and the likelihood that it will be maintained.
- Offering varieties of lists of meal plans is very helpful
- Adjustment of diet, exercise, and insulin doses according to the patient's changing lifestyle patterns is mandatory to maintain glycemic control and prevent acute and chronic complications [1,25-27].

9. Physical activity in patients with T1DM

Exercise is a significant component of diabetes management [28,29].

9.1. Benefits of exercise

- Improved glycemic control
- Weight control
- Reduction in comorbidities (hypertension, dyslipidemia, and cardiovascular disease)
- Improved mood and quality of life

9.2. General tips for physical activity in T1DM

- Patients with T1DM should engage in 30 min or more of moderate intensity physical activity on most days of the week. Individuals for whom weight loss and weight maintenance are a concern, may need 60–90 min of moderate to vigorous intensity activity 3 days a week.
- For patients who are trying to lose weight, it is preferable to adjust insulin doses rather than increase food intake to compensate for exercise.
- Timing of exercise in relation to insulin dose, type, mode of delivery, and time of injection should be considered.
- Patients with diabetes should check blood sugar levels before and after exercising, especially in the beginning of an exercise program, to evaluate glycemic response to exercise and adjust insulin regimen [28, 29].

9.3. Diabetes and sports

Athletes need additional blood glucose testing prior to exercise, during exercise (especially exercise lasting greater than 60 min), immediately after exercise, several hours after exercise, and at any time significant changes in intensity, type, or duration of exercise are made. If blood glucose is less than 100 mg/dL, CHO intake of 15–40 mg is important before exercise. If blood glucose is high, urine ketones should be tested and exercise prevented until ketones disappear by insulin and medication adjustments. In absence of ketones, exercise with caution can be allowed [28, 29].

9.4. General nutritional tips for performance of sports in T1DM

- Preactivity meals (1–2 h before exercise) should be relatively high in carbohydrate, moderate to high in protein and low in fat.
- Protein of high biological value (1 gram of protein per pound of body weight) should be used.
- Protein shake can be used before workout (a shake containing at least 6 g of amino acids—the muscle-building blocks of protein—and 35 g of carbohydrates 30–60 min before exercising increases protein synthesis more than drinking the same shake after training.
- Good-quality whey-protein powders usually contain at least 30 g of protein per serving, as well as a healthy supply of vitamins and minerals.
- Weight-gain powders can also provide a lot of high-quality protein and nutrients in each serving, but they also tend to be extremely high in calories, carbohydrates, and sugar.
- Vigorous exercise involving a muscle group shortly after having injected insulin near to that area could cause the insulin to be absorbed more rapidly than usual, increasing the chances of hypoglycemia.
- Competitive/power exercise can lead to hyperglycemia.

- Individual reactions may vary, and so it is best to verify this by checking blood glucose levels before the burst of activity and about 30 min after, to see how the body responds.
- Warming up is necessary to reduce injury

9.5. During exercise

- During exercise lasting more than 30 min, 15–30 gm CHO should be consumed every 30–60 min.
- Sport drinks, dilute juices, sport bars, and/or high fiber cookies should be carried in a food bag to be consumed during exercise.
- Keeping hydrated by drinking around 150 ml of fluid every 15 min is advised.
- CHO foods should be available during and after exercise.

9.6. After exercise

- After a period of strenuous activity or a long period of exercise, blood sugar levels can drop for up to 48 h. Management includes reducing insulin requirements or dosage of antidiabetic drugs over this period, or take more carbohydrate.
- A high-quality protein meal should be consumed after training.
- Omega-3 fatty acids are beneficial.
- Rest: a full-body workout should be followed by a day of rest or alternatively, at least 3 days of rest each week is advised [28, 29].

10. Summary and conclusion

Achieving metabolic control in patients with T1DM cannot be reached except with proper medical nutrition therapy. Nutrition advice should be customized according to age, medical condition, lifestyle, and personal factors. The nutritional goals for people with type 1 diabetes are to maintain blood glucose (BG) concentrations in a physiologically normal range as possible, by coordinating diet and physical activity patterns and insulin therapy, minimizing episodes of hypoglycemia, maintaining optimal blood pressure and lipid levels, and managing weight appropriately, and by providing adequate calories, thus also ensuring normal growth and development for children and adolescents with T1DM both physically and emotionally. Although a focus on careful carbohydrate counting is integral to insulin delivery and glycemic control for patients with T1DM, many of the other fundamental principles of nutrition management are important to be considered. The patient should be advised for adhering to the negotiated meal plan, adjusting food and/or insulin in response to hyperglycemia, as well as adjusting insulin dose for meal size and content and appropriately treating hypoglycemia. Proper estimation of energy requirements, macronutrients, and micronutrients needs as well as adjustment of MNT during exercise and sports are all of high importance. A team approach, capitalizing on the expertise of pediatric and adult dietitians, psychologists, nurses, and physicians, can best assist patients and their families overcome challenges in their care and reach their therapeutic goals.

Author details

Shereen Abdelghaffar*

Address all correspondence to: sh.abdelghaffar@gmail.com

Pediatric Diabetes and Endocrinology Cairo University, Egypt

References

[1] American Academy of Pediatrics. Pediatric Nutrition. Nutrition Therapy for Children and Adolescents with Type 1 and 2 Diabetes Mellitus. 7th edition. Chapter 31. 2013 pp 741–769

[2] Franz MJ, Bantle JP, Beebe CA, et al. Evidence-based nutrition principles and recommendations for the treatment and prevention of diabetes and related complications. Diabetes Care 2002; 25:148.

[3] American Diabetes Association. Standards of medical care in diabetes—2014. Diabetes Care 2014; 37 Suppl 1:S14.

[4] Anderson EJ, Richardson M, Castle G, et al. Nutrition interventions for intensive therapy in the Diabetes Control and Complications Trial. The DCCT Research Group. Journal of the American Dietetic Association 1993; 93:768.

[5] Brand-Miller J, Hayne S, Petocz P, Colagiuri S. Low-glycemic index diets in the management of diabetes: a meta-analysis of randomized controlled trials. Diabetes Care 2003; 26:2261.

[6] Buyken AE, Toeller M, Heitkamp G, et al. Glycemic index in the diet of European outpatients with type 1 diabetes: relations to glycated hemoglobin and serum lipids. American Journal of Clinical Nutrition 2001; 73:574.

[7] Close EJ, Wiles PG, Lockton JA, et al. The degree of day-to-day variation in food intake in diabetic patients. Diabetic Medicine 1993; 10:514.

[8] Delahanty LM, Halford BN. The role of diet behaviors in achieving improved glycemic control in intensively treated patients in the Diabetes Control and Complications Trial. Diabetes Care 1993; 16:1453.

[9] Delahanty L, Simkins SW, Camelon K. Expanded role of the dietitian in the Diabetes Control and Complications Trial: implications for clinical practice. The DCCT Research Group. J Am Diet Assoc 1993; 93:758.

[10] Delahanty LM, Nathan DM, Lachin JM, et al. Association of diet with glycated hemoglobin during intensive treatment of type 1 diabetes in the Diabetes Control and Complications Trial. American Journal of Clinical Nutrition 2009; 89:518.

[11] Dumesnil JG, Turgeon J, Tremblay A, et al. Effect of a low-glycaemic index–low-fat–high protein diet on the atherogenic metabolic risk profile of abdominally obese men. British Journal of Nutrition 2001; 86:557.

[12] Evert AB, Boucher JL, Cypress M, et al. Nutrition therapy recommendations for the management of adults with diabetes. Diabetes Care 2013; 36:3821.

[13] Franz MJ. Finding the right fit for meal planning. Diabetes Care 1993; 16:1043.

[14] Centers for Disease Control and Prevention. Clinical Growth Chart. Available at: http://www.cdc.gov/growth charts/clinical_charts.htm. Accessed December 2014.

[15] Heller SR, Clarke P, Daly H, et al. Group education for obese patients with type 2 diabetes: greater success at less cost. Diabetic Med 1988; 5:552.

[16] Jenkins DJ, Wolever TM, Taylor RH, et al. Glycemic index of foods: a physiological basis for carbohydrate exchange. American Journal of Clinical Nutrition 1981; 34:362.

[17] Johnston CS, Buller AJ. Vinegar and peanut products as complementary foods to reduce postprandial glycemia. Journal of the American Dietetic Association 2005; 105:1939.

[18] Mannucci E, Rotella F, Ricca V, et al. Eating disorders in patients with type 1 diabetes: a meta-analysis. Journal of Endocrinological Investication 2005; 28:417.

[19] Nathan DM, Cleary PA, Backlund JY, et al. Intensive diabetes treatment and cardiovascular disease in patients with type 1 diabetes. New England Journal of Medicine 2005; 353:2643.

[20] Nuttall FQ. Carbohydrate and dietary management of individuals with insulin-requiring diabetes. Diabetes Care 1993; 16:1039.

[21] Pastors JG, Waslaski J, Gunderson H. Diabetes meal-planning strategies. In: Diabetes Medical Nutrition Therapy and Education, Ross TA, Boucher JL, O'Connell BS (Eds.), American Diabetes Association, Chicago, IL; 2005.

[22] Wolever TM, Nguyen PM, Chiasson JL, et al. Determinants of diet glycemic index calculated retrospectively from diet records of 342 individuals with noninsulin-dependent diabetes mellitus. American Journal of Clinical Nutrition 1994; 59:1265.

[23] Peveler RC, Bryden KS, Neil HA, et al. The relationship of disordered eating habits citand attitudes to clinical outcomes in young adult females with type 1 diabetes. Diabetes Care 2005; 28:84.

[24] Rabasa-Lhoret R, Garon J, Langelier H, et al. Effects of meal carbohydrate content on insulin requirements in type 1 diabetic patients treated intensively with the basal-bolus (ultralente-regular) insulin regimen. Diabetes Care 1999; 22:667.

[25] Rydall AC, Rodin GM, Olmsted MP, et al. Disordered eating behavior and microvascular complications in young women with insulin-dependent diabetes mellitus. New England Journal of Medicine 1997; 336:1849.

[26] Wolever TM. Carbohydrate and the regulation of blood glucose and metabolism. Nutr Rev 2003; 61:S40.

[27] Wolever TM, Hamad S, Chiasson JL, et al. Day-to-day consistency in amount and source of carbohydrate intake associated with improved blood glucose control in type 1 diabetes. Journal of the American College of Nursing 1999; 18:242.

[28] American Diabetes Association. Physical activity/exercise and diabetes. Diabetes Care 2004; 27 Suppl 1:S58.

[29] Brooks GA, Butte NF, Rand WM, et al. Chronicle of the Institute of Medicine physical activity recommendation: how a physical activity recommendation came to be among dietary recommendations. American Journal of Clinical Nutrition 2004; 79:921S.

Permissions

All chapters in this book were first published in DIC, by InTech Open; hereby published with permission under the Creative Commons Attribution License or equivalent. Every chapter published in this book has been scrutinized by our experts. Their significance has been extensively debated. The topics covered herein carry significant findings which will fuel the growth of the discipline. They may even be implemented as practical applications or may be referred to as a beginning point for another development.

The contributors of this book come from diverse backgrounds, making this book a truly international effort. This book will bring forth new frontiers with its revolutionizing research information and detailed analysis of the nascent developments around the world.

We would like to thank all the contributing authors for lending their expertise to make the book truly unique. They have played a crucial role in the development of this book. Without their invaluable contributions this book wouldn't have been possible. They have made vital efforts to compile up to date information on the varied aspects of this subject to make this book a valuable addition to the collection of many professionals and students.

This book was conceptualized with the vision of imparting up-to-date information and advanced data in this field. To ensure the same, a matchless editorial board was set up. Every individual on the board went through rigorous rounds of assessment to prove their worth. After which they invested a large part of their time researching and compiling the most relevant data for our readers.

The editorial board has been involved in producing this book since its inception. They have spent rigorous hours researching and exploring the diverse topics which have resulted in the successful publishing of this book. They have passed on their knowledge of decades through this book. To expedite this challenging task, the publisher supported the team at every step. A small team of assistant editors was also appointed to further simplify the editing procedure and attain best results for the readers.

Apart from the editorial board, the designing team has also invested a significant amount of their time in understanding the subject and creating the most relevant covers. They scrutinized every image to scout for the most suitable representation of the subject and create an appropriate cover for the book.

The publishing team has been an ardent support to the editorial, designing and production team. Their endless efforts to recruit the best for this project, has resulted in the accomplishment of this book. They are a veteran in the field of academics and their pool of knowledge is as vast as their experience in printing. Their expertise and guidance has proved useful at every step. Their uncompromising quality standards have made this book an exceptional effort. Their encouragement from time to time has been an inspiration for everyone.

The publisher and the editorial board hope that this book will prove to be a valuable piece of knowledge for researchers, students, practitioners and scholars across the globe.

List of Contributors

Madhur Dev Bhattarai
Nepal Diabetes Association, Kathmandu, Nepal

Luis M. Román-Pintos and Geannyne Villegas-Rivera
Health & Disease Department, Tonalá University Centre, University of Guadalajara, Guadalajara, Jalisco, México

Ernesto G. Cardona-Muñoz, Adolfo D. Rodríguez-Carrizalez and Alejandra G. Miranda-Díaz
Department of Physiology, Health Sciences, Clinical and Experimental Therapeutics Institute, University Centre, Jalisco, México

Aldo Moreno-Ulloa
Biomedical Innovation Department, College Education and Scientific Research Center of Ensenada, Baja California, México

Nicole Rubin
Miltenyi Biotec Inc, Auburn, CA, USA

Andra-Iulia Suceveanu
Faculty of Medicine, Department of Gastroenterology, Emergency Hospital of Constanta, Ovidius University, Constanta, Romania

Adrian-Paul Suceveanu
Faculty of Medicine, Department of Internal Medicine, Emergency Hospital of Constanta, Ovidius University, Constanta, Romania

Andreea-Daniela Gheorghe and Laura Mazilu
Faculty of Medicine, Department of Oncology, Emergency Hospital of Constanta, Ovidius University, Constanta, Romania

Thiago Gomes Heck, Matias Nunes Frizzo and Mirna Stela Ludwig
Department of Life Sciences, Research Group in Physiology, Regional University of Northwestern Rio Grande do Sul State (UNIJUI), Ijuí, RS, Brazil
Postgraduation Program in Integral Attention to Health (PPGAIS), Regional University of Northwestern Rio Grande do Sul State (UNIJUI), Ijuí, RS, Brazil

Pauline Brendler Goettems Fiorin
Department of Life Sciences, Research Group in Physiology, Regional University of Northwestern Rio Grande do Sul State (UNIJUI), Ijuí, RS, Brazil
Postgraduation Program in Health Sciences, Federal University of Health Sciences of Porto Alegre, Porto Alegre, RS, Brazil

Maurílio de Souza Cazarim and Leonardo Régis Leira Pereira
Faculty of Pharmaceutical Sciences of Ribeirão Preto, University of São Paulo (FCFRP-USP), Ribeirão Preto, SP, Brazil

Ana Carolina de Oliveira Gonçalves and André de Oliveira Baldoni
Federal University of São João Del-Rei (UFSJ), Campus Centro-Oeste Dona Lindu (CCO), MG, Brazil

Teodoro Durá-Travé
Department of Pediatrics, School of Medicine, University of Navarre, Pamplona, Spain
Department of Pediatrics, Navarre Hospital Complex, Pamplona, Spain

Fidel Gallinas-Victoriano
Department of Pediatrics, Navarre Hospital Complex, Pamplona, Spain

Ernesto Cortes-Castell and Manuel Moya-Benavent
Department of Pediatrics, School of Medicine, University of "Miguel Hernández", Elche, Spain

Alexander S. Ametov and Dinara G. Gusenbekova
Russian Medical Academy of Postgraduate Education, Moscow, Russian Federation

Irina Sarvilina
Medical Centre "Novomeditsina,"Rostov State Medical University, Rostov-on-Don, Russia

Viduranga Y. Waisundara
Technology Degree Programme, Faculty of Applied Sciences, Rajarata University, Mihintale, Sri Lanka

Naofumi Shiomi
School of Human Sciences, Department of Biosphere Sciences, Kobe College, Hyogo, Japan

Javier Eduardo Escober Torres
Universidad Nacional Autónoma de Honduras, Tegucigalpa, Honduras

Ryosuke Takeda and Kazunobu Okazaki
Department of Environmental Physiology for Exercise, Osaka City University Graduate School of Medicine, Research Center for Urban Health and Sports, Osaka City University, Sumiyoshi, Osaka, Japan

Shereen Abdelghaffar
Pediatric Diabetes and Endocrinology Cairo University, Egypt

Index